Manual of Emergency
Airway Management

Second Edition

Manual of Emergency Airway Management

Second Edition

Editor-in-Chief

Ron M. Walls, MD, FRCPC, FACEP

Chairman, Department of Emergency Medicine
Brigham and Women's Hospital
Associate Professor of Medicine
Division of Emergency Medicine
Harvard Medical School
Boston, Massachusetts

Senior Editor

Michael F. Murphy, MD, FRCPC (EM), FRCPC (ANAES)

Attending Physician
Department of Emergency Medicine
Carolinas Medical Center
Charlotte, North Carolina
Clinical Assistant Professor of Emergency Medicine
University of North Carolina
Chapel Hill, North Carolina
Clinical Chief Anesthesiology
Lincoln Medical Center
Lincolnton, North Carolina

Contributing Editors

Robert C. Luten, MD

Professor of Emergency Medicine and Pediatrics
University of Florida Health Sciences Center
Jacksonville, Florida

Robert E. Schneider, MD

Academic Faculty
Department of Emergency Medicine
Carolinas Medical Center
Charlotte, North Carolina
Clinical Associate Professor of Emergency Medicine
University of North Carolina
Chapel Hill, North Carolina

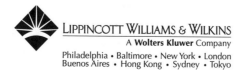

LIPPINCOTT WILLIAMS & WILKINS
A **Wolters Kluwer** Company
Philadelphia • Baltimore • New York • London
Buenos Aires • Hong Kong • Sydney • Tokyo

Acquisitions Editor: Anne M. Sydor
Developmental Editor: Maureen Iannuzzi
Production Manager: Robert Pancotti
Production Editor: Barbara Stabb, TechBooks
Manufacturing Manager: Benjamin Rivera
Cover Designer: Brian Crede
Compositor: TechBooks
Printer: Maple Press

© **2004 by LIPPINCOTT WILLIAMS & WILKINS**
530 Walnut Street
Philadelphia, PA 19106 USA
LWW.com

Printed in the USA

Library of Congress Cataloging-in-Publication Data

Manual of emergency airway management / editor-in-chief, Ron M. Walls ;
   senior editor, Michael F. Murphy ; contributing editors, Robert C. Luten,
   Robert E. Schneider.—2nd ed.
     p. ; cm.
   Includes bibliographical references and index.
   ISBN 0-7817-4764-3
   1. Respiratory emergencies—Handbooks, manuals, etc. 2. Respiratory
intensive care—Handbooks, manuals, etc. 3. Airway
(Medicine)—Handbooks, manuals, etc. I. Walls, Ron M.
   [DNLM: 1. Airway Obstruction—therapy—Handbooks. 2. Emergency
Treatment—Handbooks. 3. Intubation, Intratracheal—Handbooks.
WF 39 M2944 2004]
RC735.R48M36 2004
616.2′00425—dc22

                    2004044142

---

10 9 8 7 6 5 4 3 2

This book is dedicated to those intrepid front-line providers who are called upon time and again to save a life by rapidly and expertly establishing a definitive airway before a patient's precious intellectual function is lost. You do this quietly and without expectation of recognition, often while the nation slumbers. You are our true heroes.

Contents

Section 6. Monitoring and Mechanical Ventilation

Contributing Authors

Aaron E. Bair, M.D., F.A.A.E.M. *Assistant Professor, Division of Emergency Medicine, University of California, Davis, Sacramento, California*

Erik D. Barton, M.D., M.S. *Assistant Professor of Surgery (Emergency Medicine), University of Utah; Chief, Division of Emergency Medicine, University of Utah Health Sciences Center, Salt Lake City, Utah*

Diane M. Birnbaumer, M.D., F.A.C.E.P. *Professor of Medicine, University of California, Los Angeles; Associate Program Director, Department of Emergency Medicine, Harbor-UCLA Medical Center, Redondo Beach, California*

Kerryann B. Broderick, M.D. *Assistant Professor of Emergency Medicine, Department of Surgery, University of Colorado Health Science Center; Associate Residency Program Director, Department of Emergency Medicine, Denver Health Medical Center, Denver Colorado*

John J. Bruns, Jr., M.D. *Clinical Assistant Professor of Emergency Medicine; Attending Physician, Mount Sinai School of Medicine, New York, New York*

David A. Caro, M.D. *Assistant Professor, Associate Residency Director, Department of Emergency Medicine, University of Florida Health Science Center, Jacksonville, Florida*

Michael A. Gibbs, M.D., F.A.C.E.P. *Professor of Emergency Medicine, University of Vermont School of Medicine, Burlington, Vermont; Chief, Department of Emergency Medicine, Maine Medical Center, Portland, Maine*

Stephen A. Godwin, M.D., F.A.C.E.P. *Assistant Professor, Residency Director, Department of Emergency Medicine, University of Florida Health Sciences Center, Jacksonville, Florida*

Orlando R. Hung, M.D. *Professor, Departments of Anesthesiology, Pharmacology, and Surgery, Dalhousie University; Staff Anesthesiologist, Queen Elizabeth II Health Sciences Center, Halifax, Nova Scotia, Canada*

Andy S. Jagoda, M.D., F.A.C.E.P. *Professor of Emergency Medicine, Mount Sinai School of Medicine, New York, New York*

Niranjan Kissoon, M.B.B.S., C.P.E. *Professor, Pediatrics and Emergency Medicine, University of Florida Health Sciences Center, Jacksonville; Chief, Pediatric Critical Care Medicine, Wolfson Children's Hospital, Jacksonville, Florida*

J. Adam Law, M.D. *Associate Professor, Anesthesiology and Surgery, Dalhousie University; Staff Neuroanesthesiologist, Queen Elizabeth II Health Sciences Center, Halifax, Nova Scotia, Canada*

Robert C. Luten, M.D. *Professor of Emergency Medicine and Pediatrics, University of Florida Health Sciences Center, Jacksonville, Florida*

Gregory W. Murphy, B.Sc., R.R.T.   *Territory Manager, Bay State Anesthesia, Inc., North Andover, Massachusetts*

Michael F. Murphy, M.D., F.R.C.P.C. (EM), F.R.C.P.C. (ANAES)   *Attending Physician, Department of Emergency Medicine, Carolinas Medical Center, Charlotte, North Carolina; Clinical Assistant Professor of Emergency Medicine, University of North Carolina, Chapel Hill, North Carolina; Clinical Chief Anesthesiology, Lincoln Medical Center, Lincolnton, North Carolina*

John C. Sakles, M.D.   *Associate Professor, Department of Emergency Medicine, University of Arizona College of Medicine, Tucson, Arizona*

Robert E. Schneider, M.D.   *Academic Faculty, Department of Emergency Medicine, Carolinas Medical Center, Charlotte, North Carolina; Clinical Associate Professor of Emergency Medicine, University of North Carolina, Chapel Hill, North Carolina*

Robert J. Vissers, M.D., F.A.C.E.P., F.R.C.P.C.   *Residency Director and Assistant Professor, Department of Emergency Medicine, University of North Carolina, Chapel Hill, North Carolina*

Ron M. Walls, M.D., F.R.C.P.C., F.A.C.E.P.   *Chairman, Department of Emergency Medicine, Brigham and Women's Hospital; Associate Professor of Medicine, Division of Emergency Medicine, Harvard Medical School, Boston, Massachusetts*

Richard D. Zane, M.D.   *Medical Director, Disaster and Bioterrorism Response; Vice Chair, Department of Emergency Medicine, Brigham and Women's Hospital; Instructor, Harvard Medical School, Boston, Massachusetts*

Illustrators

Sally Johns Design
Raleigh, North Carolina
Figs. 2-1, 2-2, 2-3, 2-4, 2-5, 21-1, 32-1, and 33-1.

Kjerstan Kowack
Staff Medical Illustrator, Department of Medical Arts
Carolinas HealthCare System
Charlotte, North Carolina
Figs. 5-10, 5-12–5-15, 5-18, and 5-19.

Anne K. Olson
Staff Medical Illustrator, Department of Medical Arts
Carolinas HealthCare System
Charlotte, North Carolina
Figs. 5-1–5-9, 5-11, 5-16, 5-17, 6-2, 6-3, 15-1–15-8, 19-2, 19-3, 20-1B, and 20-2.

Robert Williams
San Francisco, California
Figs. 4-3–4-6, 9-1–9-11, 10-3–10-5, 11-3, 13-2, 13-3, and 13-5.

Preface

Airway management defines the specialty of emergency medicine. It is true that the cardiologist can care for acute pulmonary edema or cardiogenic shock as well as the emergency physician can, but if intubation is required, the cardiologist may well need to call on the emergency physician to accomplish this crucial resuscitative step. The pulmonologist can care for status asthmaticus or severe respiratory failure in chronic obstructive pulmonary disease as well as the emergency physician can, but if intubation is required, the pulmonologist's expertise may be exceeded, and the assistance of the emergency physician may be vital. Although care of these critically ill patients may require the resources of many different specialties working in concert, it is the emergency physician, and often the emergency physician alone, who can provide definitive resuscitative care to all patients, regardless of their complexity, severity, or presenting condition. And it is often the emergency physician alone who is in the hospital 24 hours each day, 365 days each year, ready to respond immediately to a life-threatening airway crisis. These truths are the genesis of the National Emergency Airway Management Course (The Airway Course) and of this book, the second edition of which we hope will continue to help front-line providers advance their airway skills.

Much has happened since we published the first edition in 2000. New airway devices have been approved that offer unparalleled access to the airway through the spectacular windows of fiberoptics and video technology. We have taught thousands more providers the skills and thought processes that drive advanced airway management, and our thinking with respect to the difficult airway, rapid sequence intubation, and various pharmacologic approaches has been widely accepted and incorporated into other important learning systems like the Advanced Cardiac Life Support Course and textbook. We have refined our thinking with respect to the approach to the difficult airway, and there are some subtle and not-so-subtle changes to the algorithms. Medical simulation has become the anchor of The Airway Course, and we find ourselves amazed, looking back at the first edition of the book, that we were ever able to function without it. In 2002, we launched a second course: The Difficult Airway Course: Anesthesia, and found that anesthesiologists and nurse anesthetists also embraced our tightly defined, algorithmic approach to airway management. Our community of instructors grew to include anesthesia specialists, and we were delighted and amazed at the synergy between the anesthesia and emergency medicine experts as they worked together to train both anesthesia and emergency medicine providers.

The book itself is significantly different from the first edition. We have added an evidence section at the end of most chapters to provide a more analytical, evidence-based discussion of the issues covered in that chapter. We have maintained the "manual" approach throughout the chapters proper, though, as our course participants and reviewers found the first edition extremely easy to use, and we did not want to impair that format. We have organized the pediatrics topics into one section, and have added new chapters to cover new devices, such as video laryngoscopy. We have also provided much more detail on the use of difficult and failed airway devices, expanding this information into a series of chapters, as both experience and published evidence provide much more information about the use of these important airway tools.

As before, we are grateful to our colleagues and teachers, and especially those gifted instructors in The Airway Course and The Difficult Airway Course: Anesthesia, an increasing number of whom have contributed to this book. Most of all, we are grateful to our students, whose questions continually push us to think critically and to keep exploring.

Acknowledgments

I have been incredibly privileged to learn from the giants of our specialty, especially John Marx and Peter Rosen, and to then have the extraordinary opportunity to give back by teaching others. My colleagues in The Airway Course and at Brigham and Women's Hospital have been precious mentors and role models, even as I tried to be the same for them. I am in awe of those practicing physicians, nurses, physician assistants, and paramedics who take precious time from their families and work to improve their airway skills in our course, and I am grateful to them for always teaching me at least as much as I teach them. My family has been the single most defining element in my adult life, and have both created my joy and shared it. My wife, Barb, and my children, Andrew, Blake, and Alexa, have unfailingly helped me keep my perspective, and have given me so much more than they will ever know.

RMW

I wish first to acknowledge my family: Deb, Amanda, Ryan, and Teddy and to thank them for their tireless support. I am also grateful to my colleagues and close friends, Ron, Bob, and Bob, whose energy and commitment has allowed us to undertake this important mission; the faculty that make it possible to deliver it; and the students who drive us to the cutting edge of emergency airway management.

MFM

To my wife and best friend, Kathleen Ann Rheingans, for her infinite love and support. To my children, Erin Elizabeth, Lauren Banuvar, and Ian Paul Harlan for their honesty and humor, which keeps me grounded and humble. To my mentor and close friend, John Andrew Marx, who continually shows me how one achieves their potential for greatness. Finally, to my fellow editors, Ron, Mike, and Bob, with great thanks for their hard work, encouragement, and friendship that made this book and the Airway Course a reality.

RES

At this point in my life I have come to realize that any contribution I make has little to do with my own limited ability, but is the product of the influence and gifts of others. First, I thank my wife Cindi for her support and for allowing me to have the joys of a family life while still enjoying the privilege of creative work. I acknowledge the students who use this information and teach me daily. To my friends Ron, Mike, and Bob who have given me this opportunity and inspire me to do the best I am able to do. And last, but most important, to my God who is responsible for all of this and has given me the wisdom to understand my role.

RCL

Manual of Emergency Airway Management

Second Edition

1

The Decision to Intubate

Ron M. Walls

Airway management is the single most important skill of the emergency physician and is one of the defining skills of emergency medicine. Loss of the airway, with resultant failure of ventilation and oxygenation, is the terminal pathway for many emergency patients. Timely, effective, and decisive management of the airway can quite literally make the difference between life and death or between ability and disability. The emergency physician has final responsibility for definitive management of the airway for patients presenting to the emergency department.

> **The emergency physician is responsible for airway management for patients in the emergency department.**

Airway management comprises a series of complex actions, each of which must be mastered. Specifically, the emergency physician must be capable of the following:

- Rapidly assessing the patient's need for intubation and the urgency of the situation
- Determining the best method of airway management for the particular circumstances at hand
- Deciding which pharmacological agents to use, in what order, and in what doses
- Managing the airway in the context of the patient's overall condition
- Using a myriad of airway devices proficiently to achieve a definitive airway while minimizing the likelihood of hypoxemia or hypercarbia
- Recognizing when the planned airway intervention has failed and an alternative (rescue) technique is required

The emergency physician must be proficient with rapid sequence intubation, which requires a thorough knowledge of the pharmacology and effects of neuromuscular blocking agents, sedative or induction agents, and other medications that are used to improve outcome or mitigate adverse effects. The entire repertoire of airway skills must be mastered, ranging from bag and mask ventilation through rapid sequence intubation, techniques for the difficult airway, and rescue maneuvers, including surgical airway techniques, in the event of airway failure. Emergency airway management requires diligent maintenance of a knowledge base, sound clinical judgment, and the decisiveness to act when action is indicated. In many cases, indecision leads to delayed intervention, increased difficulty, and a greater likelihood of a bad outcome. This chapter focuses on the decision to intubate. Subsequent chapters will describe the technique of rapid sequence intubation and its place in the emergency airway algorithm.

A greater proportion of the patient's ultimate outcome will likely rest on the timeliness of the initial decision to intubate and the appropriateness of the method selected rather than on the technical proficiency of the intubator.

The airway is rightfully allocated the "A" in the ABC of resuscitation and in all cases, the airway is paramount and takes precedence over all other clinical considerations. Establishment and protection of the airway with assurance of optimal oxygenation and ventilation constitute the foundation on which all other resuscitative measures are based. Without a secure airway and adequate oxygenation and ventilation, all other resuscitative measures are doomed to failure. With the exception of the immediate defibrillation of the cardiac arrest patient, no single resuscitative maneuver takes priority over management of the airway.

I. Indications for intubation

The decision to intubate should be based on three fundamental clinical assessments:

1. Is there a failure of airway maintenance or protection?
2. Is there a failure of ventilation or oxygenation?
3. What is the anticipated clinical course?

The results of these three evaluations will lead to a correct decision to intubate or not to intubate in virtually all conceivable cases. Although some recommend the use of a list of indications for intubation, such lists are never complete and they tend to be difficult to recall in critical situations. In any case, all conditions and circumstances for which intubation is indicated can be determined using these three fundamental clinical assessments.

A. *Is there a failure of airway maintenance or protection?*

The conscious, alert patient uses the musculature of the upper airway and various protective reflexes to maintain a patent airway and to protect against the aspiration of foreign substances, gastric contents, or secretions. The ability of the patient to phonate with a clear, unobstructed voice is strong evidence of both airway patency and protection. In the severely ill or injured patient, such airway maintenance and protection mechanisms are often attenuated or lost. A patent airway is essential for adequate oxygenation and ventilation, and protection of this airway against aspiration of gastric contents is vital. If the patient is not able to maintain an adequate airway, an artificial airway may be established by insertion of an oropharyngeal airway or a nasopharyngeal airway. Although such airway devices may establish a patent airway, they do not provide any protection against aspiration. As a general rule, any patient who requires the establishment of an airway also requires protection of that airway, and the use of an oropharyngeal or nasopharyngeal airway should be considered a temporizing measure.

> *Any patient who requires the establishment of an airway also requires protection of that airway.*

A patient with a spontaneously patent airway and adequate respirations may not be able to protect the airway against aspiration of gastric contents, which carries a significant morbidity and mortality. It has been taught that assessment of the gag reflex is a reliable method of evaluating airway protective reflexes. In fact, this concept has never been subjected to adequate scientific scrutiny, and the absence of a gag reflex is neither sensitive nor specific as an indicator of loss of airway protective reflexes. The presence of a gag reflex has similarly not been demonstrated to ensure the presence of airway protection. In addition, testing the gag reflex in a supine, obtunded patient may result in vomiting and possible aspiration.

> **The gag reflex does not correlate well with airway protection and is of no clinical value when assessing the need for intubation.**

Evaluation of the ability to swallow spontaneously and to handle secretions is probably a better clinical assessment for airway protection. Swallowing is a very complex reflex that requires the patient to sense the presence of material in the posterior oropharynx and then to execute a series of very intricate and coordinated muscular actions to direct the secretions down past a closed airway into the esophagus. Although this concept also has not been adequately studied, the assessment of spontaneous or volitional swallowing is probably a better tool for assessing the ability to protect the airway than is the presence or absence of a gag reflex. The presence of pooled secretions in the patient's oropharynx should be considered to indicate a potential failure of airway protection. In the absence of an immediately reversible condition, such as opioid overdose or reversible cardiac dysrythmia, prompt intubation is indicated for any emergency department patient who is unable to maintain and protect the airway. A common clinical error occurs when a patient is evaluated and found to be breathing on his or her own. Although it may indeed be true that the spontaneous ventilation is adequate, the patient may be at risk for serious aspiration.

B. *Is there failure of ventilation or oxygenation?*
Oxygenation of the vital organs is the primary function of the respiratory system. Although ventilation and disposal of waste product carbon dioxide (CO_2) are important for pH balance, it is oxygen that is vital for survival. If the patient is unable to ventilate adequately, or if adequate oxygenation cannot be achieved despite supplemental oxygen, then intubation is indicated. In such cases, the intubation is being performed to facilitate ventilation and oxygenation rather than simply to establish or protect the airway. An example is the patient with status asthmaticus, who will generally maintain and protect the airway even when *in extremis*. However, fatigue produces ventilatory failure and the resultant hypoxemia will lead to death without intervention. Similarly, the patient with severe pulmonary edema may again be maintaining and protecting the airway, but may have progressive oxygenation failure that can be managed only with positive pressure ventilation through an endotracheal tube. Although some of these patients can be managed with noninvasive ventilatory techniques, such as bilevel continuous positive airway pressure (BL-PAP), many still require intubation. Unless ventilatory or oxygenation failure is due to a reversible cause, such as opioid overdose, intubation is mandatory.

C. *What is the anticipated clinical course?*
Most patients who require intubation in the emergency department have one or more of the previously discussed indications: airway maintenance, airway protection, oxygenation, or ventilation. However, there is a large and important group for whom intubation is indicated even though none of these four fundamental elements is present. This is the patient whose condition can be predicted to deteriorate, either because of dynamic and progressive changes related to the presenting condition or because the work of breathing will become overwhelming in the face of catastrophic illness or injury. For example,

consider the patient who presents with a stab wound to the midzone of the anterior neck and a visible hematoma. At the time of presentation, the patient may have perfectly adequate airway maintenance and protection and be ventilating and oxygenating well. The hematoma, though, provides clear evidence of significant vascular injury. Ongoing bleeding may be clinically occult, because the blood often tracks down the tissue planes of the neck (e.g. prevertebral space) rather than causing visible expansion of the hematoma. Furthermore, the anatomical distortion caused by the enlarging internal hematoma may well thwart various airway management techniques that would have been successful if undertaken earlier. The patient inexorably progresses from awake and alert with a patent airway to a state in which the airway becomes obstructed, often quite suddenly, and the anatomy is so distorted that airway management is difficult or impossible.

> *Acute, progressive anatomical airway distortion is a potential time bomb. Intubate early, before deterioration occurs!*

Analogous considerations apply to the polytrauma patient who presents with hypotension, multiple bilateral rib fractures, a tender abdomen, pelvic fracture, femoral fracture, and mild head injury with combative behavior. Although this patient has adequate airway maintenance and protection, and ventilation and oxygenation may be acceptable, intubation is indicated as part of the management of this constellation of injuries. The reason for the intubation becomes clear when one examines the anticipated clinical course of this patient. The hypotension mandates aggressive fluid resuscitation and evaluation for the source of the blood loss, including diagnostic peritoneal lavage, abdominal ultrasound, or abdominal computed tomography (CT) scan. Any of these maneuvers will require a significant degree of patient cooperation. The pelvic fracture, if unstable, requires immobilization and likely embolization of bleeding vessels. The femoral fracture will certainly require operative intervention. Chest tubes may be required for one or both hemithoraces to treat hemopneumothorax or in preparation for positive pressure ventilation during surgery. The combative behavior pertaining to the head injury may mandate a head CT scan or placement of an intracranial pressure monitor depending on other injury priorities. Throughout all of this, the patient's shock state leads to inadequate tissue perfusion and increasing metabolic debt. This debt significantly affects the muscles of respiration, and progressive respiratory fatigue and failure often supervene. With the patient's ultimate destination certain to include the operating room and the complex and potentially painful series of procedures and diagnostic evaluations required, this patient is best served by early intubation. In addition, intubation improves tissue oxygenation during shock and helps reduce the increasing metabolic debt burden.

Sometimes, the clinical course may be uncertain and the patient may be exposed to a period of increased risk. For example, the patient who appears relatively stable with a series of injuries might be appropriately managed without intubation in the emergency department. If that same patient requires CT scan, angiography, or any other prolonged diagnostic procedure, it may be more appropriate to intubate the patient prior to allowing him or her to leave the department so that an airway crisis will not ensue in the radiology suite, where recognition may be delayed and response may not be optimal. Similarly, if such a patient were to be transferred from one hospital to another, airway management may be mandated on the basis of the increased risk to the patient during that transfer. This is not to say that every trauma patient or every patient with a serious medical disorder requires intubation, but in general, it is better to err on the side of performing an intubation that might not, in retrospect, have been required, rather than to expose the patient to a potentially disastrous deterioration. It is important for the physician to consider the patient's presenting condition in the context of the clinical course of subsequent care. If the patient will be leaving the relative safety of the emergency department for a prolonged period and the airway is potentially at risk, steps must be taken to ensure the airway will be preserved and protected and that ventilation and oxygenation will be maintained throughout.

If the anticipated clinical course is one of deterioration or if the critically ill or injured patient will be leaving the relatively safe confines of the emergency department, intubate early before deterioration and airway compromise occur.

II. Approach to the patient

When the patient presents to the emergency department, the first assessment should be of the patency and adequacy of the airway. In many cases, the adequacy of the airway is confirmed by having the patient speak. Questions such as "What is your name?" or "Do you know where you are?" provide information about the neurological status and valuable information about the airway. A normal voice, the ability to inhale and exhale in the modulated manner required for speech, and the ability to comprehend the question and follow instructions are strong evidence of adequate upper airway function. Although such an evaluation should not be taken as proof that the upper airway is intact and functioning, it is strongly suggestive that the airway is adequate for the time being. More important, inability of the patient to phonate properly, stridor, or altered mental status precluding response to the questions mandates more detailed assessment of the adequacy of airway function and ventilation. Following this preliminary evaluation, a more detailed examination of the mouth and oropharynx is required. The mouth should be examined for bleeding, swelling of the tongue or uvula, abnormalities of the oropharynx, such as peritonsillar abscess, or any other abnormalities that might interfere with the free passage of air through the mouth and oropharynx. The mandible and central face should be examined briefly for integrity. Careful examination of the anterior neck requires both visual inspection for deformity, asymmetry, or abnormality and palpation of the anterior neck, including the larynx and trachea. During palpation, the presence of subcutaneous air should be sought. This is identified by a crackling feeling on compression of the cutaneous tissues of the neck, much as if a sheet of wrinkled tissue paper were lying immediately beneath the skin. When only a small amount of subcutaneous air is present, this physical finding may be subtle and transient and must be sought carefully. Presence of subcutaneous air indicates disruption of an air-filled passage; often the airway itself, especially in the setting of blunt or penetrating chest or neck trauma. Subcutaneous air in the neck can also be caused by esophageal rupture, or rarely, by gas-forming infections. Although these latter two conditions are not immediately threatening to the airway, patients may nevertheless rapidly deteriorate, requiring subsequent airway management in any case.

After inspection and palpation of the upper airway, the respiratory pattern of the patient should be noted. The presence of respiratory stridor, however slight, indicates some degree of upper airway obstruction. Stridor is audible without a stethoscope and should not be confused with intermittent expiratory moaning, which is often exhibited by patients in pain. Careful auscultation of the neck with a stethoscope can reveal subclinical stridor that indicates mild airway compromise. Significant airway compromise may develop before any sign of stridor is evident. When evaluating the respiratory pattern, the chest should also be observed. Symmetrical, concordant chest movement is the expected finding. In cases where there is significant injury, paradoxical movement of a flail segment of the chest may be observed. If spinal cord injury has disturbed intercostal muscle functioning, diaphragmatic breathing may be present. In this form of breathing, there is little movement of the chest wall and inspiration is evidenced by apparent increase in abdominal volume caused by descent of the diaphragm. Auscultation of the chest will provide clues as to the adequacy of the air exchange. Decreased breath sounds caused by pneumothorax, hemothorax, or other pulmonary pathology are detected. Acute pneumothorax rarely causes any significant degree of tracheal deviation until the patient is *in extremis* or arrested, and tracheal deviation, when found, will likely represent a chronic process.

The assessment of ventilation and oxygenation is a clinical one. Arterial blood gas determination provides little additional information to assess whether intubation is necessary and may be misleading. The clinical impression of the patient's mentation, degree of fatigue, and severity of concomitant injuries or conditions is more important than isolated or even serial determination of arterial oxygen or CO_2 tension. With the advent of pulse oximetry, oxygen saturation can be measured transcutaneously and arterial blood gases are rarely indicated for the purpose of determining arterial oxygen tensions. In certain circumstances oxygen saturation monitoring is unsuccessful because of abnormal peripheral perfusion, and arterial blood gases may then be required to assess oxygenation or to provide correlation with pulse oximetry measurements. Measurement of arterial CO_2 tension will contribute little useful information to a decision regarding the need for intubation. In patients with obstructive lung disease, such as asthma or chronic obstructive pulmonary disease, intubation may be required with relatively low CO_2 tensions because of patient fatigue. Other times, extremely high CO_2 tensions may be managed successfully without intubation.

> *Arterial blood gas values are rarely helpful in the decision to intubate and may lead to faulty decision making.*

Finally, after assessment of the upper airway and the patient's ventilatory status, including pulse oximetry and mentation, an evaluation of the patient's anticipated clinical course is required. If the patient's condition is such that intubation is inevitable and a series of interventions is required, early intubation is preferable. Similarly, if the patient has a condition that is likely to worsen over time, especially if such worsening is likely to compromise the airway itself, early airway management is indicated. The same consideration applies to patients who require interhospital transfer by air or ground. Intubation before transfer is vastly preferable to a difficult, uncontrolled intubation during transfer when the condition has worsened. In all circumstances, the decision to intubate should be given precedence. If doubt exists as to whether the patient requires intubation, error should occur on the side of intubating the patient. It is preferable to intubate the patient and ensure the integrity of the airway than to leave the patient without a secure airway and have an irreversible catastrophe occur.

EVIDENCE

1. The gag reflex is not a useful indicator of the need to intubate. In a study of 111 patients requiring neurological observation in the emergency department, Moulton et al. found no correlation between the Glasgow Coma Scale (GCS) and the presence or absence of a gag reflex. The gag reflex was noted to be variably present across the range of GCS from 6 to 15, independent of the patient's perceived need for intubation (1). The gag reflex is not involved in laryngeal closure or protection of the airway. Bleach found an absent gag reflex in 27% of fully conscious patients who had undergone speech therapy and videofluoroscopy to assess for possible aspiration after neurological events. There was no correlation between aspiration and the presence (or absence) of the gag reflex (2). Davies et al. studied 140 healthy adults, half of whom were elderly, and found that 37% lacked any gag reflex (3). Chan et al. studied 414 patients with acute poisoning and noted absence of the gag reflex to be only 70% sensitive in identifying patients who required intubation. Contrary to those studies that find the gag reflex frequently absent in the normal population, absence of a gag reflex was 100% specific in identifying patients requiring intubation; however, the use of a GCS score of 8 or less outperformed the gag reflex, and evaluation of the gag reflex added nothing to the assessment of the GCS score alone (4).

REFERENCES

1. Moulton C, Pennycook A, Makower A. Relation between the Glasgow Coma Scale and the gag reflex. *BMJ* 1991;303:1240–1241.
2. Bleach N. The gag reflex and aspiration; a retrospective analysis of 120 patients assessed by videofluoroscopy. *Clin Otolaryngol* 1993;18:303–307.
3. Davies AE, Kidd D, Stone SP, et al. Pharyngeal sensation and gag reflex in healthy subjects. *Lancet* 1995;345: 487–488.
4. Chan B, Gaudry P, Grattan-Smith TE, et al. The use of Glasgow Coma Score in poisoning. *J Emerg Med* 1993; 11:579–582.

2

The Emergency Airway Algorithms

Ron M. Walls

Attempts to define a unified approach to airway management have met with mixed success. The American College of Surgeons' Committee on Trauma developed an algorithmic approach to airway management for trauma patients for the Advanced Trauma Life Support Course. Although fundamentally reasonable, the role of neuromuscular blockade in airway management is inadequately addressed, and this algorithm is not applicable to patients with medical disorders requiring intubation. This chapter will present and discuss the emergency airway algorithm and the specialized algorithms that supplement it. Together, these algorithms comprise a fundamental, reproducible approach to the emergency airway. The specialized algorithms all build from concepts found in the main emergency airway algorithm, which details the evaluation of the patient for the presence of a crash airway, a difficult airway, or a failed airway. The algorithms do not attempt to define the need for intubation and do not deal with the decision to intubate. These are covered in Chapter 1. Therefore, the entry point for the emergency airway algorithm is immediately after the decision to intubate has been made.

The algorithms are intended as guidelines in the approach to the emergency airway. They are designed to present distinct, recognizable patterns and to guide the action to be taken once the pattern is recognized. The goal is to help to demystify some of the difficulties encountered during emergency airway management and to aid in the recognition and management of distinct classes of airway problems. By separating out those patients who are essentially dead (i.e., unresponsive, agonal) and managing them using a distinct pathway, customization of airway management is facilitated. Similarly, serious problems can ensue if a patient with a difficult airway undergoes rapid-sequence intubation (RSI), unless the difficulty was identified and planned for. The algorithms assist the clinician in applying basic notions of pattern recognition so that in relatively uncommon circumstances, the response is predefined rather than requiring improvisation. Thus, in the case of a difficult airway, the algorithms facilitate recognition of the problem and formulation of a distinct, but reproducible, approach. Algorithms are best thought of as a series of key questions and critical actions, with the answer to each question guiding the next critical action.

> *In uncommon situations, failure of pattern recognition is often a precursor to medical error.*

A brief overview algorithm (Fig. 2-1) defines the overall approach to the emergency airway as follows: When a patient requires intubation, the first evaluation regards whether the

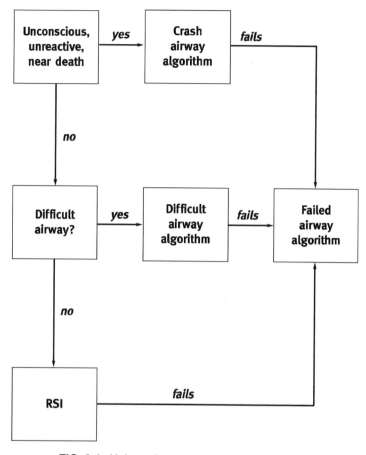

FIG. 2-1. Universal emergency airway algorithm.

patient represents a crash scenario (unconscious, near death, agonal or no respirations, expected to be unresponsive to laryngoscopy). If so, the patient is managed as a crash airway (see Fig. 2-3). If not, the next determination regards whether the patient represents a difficult airway (see Chapter 6). If so, the patient is managed as a difficult airway (see Fig. 2-4). If neither a crash airway nor a difficult airway is present, then RSI is recommended. Regardless of the algorithm used initially (main, crash, or difficult), if airway failure occurs, the failed airway algorithm (see Fig. 2-5) is immediately invoked. The definition of the failed airway is important and is explained in much more detail in the following sections.

I. The emergency airway management algorithm (main algorithm)

The main algorithm is shown in Fig. 2-2. It begins after the decision to intubate and ends with postintubation management, which may be reached directly or via one of the other algorithms, depending on patient circumstances. The algorithm is navigated by following a series of defined steps with decisions driven by the answers to a series of key questions:

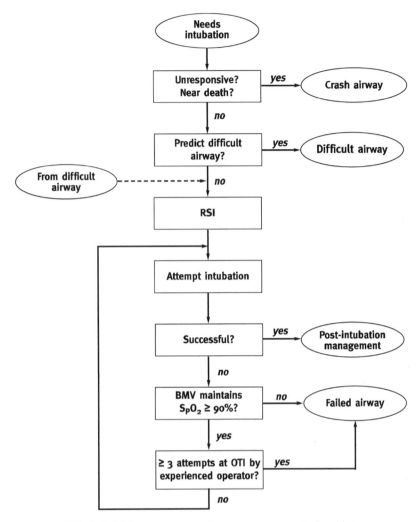

FIG. 2-2. Main emergency airway management algorithm.

- **Key question 1: Is this a crash airway?** If the patient presents in an essentially unresponsive state and is deemed to be unlikely to respond in any way to direct laryngoscopy, then the patient is said to have a crash airway. Here, we are identifying patients who are in full cardiac arrest, respiratory arrest, or have only agonal cardiorespiratory activity (e.g., agonal, ineffective respirations at 6/minute, pulseless idioventricular rhythm at 26/minute). These patients, who have been referred to as the nearly dead or the newly dead, are managed in a manner appropriate for their *extremis* condition. If a crash airway is identified, exit this main algorithm and enter the crash airway algorithm (Fig. 2-3). Otherwise, continue on the main algorithm.
- **Key question 2: Is this a difficult airway?** If the airway is not identified as a crash airway, the next task is to determine whether it is a difficult airway. The assessment of the patient for potentially difficult intubation using the LEMON mnemonic is described in Chapter 6. It is understood that virtually all emergency intubations are difficult to some extent. However, the evaluation of the patient for attributes that will predict difficult intubation is extremely important. If the patient represents a particularly difficult airway

situation, then he or she is managed as a difficult airway, using the difficult airway algorithm (Fig. 2-4), and one would exit the main algorithm. Otherwise, continue on the main algorithm to the next step, which is to perform RSI.

- **Critical action: Perform rapid sequence intubation (RSI).** In the absence of an identified crash or difficult airway, RSI is the method of choice for airway management in the emergency department. RSI is described in detail in Chapter 3 and affords the best opportunity for success with the least opportunity for adverse outcome of any possible airway method, when applied to appropriately selected patients. This step assumes that the appropriate sequence of RSI (the seven Ps) will be followed as described in Chapter 3. If the patient is in extreme respiratory distress, or if haste is indicated for any reason, an accelerated or immediate RSI protocol can be used (see Chapter 3).

  During RSI, intubation is attempted. *An attempt is defined as activities occurring during a single continuous laryngoscopy maneuver.* In other words, if several attempts are made to pass an endotracheal tube through the glottis during the course of a single laryngoscopy, these aggregate efforts count as one attempt. This distinction is important because of the definition of the failed airway below.

- **Key question 3: Was intubation successful?** If the first oral intubation that is attempted during RSI is successful, the patient is intubated, postintubation management is indicated, and the algorithm terminates. If the intubation attempt is not successful, continue on the main pathway.

- **Key question 4: Can the patient's oxygenation be maintained?** When the first attempt at intubation is unsuccessful, the appropriate first maneuver is bag and mask ventilation of the patient. This approach underscores the importance of assessing the likelihood of successful bag and mask ventilation before beginning the intubation sequence. In the vast majority of cases, especially when neuromuscular blockade has been used, bag and mask ventilation will provide adequate ventilation and oxygenation for the patient, defined as maintenance of the oxygen saturation at 90% or higher. If bag and mask ventilation is not capable of maintaining the oxygen saturation above 90%, better technique, including oral and nasal airways, two-person–two-handed technique, and optimal positioning of the patient will usually result in effective ventilation (see Chapter 5). If bag and mask ventilation fails despite optimal technique, the airway is considered a failed airway and one must exit this algorithm and go directly to the failed airway algorithm (Fig. 2-5). If not, the airway is not failed, and repeated attempts at intubation are indicated. Recognition of the failed airway is crucial, for delays caused by persistent, futile attempts at intubation will lose critical seconds or minutes and may sharply reduce the time remaining for a rescue technique to be successful before brain injury ensues. There are two essential definitions of the failed airway:
  - "Can't intubate, can't oxygenate."
  - Three failed attempts by an experienced operator

  In either case, the failed airway algorithm (Fig. 2-5) will provide the appropriate guidance, once the failed airway pattern has been recognized. The failed airway is discussed in more detail in Chapter 6.

- **Key question 5: Have three attempts at orotracheal intubation been made by an experienced operator?** If three separate attempts at orotracheal intubation by direct laryngoscopy by an experienced operator have been unsuccessful, then the airway again is defined as a failed airway despite the ability to adequately oxygenate the patient using a bag and mask. If an experienced operator has had three attempts at intubation without success, the likelihood of success with further attempts is very small. The airway must be recognized as a failed airway and managed as such using the failed airway algorithm. If there have been fewer than three unsuccessful attempts at intubation, but bag ventilation is successful, then it is appropriate to attempt orotracheal intubation again after a brief period of bag-mask ventilation to ensure adequate oxygenation of the patient. Similarly, if the initial attempts were made by an inexperienced operator, such as a trainee, and the patient is adequately ventilated and oxygenated between attempts, then it is appropriate to reattempt oral intubation until three attempts by an *experienced* operator have been unsuccessful. Thus, if fewer than three attempts have been made, branch back up to again attempt oral intubation. In some circumstances, it is clear to an *experienced* operator that intubation will not be possible after only a single attempt at laryngoscopy. In such cases, if the patient has been optimally placed in the sniffing position, good relaxation has been achieved, the BURP maneuver has been used, and the operator is convinced that further attempts at laryngoscopy would be futile, the airway should be immediately regarded as a failed airway and appropriate steps should be taken.

> *It is not essential to make three laryngoscopic attempts before labeling an airway as failed, but three failed attempts by an experienced operator should always be considered a failed airway, unless the laryngoscopist identifies a particular opportunity for success during the last attempt.*

II. The crash airway algorithm

Entering the crash airway algorithm (Fig. 2-3) indicates that one has identified an unconscious, unresponsive patient with immediate need for airway management. It is assumed throughout that bag/mask ventilation is occurring as indicated as preparations are made to intubate.

- **Critical action: Intubate immediately:** The first step in the crash algorithm is to attempt oral intubation immediately by direct laryngoscopy without pharmacological assist. In these patient circumstances, direct oral intubation has success rates that approach those of RSI, presumably because the patients are relaxed and unresponsive in a manner similar to that achieved by RSI.
- **Key question 1: Was intubation successful?** If yes, carry on with postintubation management and general resuscitation. If intubation was not successful, resume bag and mask ventilation and proceed to the next step.
- **Key question 2: Is bag and mask ventilation adequate?** If bag ventilation is successful, then further attempts at oral intubation are possible. If bag ventilation is unsuccessful in the context of a single failed oral intubation attempt with a crash airway, then a failed airway is present. One further attempt at intubation may be rapidly tried, but no more than one, because intubation has failed and the failure of bag ventilation places the patient in serious and immediate jeopardy. This is a can't intubate, can't oxygenate scenario, analogous to that described previously. Exit here and proceed directly to the failed airway algorithm.

> *Adequacy of bag mask ventilation with a crash airway is usually not determined by pulse oximetry, but by assessment of chest rise, bag compliance, mask seal, and patient color.*

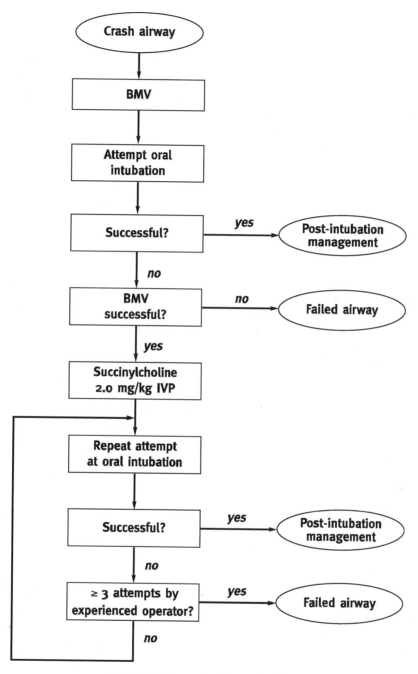

FIG. 2-3. The crash airway algorithm.

- **Critical action: Administer succinylcholine 2.0 mg/kg IV push:** If intubation is not successful, it must be assumed that the patient is not optimally relaxed. The dose of the succinylcholine is increased here because these patients often have severe circulatory compromise, impairing the effectiveness and rapidity of the succinylcholine. Bag and mask ventilation continues for 60 seconds to allow the succinylcholine to distribute.

- **Critical action: Attempt intubation:** After allowing time for the succinylcholine to circulate, another attempt is made at oral intubation.
- **Key question 3: Was the intubation successful?** If intubation is achieved, then proceed to postintubation management. If not, another attempt is indicated, unless there have already been three failed attempts after the administration of the succinylcholine.
- **Key question 4: Have there been three or more attempts at intubation by an experienced operator?** If the answer to this question is yes, then consistent with the previous definition, the situation represents a failed airway. If fewer than three attempts have been made by an experienced operator, then repeated attempts at oral intubation are justified and one cycles through another intubation attempt. After each unsuccessful intubation attempt, defined by a single laryngoscopy, the patient should receive ventilation and oxygenation through a bag and mask, and this ventilation must be effective.

> *If succinylcholine has been administered to a crash patient, count the subsequent intubation attempt as attempt 1.*

III. The difficult airway algorithm

Assessment and management of the difficult airway is discussed in detail in Chapter 6. This algorithm (Fig. 2-4) represents the clinical approach that should be used in the event of an anticipated difficult airway.

- **Critical action: Call for assistance:** The "call for assistance" box is linked as a dotted line because this is an optional step, dependent on the clinical circumstances, the skill of the physician, available resources, and the availability of additional personnel. In circumstances where two emergency physicians are on duty, this call for assistance might simply be to notify the second emergency physician of the intubation so that help might be readily available, if required. Assistance might include personnel, special airway equipment, or both.
- **Key question 1: Is there adequate time?** If ventilation and oxygenation are adequate and oxygen saturation is over 90%, then a careful assessment and a methodical, planned approach can be undertaken, even if significant preparation time is required. However, if ventilation and oxygenation are inadequate, then immediate action is indicated to ensure adequate ventilation and oxygenation by the administration of supplemental oxygenation, bag and mask ventilation, or both. Supplemental oxygen and bag assisted ventilation may provide adequate oxygenation and ventilation to allow a more methodical and planned approach to the difficult airway. If so, remain on the main path down the algorithm. If not, the situation is equivalent to a can't intubate (identified difficult airway is a surrogate for can't intubate), can't oxygenate (adequate oxygenation saturation cannot be achieved) failed airway, and a decision must be rapidly made to move to the failed airway algorithm. Certain difficult airway patients will have chronic pulmonary disease and may not be able to reach oxygen saturation of 90%, but can be kept stable and viable at, say, 86%. Whether to call this case a failed airway is a matter of judgment, but if a decision is made to proceed down the difficult airway algorithm rather than switching to the failed airway algorithm, it is essential to be aware of the rapid desaturation that will occur during intubation attempts (see Chapter 3) and to be vigilant with respect to hypoxemia.
- **Key question 2: Despite the presence of the difficult airway, is RSI indicated?** Because we have identified that the patient can be adequately oxygenated, the next step is to consider RSI. This decision hinges on two key questions. The first, and most important,

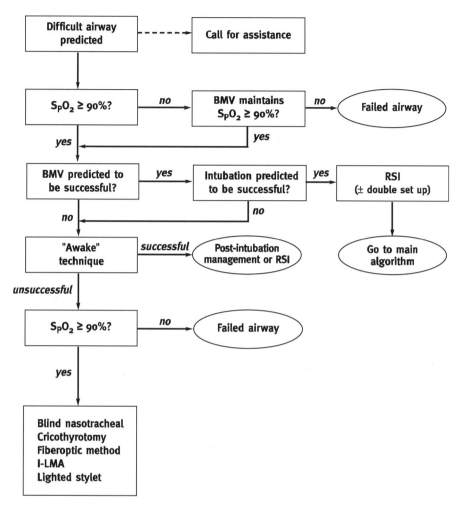

FIG. 2-4. The difficult airway algorithm.

is whether bag-mask ventilation is predicted to be successful. This answer may already be known if bag-mask ventilation is required to maintain the patient's adequate oxygenation. If the patient has been breathing spontaneously and oxygenating adequately to this point, bag-mask ventilation may have not been attempted. It is necessary to make an assessment as to whether bag-mask ventilation is likely to be successful as this is a virtually essential prerequisite for RSI. The assessment of a patient with respect to predicting difficult bag-mask ventilation is described in Chapter 6. In some cases, it may be desirable to attempt a trial of bag-mask ventilation, but this approach does not reliably predict the ability to bag-mask ventilate the patient after paralysis. If bag-mask ventilation is predicted to be successful, then the next consideration is whether intubation is reasonably likely to be successful, despite the difficult airway attributes. In reality, many patients with identified difficult airways are successfully intubated in the emergency department using RSI, so if there is a reasonable likelihood of success with oral intubation, *despite the difficult airway,* then rapid sequence intubation may be undertaken. In some cases, the RSI may be done under a double setup, in which the patient is evaluated and prepped for cricothyrotomy and the surgical instruments are open and ready before the RSI is initiated. In most cases, though, when RSI is undertaken despite identification of difficult airway attributes, appropriate care during the technique and planning related to the particular difficulties present will result in success. If bag-mask ventilation is unlikely to succeed in the context of difficult intubation or if the chance of successful oral intubation is felt to be poor, then RSI is not recommended.

> *RSI is often both safe and effective even in a patient with an identified difficult airway, but identifying the difficult airway in advance permits careful planning and use of a double setup when indicated.*

- **Critical action: Perform "awake" laryngoscopy:** Just as RSI is the cornerstone of emergency airway management overall, awake laryngoscopy is the cornerstone of management of the difficult airway. This technique, which is discussed in detail in Chapter 7, requires sedation of the patient to a depth of sedation similar to that used for a painful procedure, such as reduction of a dislocated shoulder, and liberal use of local anesthesia (usually topical) to permit a laryngoscopy to be performed without paralyzing and inducing the patient. Thus, "awake" is a misnomer because the patient is sedated, but the principle involves allowing the patient to maintain spontaneous respirations until such time as it has been ascertained that the trachea can be successfully intubated. The laryngoscopy can be done with a standard laryngoscope, flexible fiberoptic scope, or any of a variety of other devices (semirigid fiberoptic scope, video scope, etc.) that facilitates an optimal view of the glottis. These devices are discussed in detail in Chapters 12–14. Two possible outcomes are possible from this awake examination. Firstly, the glottis may be adequately visualized, informing the operator that oral intubation using that device will succeed. If the difficult airway is static (i.e., chronic), then the best approach might be to proceed with RSI, now that it is known that the trachea can be intubated, using that same device. If, however, the difficult airway is dynamic (i.e., acute), then it is the judgment of the operator whether to proceed directly with intubation during this awake laryngoscopy or to back out and perform RSI. This decision is predicated on the likelihood that the airway may deteriorate further in the intervening time, arguing in favor of immediate intubation during the awake examination. In general, it is probably advisable to proceed directly with intubation when the difficult airway problem is acute and evolving, rather than simply assuming that the glottis will be visualized with equal ease a few minutes later during an RSI. Intervening deterioration, possibly contributed to by the laryngoscopy itself, might make a subsequent laryngoscopy more difficult or even impossible (see Chapter 7). The second possible outcome during the awake laryngoscopic examination is that the glottis is not adequately visualized to permit intubation. In this case, the examination has confirmed the suspected difficult intubation and reinforced the decision to perform the awake laryngoscopy rather than to proceed with RSI. A failed airway has been avoided and several options remain. Oxygenation should be maintained as necessary at this point.

> *Awake laryngoscopy is the cornerstone of management of the difficult airway when RSI is not felt sufficiently likely to result in successful intubation.*

- **Key question 3: Is the oxygenation still adequate?** If no, and bag and mask ventilation is not successful in restoring adequate oxygen tension, the situation has transformed into a failed airway as described previously. If oxygenation remains adequate, several options remain.
- **Critical action: Consider alternative airway approaches:** At this point, we have clarified that we have a patient with difficult airway attributes, who has proven to be a poor candidate for laryngoscopy, and thus is inappropriate for RSI. There are a number of options available here, including cricothyrotomy (open or Seldinger technique), fiberoptic methods, the intubating laryngeal mask airway, a lighted stylet, or blind nasotracheal intubation. The choice of which of these to use will depend on the operator's experience, the particular difficult airway attributes the patient possesses, and the urgency of the intubation. The devices and techniques are described in Section 2. Whichever technique is used, the goal is to place a cuffed endotracheal tube in the trachea, so any device that does not result in an intubated, protected airway should not be used.

IV. The failed airway algorithm

At several points in the preceding algorithms, it may be determined that airway management has failed. The definition of the failed airway (see discussion earlier in this chapter and in Chapter 6) is based on one of two criteria being satisfied:
- Has there been a failure of an intubation attempt in a patient for whom oxygenation cannot be adequately maintained with a bag and mask, or
- Have there been three unsuccessful intubation attempts by an experienced operator?

Unlike the difficult airway, where the standard of care would dictate the placement of a cuffed tube in the trachea providing a definitive, protected airway, the failed airway calls for action to provide emergency oxygenation sufficient to prevent patient morbidity (especially hypoxic brain injury) by whatever appropriate means are available, regardless of whether this treatment results in a secure, protected airway. Thus the devices considered for the failed airway are somewhat different from, but inclusive of, the devices used for the difficult airway (see Chapter 6). When a failed airway has been determined to occur, the response is dictated by whether bag-mask ventilation is possible and adequate. A recommended approach to the failed airway is described in the following discussion and shown in Fig. 2-5.
- **Critical action: Call for assistance:** As is the case with the difficult airway, it is best to call for any available and necessary assistance as soon as a failed airway is identified. Again, this action may be a stat consult to anesthesia, surgery, or ENT, a request for a respiratory therapist, a call for special equipment, or recruitment of an emergency physician colleague from another section of the department.
- **Key question 1: Is oxygenation adequate?** As is the case for the difficult airway, this question addresses the time available for a rescue airway. If the patient is a failed airway because of three failed attempts by an experienced operator, in most cases, oxygen saturation will be adequate and there is time to consider various approaches. If, however, the failed airway is because of a can't intubate, can't oxygenate (CICO) situation, then there is very little time left before cerebral hypoxia will result in permanent deficit, and immediate cricothyrotomy is indicated. There may be rare circumstances when cricothyrotomy is contraindicated, for example, by a large hematoma across the anterior neck in an anticoagulated patient. Even in such cases, though, the contraindications are relative, and cricothyrotomy remains the first consideration, unless it is the opinion of the operator that cricothyrotomy would not be successful in the particular circumstance at hand. It must be restressed that such circumstances are rare indeed. The only partial

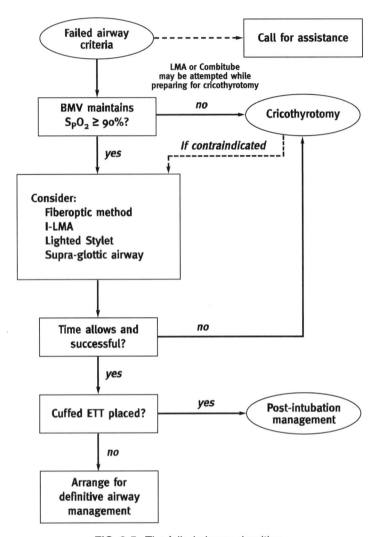

FIG. 2-5. The failed airway algorithm.

exception to the rule that a CICO situation mandates immediate cricothyrotomy as the first rescue step is when the operator makes a single attempt to insert a rapidly placed alternative device, such as the Combitube or I-LMA, *simultaneously with the preparation for a cricothyrotomy.* In other words, when the attempt with this alternative device is in parallel with, and not instead of, preparation for immediate cricothyrotomy, it may be prudent and reasonable to attempt a single placement of a rapid, reliable rescue device, which, if successful, converts the **can't** intubate, **can't** oxygenate situation into a **can't** intubate, **can** oxygenate situation, allowing time for consideration of a number of different approaches to securing the airway.

> *Can't intubate, can't oxygenate = cricothyrotomy in the vast majority of circumstances!*

- **Critical action: Achieve oxygenation using fiberoptic method, intubating laryngeal mask airway, lighted stylet, or supraglottic airway:** In the can't intubate, but can oxygenate situation, various devices are available to provide ongoing oxygenation, and most of these also provide a protected airway. In addition to fiberoptic intubation and the lighted stylet, both of which establish a cuffed endotracheal in the trachea, the intubating laryngeal mask airway has a very high likelihood of providing ventilation and will usually permit intubation through the device. In addition to these approaches, there are a number of supraglottic airways (e.g., Combitube) and these are discussed in detail in Chapter 10. In practical terms, if the patient is able to be successfully ventilated and oxygenated with a bag and mask, the preference is to use a device that places a cuffed endotracheal tube in the trachea (e.g. fiberoptic method, lighted stylet) rather than a nondefinitive temporizing device (e.g., Combitube).
- **Key question 2: Does the device used establish a working airway and provide adequate oxygenation?** If at any time during management of the failed airway, the patient experiences oxygen desaturation and cannot be adequately oxygenated with either a bag and mask or with the rescue device that has been placed, the fallback rescue technique is always cricothyrotomy. In other words, cricothyrotomy is the final rescue for a failed airway in a patient with inadequate oxygen saturation. As long as the device that has been placed is successful in maintaining oxygen saturation, however, cricothyrotomy may not be necessary.
- **Key question 3: Does the device used result in a definitive airway?** If the device used results in a definitive airway, i.e., a cuffed endotracheal tube in the trachea, then one can move on to postintubation management. If a supraglottic device has been used, such as a Combitube or an intubating laryngeal mask airway, without successful intubation, then arrangements must still be made to provide a definitive airway. A definitive airway may be provided in the operating room, intensive care unit, or in the emergency department, once the necessary personnel and equipment are available. Until then, constant surveillance is required to ensure that the airway, as placed, continues to provide adequate oxygenation, with cricothyrotomy always available as a backup.

V. Conclusions

The algorithms presented in this chapter represent a recommended approach to airway management in the emergency department. The algorithms are intended as guidelines only. Individual decision making, clinical circumstances, skill of the physician, and available resources will determine the final, best approach to airway management in any individual case. Understanding the fundamental concepts of the difficult and failed airway, recognition of the crash circumstances that mandate immediate airway management and the use of RSI as the airway management method of choice for most emergency department patients, however, will result in successful airway management with minimal morbidity in the vast majority of circumstances.

EVIDENCE

1. RSI is superior to sedation alone for intubation. Blinded anesthesia studies comparing intubating conditions and success under conditions of deep general anesthesia with various neuromuscular blocking agents have included a control group that received no neuromuscular blocking agent. Despite the deep level of anesthesia, much deeper than that existing in the ED during conditions of RSI, the intubating conditions in the no neuromuscular blockade group were so inferior that both authors subsequently advised against including such a control group in the future (1,2). Recently, 70% of patients undergoing general anesthesia with fentanyl 2 mcg/kg and propofol 2 mg/kg but without succinylcholine demonstrated unacceptable intubating conditions with vocal cords either adducted or closing, excessive patient movement, or sustained coughing, compared to only 2% of patients receiving 1.0 mg/kg of succinylcholine (3). Increasing the dose of succinylcholine from 0.5 to 1.5 mg/kg increases the incidence of excellent intubating conditions from 56% to 85% (4). In two other studies, 19 of 20 and 10 of 10 patients had poor intubating conditions or impossible intubation when neuromuscular blocking agents were not used, despite appropriate doses of anesthetic agents (5,6).

2. RSI has a high success rate in the ED. Sakles et al. prospectively studied 610 emergency department intubations from one high-volume center. In this series, RSI was used in 515 (84%) with a success rate of 98.9%; seven patients underwent cricothyrotomy. The overall complication rate was 8.0%; 95% confidence interval [CI], 6% to 11%) (7). Tayal et al. reported on RSI in 417 of 596 (70%) critically ill patients requiring emergent intubation. Intubations by residents and attendings were successfully completed within two attempts in 97% of the patients. Major immediate adverse events (hypotension, hypoxemia, dysrhythmia) were uncommon (1.4%) and there was no death attributable to RSI. Ninety-six percent of intubations required two or fewer attempts and were completed without major immediate adverse event (8). Initial reports from the National Emergency Airway Registry project, a multicenter study of emergency department intubations that has now gathered data on over 10,000 ED intubations, show very high success rates with a low incidence of adverse events. Sivilotti et al. reported on 3407 ED intubations, of which 2380 (70%) were intubated using RSI. 95% of the patients were intubated in the first two laryngoscopic attempts and 98.5% were successfully intubated without requiring a second (rescue) method. Emergency medicine physicians performed the initial intubation in 2118 (89%) cases (9). Similar success is reported for pediatric intubations in the NEAR I project (10). RSI is the method of choice for most intubations and is also the most common rescue maneuver when another intubation method fails (11).

3. The alternate airway devices as rescue devices. Parr et al. reported on the use of the intubating laryngeal mask airway (ILMA) for two anesthesia patients with failed oral intubation due to impossible laryngoscopic visualization of the glottis (12). Both patients were successfully ventilated with a bag and mask, had the ILMA placed, then were intubated through the ILMA. One hundred per cent of 254 patients with identified difficult airways were successfully ventilated with the ILMA and 96.5% of those on whom intubation was attempted ($n = 200$) were successfully intubated within 5 attempts through the ILMA (13). One hundred patients with identified difficult airways were randomized to undergo intubation either using an ILMA or with a fiberoptic (FO) scope. Success required intubation within three attempts, and success rates were 45/49 (92%) for FO and 48/51 (94%) for ILMA. When the first method of intubation failed (seven patients total), all patients were successfully intubated within two attempts using the other method (14). Both the Combitube and the LMA appear to be easy to place and ventilate with, even by inexperienced personnel (15). All of these devices are discussed in more detail in the relevant chapters.

4. Evidence for the algorithms. Unfortunately, there are no systematized data supporting the algorithmic approach presented in this chapter. The algorithms are the result of careful review of the American Society of Anesthesiologists (ASA) difficult airway algorithm and composite knowledge and experience of the editors, who functioned as an expert panel in this regard. There has not been, and likely never will be, a study comparing, for example, the outcomes of cricothyrotomy versus alternate airway devices in the can't intubate, can't ventilate situation, and clearly randomization of such patients is not ethical. Thus, the algorithms are derived from a rational body of knowledge (described previously) and represent a recommended approach but cannot be considered to be scientifically proven as the only or even necessarily the best way to approach any one clinical problem or patient. Rather, they are designed to help guide a consistent approach to both common and uncommon airway management situations.

REFERENCES

1. Cicala R., Westbrook L. An alternative method of paralysis for rapid-sequence induction. *Anesthesiology* 1988;69:983–986.
2. Baumgarten RK, Carter CE, Reynolds WJ, et al. Priming with nondepolarizing relaxants for rapid tracheal intubation: a double-blind evaluation. *Can J Anaesth* 1988;35:5–11.
3. Naguib M, Samarkandi A, Riad W, et al. Optimal dose of succinylcholine revisited. *Anesthesiology* 2003;99:1045–1049.
4. Stewart KG, Hopkins PM, Dean SG. Comparison of high and low doses of suxamethonium. *Anaesthesia* 1991;46:833–836.
5. Kahwaji R, Bevan DR, Bikhazi G, et al. Dose-ranging study in younger adult and elderly patients of ORG 9487, a new rapid-onset, short duration muscle relaxant. *Anesth Analg* 1997;84:1011–1018.
6. Pino RM, Ali HH, Denman WT, et al. A comparison of the intubation conditions between mivacurium and rocuronium during balanced anesthesia. *Anesthesiology* 1998;88:673–678.
7. Sakles JC, Laurin EG, Rantapaa AA, et al. Airway management in the emergency department: a one-year study of 610 tracheal intubations. *Ann Emerg Med* 1998;31:325–332.
8. Tayal VS, Riggs RW, Marx JA, et al. Rapid-sequence intubation at an emergency medicine residency: success rate and adverse events during a two-year period. *Acad Emerg Med* 1999;6:31–37.
9. Sivilotti MA, Filbin MR, Murray HE, et al. on behalf of the NEAR investigators. Does the sedative agent facilitate emergency rapid-sequence intubation? *Acad Emerg Med* 2003;10:612–620.
10. Sagarin MJ, Chiang V, Sakles JC, et al. on behalf of the NEAR investigators. Rapid sequence intubation for pediatric emergency airway management. *Ped Emerg Care* 2002;18:417–423.
11. Bair AE, Filbin MR, Kulkarni R, et al. on behalf of the NEAR investigators. Failed intubation in the emergency department: analysis of prevalence, rescue techniques, and personnel. *J Emerg Med* 2002;23:131–140.
12. Parr MJA, Gregory M, et al: The intubating laryngeal mask: use in failed and difficult intubations. *Anaesthesia* 1998;53:343–348.
13. Ferson DF, et al. Use of the intubating LMA-Fastrach in 254 patients with difficult airways. *Anesthesiology* 2001;95:1175–1181.
14. Langeron O, et al. Comparison of the Intubating Laryngeal Mask Airway with the Fiberoptic Intubation in Anticipated Difficult Airway Management. *Anesthesiology* 2001;94:968–972.
15. Yardy N. A comparison of two airway aids for emergency use by unskilled personnel. The Combitube and laryngeal mask. *Anaesthesia* 1999;54:179–183.

3

Rapid Sequence Intubation

Ron M. Walls

I. Definition

Rapid sequence intubation (RSI) is the administration of a potent induction agent followed immediately by a rapidly acting neuromuscular blocking agent to induce unconsciousness and motor paralysis for tracheal intubation. The technique is predicated on the fact that the patient has not fasted before intubation and is, therefore, at risk for aspiration of gastric contents. Administration of the drugs is preceded by a preoxygenation phase to permit a period of apnea to occur safely between the administration of the drugs and intubation of the trachea *without interposed assisted ventilation*. In other words, the purpose of RSI is to render the patient unconscious and paralyzed and then to intubate the trachea without the use of bag and mask ventilation, which may cause gastric distention and increase the risk of aspiration. Sellick's maneuver (posterior pressure on the cricoid cartilage) is used to occlude the esophagus and prevent passive regurgitation.

> *Rapid sequence intubation is the virtually simultaneous administration, after preoxygenation, of a potent sedative agent and a rapidly acting neuromuscular blocking agent to facilitate rapid tracheal intubation without interposed mechanical ventilation.*

II. Indications and contraindications

RSI is the cornerstone of emergency airway management. Other techniques, such as blind nasotracheal intubation or intubation using sedation and topical anesthesia, may be useful in certain patients presenting with a difficult airway. However, the superiority of RSI in terms of success rates, complication rates, and control of adverse effects makes it the procedure of choice for the majority of emergency department intubations. Contraindications to RSI are relative. Difficult intubation per se is not a contraindication to RSI; rather, it indicates to the physician that a careful preintubation plan must be made with a particular emphasis on the ability to ventilate the patient should intubation prove unsuccessful (see Chapter 2). The cardinal principle in assessing the patient with a difficult airway for RSI is the determination of whether the patient is likely to be adequately ventilated with a bag and mask; then, if ventilation is felt ensured, the decision to proceed with an attempt is guided by the likelihood of successful oral

---

Box 3-1. The Seven Ps of RSI

1. **P**reparation
2. **P**reoxygenation
3. **P**retreatment
4. **P**aralysis with induction
5. **P**rotection and positioning
6. **P**lacement with proof
7. **P**ostintubation management

---

intubation. This approach is discussed in detail in Chapter 2. Other relative contraindications pertain more to the choice of individual agents for the intubation rather than to the use of a rapid sequence technique. These relative contraindications are discussed in various places throughout this text and within the discussions of the pharmacology of each agent.

III. Description of the technique

RSI can be thought of as a series of discrete steps, the seven Ps. These are shown in Box 3-1.

A. Preparation

Before initiating the sequence, the patient must have been thoroughly assessed for difficulty of intubation and all preparations must be made (Chapters 2 and 6). Fallback plans in the event of failed intubation must be established and the necessary equipment must be close at hand. In some cases, evaluation of the potential difficulty of the intubation will mandate a double setup with surgical airway instruments open and ready and the patient's neck prepared for cricothyrotomy. The patient should be in an area of the emergency department that is organized and equipped for resuscitation. Cardiac monitoring, blood pressure monitoring, and pulse oximetry should be used in all cases. The patient should have at least one secure, well-functioning intravenous line. It is prudent for the physician to assess the patency of this intravenous line personally. It is advisable, when possible, to have a second intravenous line established and running well before initiation of the sequence, in the event the primary intravenous access is compromised. The patient should be positioned on the stretcher and the stretcher positioned within the room in such a way as to optimize the access for intubation (Chapter 5). The sequence of pharmacologic agents should be determined and all agents drawn up in properly labeled syringes. Possible contraindications to any of the planned agents, especially succinylcholine, should be reviewed one last time. All equipment should be tested. There should be at least two functioning laryngoscope handles and a variety of blades, usually two sizes each of curved and straight blades. A good, basic set of airway equipment consists of two laryngoscope handles, nos. 3 and 4 MacIntosh laryngoscope blades, nos. 3 and 4 Miller laryngoscope blades. The blade of choice should be affixed to the laryngoscope handle and clicked into the "On" position to ensure that the light functions and is bright. The light bulbs on each of the laryngoscope blades should be hand-tightened to ensure that they are firmly seated. The endotracheal tube (ETT) size should be chosen based on the patient's anatomy. In general, an 8- or 8.5-mm ETT should be used for men and a 7.5- or 8.0-mm tube for women. If difficult intubation is anticipated, a smaller tube (6.0 mm or 6.5 mm) should be prepared as well. Pediatric tube sizes are discussed in Chapter 19. The ETT cuff should be tested by inflation of air and then gentle palpation of the cuff to ensure that there is no air leak. This test can be done within the ETT package to maintain sterility without the necessity of wearing sterile gloves. The cuff should then be deflated. A stylet should be used for all intubations. With the tube configured in the desired manner for intubation, the proximal tip of the ETT is held and the stylet is pulled back to ensure that it can be successfully removed after intubation. After the stylet is appropriately shaped and placed, the proximal end of the stylet should be bent at a sharp angle over the proximal ETT adapter. This step will prevent any tendency of the stylet to slide distally in the ETT, possibly leading to protrusion of the tip and damage to the airway. Throughout this preparatory phase, the patient should be receiving preoxygenation as described in the next section. Care and time taken during this preparation and assessment phase of intubation pay great dividends when the sequence is initiated.

B. Preoxygenation

Preoxygenation is essential to the no bagging principle of RSI. Preoxygenation is the establishment of an oxygen reservoir within the lungs and body tissue to permit several minutes of apnea to occur without arterial oxygen desaturation. The principle reservoir is the functional residual capacity in the lungs, which is approximately 30 mL/kg. Administration of 100% oxygen for 3 minutes replaces this predominantly nitrogenous mixture of room air with oxygen, allowing several minutes of apnea time before hemoglobin saturation decreases to less than 90%. (see Fig. 3-1) Similar preoxygenation can be achieved much more rapidly by having the patient take eight vital capacity breaths (the greatest volume breaths the patient can take) while receiving 100% oxygen. Although only 3 minutes is required for preoxygenation, it is advisable to start the preoxygenation as early as possible and preferably 5 minutes before the neuromuscular blocking agent is pushed to ensure optimal oxygenation.

Preoxygenation is not simply the establishment of an oxygen reservoir within the lungs; it also involves creating an oxygen surplus in blood and body tissue. A combination of these factors permits prolonged apnea without significant oxygen desaturation. Time to desaturation varies, depending on the patient.

Note the bars indicating recovery from succinylcholine paralysis on the bottom right of Fig. 3-1. This demonstrates the fallacy of the oft-cited belief that a patient will quite likely recover sufficiently from succinylcholine-induced paralysis to breathe on his or her own before dying from hypoxemia even if intubation and mechanical ventilation are both impossible.

A healthy, fully preoxygenated 70-kg adult will maintain oxygen saturation over 90% for 8 minutes, whereas an obese (127-kg) adult will desaturate to 90% in less than 3 minutes. A 10-kg child will desaturate to 90% in less than 4 minutes. The time for desaturation from 90% to 0% is even more important and is much shorter. The healthy 70-kg adult desaturates from 90% to 0% in less than 120 seconds and the small child does so in 45 seconds. A term pregnant woman is a high oxygen user and has an increased body mass, so she desaturates quickly in a manner analogous to that of the obese patient. Particular caution is required in this circumstance, because both the obese patient and the pregnant woman are also difficult to intubate and to bag/mask ventilate.

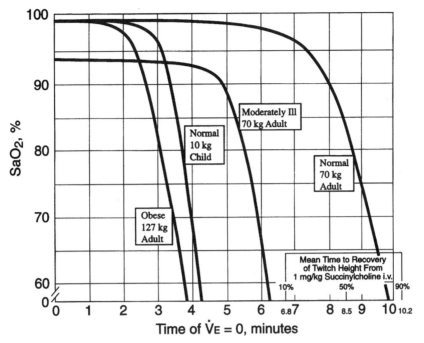

FIG. 3-1. Time to desaturation for various patient circumstances. From Benumof J, Dagg R, Benumof R. Critical hemoglobin desaturation will occur before return to an unparalyzed state following 1 mg/kg intravenous succinylcholine. *Anesthesiology* 1997;87:979.

The time to desaturate from 90% to 0% is dramatically less than the time to desaturate from 100% to 90%.

Most emergency departments do not use systems that are capable of delivering 100% oxygen. Typically, emergency department patients are preoxygenated using the 100% nonrebreather mask, which delivers approximately 65% to 70% oxygen (Chapter 5). In physiologically well patients in whom difficult intubation is not anticipated, this percentage is often sufficient. However, higher inspired fractions of oxygen are desirable for ill patients and can be delivered by active breathing through the demand valve of certain bag/mask systems or by specially designed high oxygen delivery devices. Oxygen delivery is discussed in detail in Chapter 5. The use of pulse oximetry throughout intubation enables the physician to monitor the level of oxygen saturation, thus eliminating guesswork.

The old recommendation that an intubator should hold his or her breath during the laryngoscopy to determine the maximal time that the patient should be without ventilation predated pulse oximetry and has no place in modern airway management.

Box 3-2. Pretreatment Drugs for RSI

Lidocaine — for reactive airways disease or ↑ICP

Opioid (fentanyl) — when sympathetic responses should be blunted (↑ICP, aortic dissection, intracranial hemorrhage, ischemic heart disease)

Atropine — for children ≤10 years old who will receive succinylcholine

Defasciculation — before succinylcholine if patient has ↑ICP, penetrating globe injury

---

C. Pretreatment

Pretreatment is the administration of drugs to mitigate adverse effects associated with the intubation. These adverse effects include the bronchospastic reactivity of the airways to the ETT in patients with reactive airways disease and the intracranial pressure (ICP) response to intubation in cases of elevated ICP. Pretreatment drugs also can be used to blunt the sympathetic discharge that accompanies laryngoscopy and intubation and to modulate the increase in ICP that can occur when succinylcholine is administered to a patient with elevated ICP. These clinical circumstances and the drugs used to manage them are discussed in detail in Chapter 16 and in various sections throughout this manual. The drugs themselves can be remembered using the mnemonic LOAD as shown in Box 3-2.

D. Paralysis with induction

In this phase, a rapidly acting induction agent is given in a dose adequate to produce prompt loss of consciousness (see Chapter 17). Administration of the induction agent is immediately followed by the neuromuscular blocking agent, usually succinylcholine (see Chapter 18). Both of these medications are given by intravenous push. The concept of RSI does not involve the slow administration of the induction agent, nor does it involve a titration-to-end-point approach. The sedative agent and dose should be selected with the intention of rapid intravenous administration of the drug. Although rapid administration of these induction agents can increase the likelihood and severity of side effects, especially hypotension, the entire technique is predicated on rapid loss of consciousness, rapid neuromuscular blockade, and a brief period of apnea without interposed assisted ventilation before intubation. Therefore, the induction agent is given as a rapid push followed immediately by a rapid push of the succinylcholine. Within a few seconds of the administration of the induction agent and succinylcholine, the patient will begin to lose consciousness and respirations will decline, then cease.

E. Protection and positioning

After 20 to 30 seconds, apnea will virtually universally be present. If succinylcholine has been used as the neuromuscular blocking agent, fasciculations will be observed during this time. Sellick's maneuver, the application of firm pressure (Chapter 5) on the cricoid cartilage to prevent passive regurgitation of gastric contents, should be initiated immediately on the observation that the patient is losing consciousness. Sellick's maneuver should be maintained throughout the entire intubation sequence until the ETT has been correctly placed, the position verified, and the cuff inflated.

It is often stated that Sellick's maneuver must be discontinued immediately on the initiation of active vomiting by the patient to prevent the possibility of esophageal rupture. This recommendation, although probably correct, has little bearing on the performance of RSI during which the patient is paralyzed, because vomiting requires coordinated neuromuscular activity.

Sellick's maneuver is an essential part of the protection of the airway during RSI and must be performed properly by trained personnel. Also central to protection against aspiration is the avoidance of bag/mask ventilation during the intubation sequence. Some patients, as discussed in the Special Clinical Circumstances section later in this manual, will be sufficiently compromised that they require assisted ventilation to maintain oxygen saturations over 90% before, during, and after the intubation. Such patients, especially those with profound hypoxemia, should be bag/mask ventilated throughout the sequence to prevent worsening hypoxemia. However, most patients will not require such oxygen supplementation and will be fully protected by a properly conducted preoxygenation phase. In the event that bag/mask ventilation is necessary, Sellick's maneuver should be continuously applied to minimize the likelihood of gastric distention and the risk of regurgitation with aspiration.

F. Placement and proof

Approximately 45 seconds after the administration of the succinylcholine, or 60 seconds if rocuronium is used, the patient's jaw should be tested for flaccidity and intubation should be undertaken. Because of the *minutes* of safe apnea time permitted by the preoxygenation, the intubation can be performed gently and carefully with due attention to the patient's dentition and proper attention to technique to minimize the potential for trauma to the airway. The glottic aperture should be visualized and the ETT should be placed. The stylet should be removed and the endotracheal tube cuff should be inflated. Tube placement should be confirmed as described in Chapter 5 to prove that the tube is correctly placed within the trachea. End-tidal carbon dioxide (CO_2) detection is mandatory. Sellick's maneuver can then be discontinued on the order of the intubator.

G. Postintubation management

After placement is confirmed, the ET tube must be taped or tied in place. Mechanical ventilation should be initiated as described in Chapter 34. A chest radiograph should be obtained to assess pulmonary status and ensure that mainstem intubation has not occurred. Hypotension is common in the postintubation period and is often caused by diminished venous blood return as a result of the increased intrathoracic pressure that attends mechanical ventilation, aggravated by the hemodynamic effects of the induction agent. Although this form of hypotension is often self-limited and responds to intravenous fluids, more ominous causes should be sought. Blood pressure should be measured, and if significant hypotension is present, the management steps in Table 3-1 should be undertaken.

Long-term sedation and paralysis should be administered using a benzodiazepine (e.g., lorazepam 0.03 to 0.05 mg/kg) and a competitive neuromuscular blocking agent (e.g., pancuronium 0.1 mg/kg or vecuronium 0.1 mg/kg). An opioid analgesic, such as morphine 0.1 to 0.2 mg/kg or fentanyl 1–2 mcg/kg, should be added to improve patient comfort in hemodynamically stable patients. Meperidine should not be used. The benzodiazepine and opioid should be repeated in approximately one-third to one-half of the initial dose when any signs of patient awareness are detected (especially tachycardia or hypertension), or not less frequently than hourly until it is desirable to allow the patient to recover consciousness. Alternative agents, such as

TABLE 3-1. *Hypotension in the post-intubation period*

Cause	Detection	Action
Pneumothorax	Increased peak inspiratory pressure (PIP), difficulty bagging, decreased breath sounds	Immediate thoracostomy
Decreased venous return	Worst in patients with high PIPs secondary to high intrathoracic pressure or those with marginal hemodynamic status before intubation	Fluid bolus, treatment of airway resistance (bronchodilators); increase inspiratory flow rate to allow increased expiratory time; try $\downarrow V_T$, respiratory rate, or both if S_pO_2 is adequate
Induction agents	Other causes excluded	Fluid bolus, expectant
Cardiogenic	Usually in compromised patient; ECG; exclude other causes	Fluid bolus (caution), pressors

propofol by infusion, are also useful in this regard. The neuromuscular blocking agent should be repeated as a dose of one-third the original dose (generally 2 to 3 mg in an adult patient) every 45 to 60 minutes or when any motor activity is detected.

IV. Timing the steps of rapid sequence intubation

Successful RSI requires a detailed knowledge of the precise steps to be taken and also of the time required for each step to achieve its purpose. Preoxygenation requires 3 minutes for maximal effect. In hurried circumstances, eight vital capacity breaths (if possible) can accomplish equivalent preoxygenation in less than 30 seconds. It is recommended that pretreatment drugs be given 3 minutes before the administration of the sedative and neuromuscular blocking agent. The pharmacokinetics of the sedatives and neuromuscular blockers would suggest that a 45-second interval between administration of these agents and initiation of endotracheal intubation is optimal, extending to 60 seconds if rocuronium is used. Thus the entire sequence of RSI can be described as a series of timed steps. For the purposes of discussion, time zero is the time at which the succinylcholine is pushed. The recommended sequence is shown in Table 3-2.

TABLE 3-2. *The sequence of RSI*

Time	Action (seven Ps)
Zero minus 10 min	**P**reparation: *Assemble all necessary equipment, drugs, etc.*
Zero minus 5 min	**P**reoxygenation
Zero minus 3 min	**P**retreatment (LOAD)
Zero	**P**aralysis with induction: *Administer induction agent by IV push, followed immediately by paralytic agent by IV push*
Zero plus 20–30 sec	**P**rotection: *Apply Sellick's maneuver; position patient for optimal laryngoscopy*
Zero plus 45 sec	**P**lacement: *Assess mandible for flaccidity, perform intubation; confirm placement*
Zero plus 1 min	**P**ostintubation management: *See text for details*

TABLE 3-3. *RSI for healthy 80-kg patient*

Time	Action (seven Ps)
Zero minus 10 min	**P**reparation
Zero minus 5 min	**P**reoxygenation
Zero minus 3 min	**P**retreatment—none indicated
Zero	**P**aralysis with induction: Etomidate 24 mg IV push; Succinylcholine 120 mg IV push
Zero plus 20–30 sec	**P**rotection: Sellick's maneuver; position patient
Zero plus 45 sec	**P**lacement: Confirm with ETCO$_2$*, Px[†]
Zero plus 1 min	**P**ostintubation management: Long-term sedation/paralysis as indicated

*ETCO$_2$; End tidal CO$_2$ detection.
[†] Px: Physical examination.

An example of RSI performed for a generally healthy 40-year-old, 80-kg patient is shown in Table 3-3. Other examples of RSI for particular patient conditions are in the corresponding sections throughout the text.

V. Success rates and adverse events

RSI has a very high success rate in the emergency department, approximately 99% in most modern series. The National Emergency Airway Registry (NEAR), an international multicenter study of over 10,000 emergency department intubations, reported >99% success for RSI when used on patients with medical emergencies and over 97% for trauma patients. RSI success rates are higher than those for other emergency airway management methods, and RSI is the main rescue technique when other methods, such as blind nasotracheal intubation, fail. The NEAR investigators classify events related to intubation as follows:

- Immediate (true) complications, such as witnessed aspiration, broken teeth, airway trauma, undetected esophageal intubation
- Technical problems, such as mainstem intubation, cuff leak, recognized esophageal intubation
- Physiological alterations, such as pneumothorax, pneumomediastinum, cardiac arrest, dysrhythmia

This system allows true complications to be identified and all adverse events to be captured, but avoids the incorrect attribution of various technical problems (such as recognized esophageal intubation) or physiological alterations (such as cardiac arrest in a patient who was *in extremis* before intubation was undertaken and which may or may not be attributable to the intubation) as complications. Overall, event rates were low in the NEAR studies; likewise, true complications are seen in approximately 3% of RSI patients. Hypotension and alterations in heart rate can result from the pharmacologic agents used or from stimulation of the larynx with resultant reflexes. Other studies have reported consistent results. The most catastrophic complication of RSI is unrecognized esophageal intubation, which is rare in the emergency department but occurs with alarming frequency in some prehospital studies. This situation underscores the importance of the confirmation of tube placement described in Chapter 5. It is incumbent on the person who administers neuromuscular blocking agents and potent sedatives to the patient to be able to establish an airway and maintain mechanical ventilation. This process may require a surgical airway as a final rescue for a failed oral intubation attempt. Aspiration of gastric contents can occur but is uncommon. Overall, the true complication rate of rapid sequence intubation in the emergency department is low and the success rate is exceedingly high, especially when one considers the serious nature of the illnesses for which patients are intubated and the limited time and information available to the clinician performing the intubation.

VI. **Accelerated and immediate RSI**

When time is of the essence, the RSI sequence can be compressed so that the steps are conducted much more rapidly than the standard RSI outlined previously.

1. Accelerated RSI

   More rapid intubation can be achieved by:
   - Shortening preoxygenation to 15 seconds by using the eight-vital-capacity-breath method
   - Shortening the pretreatment interval to 2 minutes from 3 minutes

2. Immediate RSI
   - Eliminate pretreatment
   - Preoxygenate with eight vital capacity breaths

EVIDENCE

1. Preoxygenation: Standard preoxygenation has traditionally been achieved by 3 minutes of normal tidal volume breathing of 100% oxygen. Panditt et al. showed that eight vital capacity breaths achieves similar oxygen intake to that of 3 minutes of normal tidal volume breathing and that both of these methods are superior to four vital capacity breaths (1). The time to desaturation of oxyhemoglobin to 95% is 5.2 minutes after eight vital capacity breaths versus 3.7 minutes after 3 minutes of tidal volume breathing versus 2.8 minutes after four vital capacity breaths (2,3). Preoxygenation of normal healthy patients can produce an average of 8 minutes of apnea time before desaturation to 90% occurs, but the times are much less (as little as 3 minutes) in patients with cardiovascular disease, obese patients, and small children (4). Sufficient recovery from succinylcholine paralysis cannot be relied on before desaturation occurs, even in properly preoxygenated healthy patients (4,5). Term pregnant women also desaturate more rapidly than nonpregnant women and desaturate to 95% in less than 3 minutes, compared with 4 minutes for nonpregnant controls. Preoxygenating in the upright position prolongs desaturation time in nonpregnant women to $5^{1}/_{2}$ minutes, but does not favorably affect the term pregnant patients (6,7).

2. Evidence regarding the use of pretreatment drugs, induction agents, and neuromuscular blocking agents are discussed in the Evidence sections of the relevant chapters.

3. Sellick's Maneuver: A metaanalysis of the studies of Sellick's maneuver by Brimacombe and Berry concluded that there is no hard evidence supporting its routine use during RSI, but the practice remains firmly entrenched in practice (8). Sellick's maneuver may be applied improperly or not at all during a significant proportion of emergency department RSIs (9). Even when applied by experienced practitioners, Sellick's maneuver can increase peak inspiratory pressure and decrease tidal volume or even cause complete obstruction during bag/mask ventilation (10). Cricoid pressure appears to enhance the success rate of fiberoptic intubation, increasing rapid insertion success from 33% to over 60% in one series (11). Properly applied, cricoid pressure tends to improve laryngoscopic view during conventional direct laryngoscopy, but it may interfere with both insertion of and ventilation through the laryngeal mask airway (12,13). Cricoid pressure is capable of moving the cervical spine approximately 5 mm in normal subjects, which suggests that it might present a hazard in patients with unstable cervical spine injuries; however, its use in patients with cervical spine injuries has never been assessed (14). A two-handed technique has been advocated, but has never been shown to be superior to the one-handed technique in terms of prevention of aspiration and results in a worse laryngoscopic view (15).

4. Rapid Sequence Intubation: The largest published series of emergency department intubations is that of Sakles, who analyzed 610 intubations from one high-volume emergency department over a one-year period (16). 84% of the patients were intubated using RSI, and overall, 98.9% of patients were successfully intubated; the remainder underwent emergency cricothyrotomy. Immediate complications were identified in 8% of patients. Bozeman et al. compared the use of etomidate alone to etomidate plus succinylcholine in a prehospital flight paramedic program and found that RSI outperformed etomidate-alone intubations by all measures of ease of intubation (17). An analysis of 200 prehospital intubations performed before and after institution of an RSI protocol found that intubation success increased from 73% before RSI was used to 96% with RSI (18). Li et al. found similar improvement when RSI was introduced in the emergency department (19). The only direct comparison between RSI and blind nasotracheal intubation showed that higher success rates and more rapid intubation is achieved by RSI in poisoned patients (20). Dufour et al. reported very high success and low complication rates in 219 patients undergoing RSI in a community hospital in Canada (21). Pediatric RSI has also been studied. A multicenter report of pediatric intubation by the NEAR I investigators identified 156 pediatric intubations from among 1,288 total intubations, with 81% of pediatric intubations having been done using RSI (22). A study of 105 children under 10 years old (average age 3 years) who underwent RSI with etomidate as the induction dose showed stable hemodynamics and high success and safety profiles (23). Bair et al. analyzed 207 (2.7%) failed intubations among 7,712 intubations in the NEAR project and found that the greatest proportion of rescue procedures (49%) involved the use of RSI to achieve intubation after failure of oral or nasotracheal intubation by non-RSI methods (24).

REFERENCES

1. Pandit JJ, Duncan T, Robbins PA. Total oxygen uptake with two maximal breathing techniques and the tidal volume breathing technique: a physiologic study of preoxygenation. *Anesthesiology* 2003;99:841–846.
2. Baraka AS, Taha SK, Aouad MT, et al. Preoxygenation: comparison of maximal breathing and tidal volume breathing techniques. *Anesthesiology* 1999;91:612–616.
3. Ramez Salem M, Joseph NJ, Crystal GJ, et al. Preoxygenation: comparison of maximal breathing and tidal volume techniques. *Anesthesiology* 2000;92:1845–1847.
4. Benumof JL, Dagg R, Benumof R. Critical hemoglobin desaturation will occur before return to an unparalyzed state following 1 mg/kg intravenous succinylcholine. *Anesthesiology* 1997;87:979–982.
5. Hayes AH, Breslin DS, Mirakhur RK, et al. Frequency of haemoglobin desaturation with the use of succinylcholine during rapid sequence induction of anaesthesia. *Acta Anaesthesiologica Scandinavica* 2001;45:746–749.
6. Heier T, Feiner JR, Lin J, et al. Hemoglobin desaturation after succinylcholine-induced apnea: a study of the recovery of spontaneous ventilation in healthy volunteers. *Anesthesiology* 2001;94:754–759.
7. Baraka AS, Hanna MT, Jabbour SI, et al. Preoxygenation of pregnant and nonpregnant women in the head-up versus supine position. *Anesth Analg* 1992;75:757–759.
8. Brimacombe JR, Berry AM. Cricoid pressure. *Can J Anaesth* 1997;44:414–425.
9. Olsen JC, Gurr DE, Hughes M. Video analysis of emergency medicine residents performing rapid-sequence intubations. *J Emerg Med* 2000;18:469–472.
10. Allman KG. The effect of cricoid pressure application on airway patency. *J Clin Anesth* 1995;7:197–199.
11. Asai T, Murao K, Johmura S, et al. Effect of cricoid pressure on the ease of fibrescope-aided tracheal intubation. *Anaesthesia* 2002;57:909–913.
12. Vanner RG, Clarke P, Moore WJ, et al. The effect of cricoid pressure and neck support on the view at laryngoscopy. *Anaesthesia* 1997;52:896–900.
13. Aoyama K, Takenaka I, Sata T, et al. Cricoid pressure impedes positioning and ventilation through the laryngeal mask airway. *Can J Anaesth* 1996;43:1035–1040.
14. Gabbott DA. The effect of single-handed cricoid pressure on neck movement after applying manual in-line stabilization. *Anaesthesia* 1997;52:586–588.
15. Cook TM. Cricoid pressure: are two hands better than one? [Comment]. *Anaesthesia* 1996;51:365–368.

16. Sakles JC, Laurin EG, Rantapaa AA, et al. Airway management in the emergency department: a one-year study of 610 tracheal intubations. *Ann Emerg Med* 1998;31:325–332.
17. Bozeman WP, Kleiner DM, Huggett V. Intubating conditions produced by etomidate alone vs. rapid sequence intubation in the prehospital aeromedical setting. *Acad Emerg Med* 2003;10:445–456.
18. Rose WD, Anderson LD, Edmond SA. Analysis of intubations. Before and after establishment of a rapid sequence intubation protocol for air medical use. *Air Med J* 1994;13:475–478.
19. Li J, Murphy-Lavoie H, Bugas C, et al. Complications of emergency intubation with and without paralysis. *Am J Emerg Med* 1999;17:141–143.
20. Dronen SC, Merigian KS, Hedges JR, et al. A comparison of blind nasotracheal and succinylcholine-assisted intubation in the poisoned patient. *Ann Emerg Med* 1987;16:650–652.
21. Dufour DG, Larose DL, Clement SC. Rapid sequence intubation in the emergency department. *J Emerg Med* 1995;13:705–710.
22. Sagarin MJ, Chiang V, Sakles JC, et al. National Emergency Airway Registry (NEAR) investigators. Rapid sequence intubation for pediatric emergency airway management. *Pediatr Emerg Care* 2002;18:417–423.
23. Guldner G, Schultz J, Sexton P, et al. Etomidate for rapid-sequence intubation in young children: hemodynamic effects and adverse events. *Acad Emerg Med* 2003;10:134–139.
24. Bair AE, Filbin MR, Kulkarni RG, et al. The failed intubation attempt in the emergency department: analysis of prevalence, rescue techniques, and personnel. *J Emerg Med* 2002;23:131–140.

4

Applied Functional Anatomy of the Airway

Michael F. Murphy

There are many salient features of the anatomy and physiology of the airway to consider with respect to airway management maneuvers. This chapter will discuss the anatomical features most involved in the act of intubation, the important vascular structures, and the innervation of the upper airway. Chapter 7 builds on these anatomical and functional relationships to describe anesthesia techniques for the airway. Chapter 19 addresses developmental and pediatric anatomical features of the airway.

We will consider each anatomical structure in the order in which it appears as we enter the airway: the nose, the mouth, the pharynx, the larynx, and the trachea (Fig. 4-1).

THE NOSE

The external nose consists of a bony vault, a cartilaginous vault, and a lobule. The bony vault comprises the nasal bones, the frontal processes of the maxillae, and the nasal spine of the frontal bone. The nasal bones are buttressed in the midline by the perpendicular plate of the ethmoid bone that forms part of the bony septum. The cartilaginous vault is formed by the upper lateral cartilages that meet the cartilaginous portion of the septum in the midline. The nasal lobule consists of the tip of the nose, the lower lateral cartilages, the fibrofatty alae that form the lateral margins of the nostril, and the columella. The cavities of each nostril are continuous with the nasopharynx posteriorly.

Important Anatomical Considerations

- Kiesselbach's plexus (Little's area) is a very vascular area located on the anteromedial aspect of the septum of each nostril. Epistaxis most often originates from this area. During the act of inserting a nasal trumpet or a nasotracheal tube, it is generally recommended that the device be inserted in the nostril such that the leading edge of the bevel (the pointed tip) is away from the septum. The goal is to minimize the chances of trauma and bleeding from this very vascular area. This means that the device is inserted 'upside down' in the left nostril and rotated 180 degrees after the tip has proceeded beyond the cartilagenous septum. Although some authors have recommended the opposite, i.e., that the bevel tip approximate the nasal septum to minimize the risk of damage and bleeding from the turbinates, the bevel away from the septum approach makes more sense and is the recommended method.
- The major nasal airway is between the laterally placed inferior turbinate, the septum, and the floor of the nose. The floor of the nose is tilted slightly downward front to back,

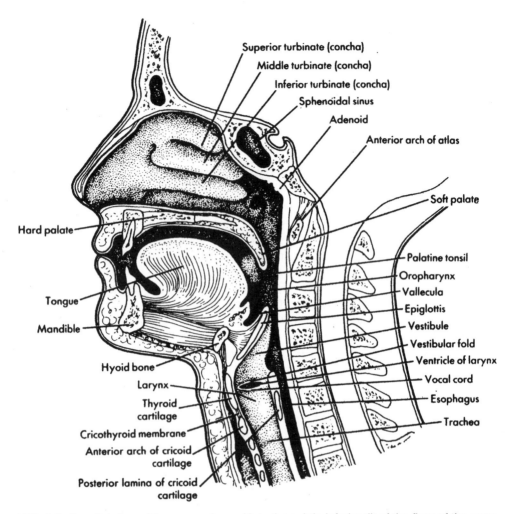

FIG. 4-1. Saggital view of the upper airway. Note the subtle inferior tilt of the floor of the nose from front to back, the location of the adenoid, the location of the vallecula between the base of the tongue and the epiglottis, and the location of the hyoid bone in relation to the posterior limit of the tongue. (From Kastendieck JG. Airway management. In: Rosen P, ed. *Emergency medicine: concepts and clinical practice*, 2nd ed. St. Louis: Mosby, 1988, with permission.)

approximately 10 to 15 degrees. Thus when a nasal tube, trumpet, or fiberscope is inserted through the nose, it ought not to be directed upward or even straight back. It should be directed slightly inferiorly to follow this major channel. Before nasal intubation of an unconscious adult patient, some authorities recommend gently but *fully* inserting one's gloved and lubricated little finger to ensure patency and to maximally dilate this channel before the insertion of the nasal tube. In addition, placing the endotracheal tube (preferably an Endotrol tube) in a warm bottle of saline or water softens the tube and attenuates its damaging properties.

- The nasal mucosa is exquisitely sensitive to topically applied vasoconstricting medications such as phenylephrine, epinephrine, oxymetazoline, or cocaine. Cocaine has the added advantage of providing profound topical anesthesia and is the only local anesthetic agent that produces vasoconstriction; all of the others cause vasodilatation. Shrinking the nasal mucosa

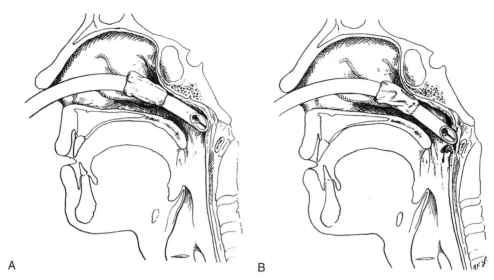

FIG. 4-2. Mechanism of nasopharyngeal perforation and submucosal tunneling of the naso-tracheal tube. **A:** The NTT entering the pit of the adenoid where the eustacean tube enters the nasopharynx. **B:** The tube perforating the mucous membrane. (From Tintinalli JE, Claffey J. Complications of nasotracheal intubation. *Ann Emerg Med* 1981;10:142–144, with permission.)

with a vasoconstricting agent can increase the caliber of the nasal airway by as much as 50% to 75% and may substantially reduce epistaxis incited by nasotracheal intubation. Cocaine has been implicated in coronary vasoconstriction when applied to the nasal mucosa, so should be used with caution in patients with coronary artery disease. (See Evidence section at the end of this chapter.)

- The nasal cavities are bounded posteriorly by the nasopharynx. The adenoids are placed slightly laterally at the back of each nostril and just behind the soft palate. The adenoids partially surround a depression in the mucosal membrane where the eustacean tube enters the nasopharynx. During insertion, the nasotracheal tube often enters this depression and resistance is encountered. Continued aggressive insertion can cause the nasotracheal tube to penetrate the mucosa and pass submucosally deep to the naso- and oropharyngeal mucous membrane (Fig. 4-2). Though alarming when one recognizes that this has occurred, no specific treatment is advised, except that withdrawing the tube and trying the opposite nostril is advised. Despite the theoretical risk of infection, there is no literature to suggest that this occurs. Documentation of the complication and communication to the accepting team on admission is mandatory.
- The soft palate rests on the base of the tongue during quiet nasal respiration, sealing the oral cavity anteriorly.
- The contiguity of the paranasal sinuses with the nasal cavity is thought to be responsible for the infections of the paranasal sinuses that may be associated with prolonged nasotracheal intubation. Although this fact has led some physicians to condemn nasotracheal intubation, considerations of later infections should not deter the emergency physician from considering nasotracheal intubation when indicated. Securing the airway in an emergency takes precedence over possible later infective complications, and in any case, the intubation can always be changed to an oral tube or tracheostomy if necessary.
- A nasotracheal intubation is relatively contraindicated in patients with basal skull fractures, i.e., when the maxilla is fractured away from its attachment to the base of the skull, because

of the risk of penetration into the cranial vault (usually through the cribiform plate) with the endotracheal tube. Careful technique avoids this complication, however, as the cribiform plate is located cephalad of the nares, and tube insertion should be directed slightly caudad (see earlier discussion). Maxillary fractures (e.g., Leforte fractures) may disrupt the continuity of the nasal cavities and are a relative contraindication to blind nasal intubation. Again cautious insertion, particularly using a fiberscope, can mitigate the risk.

THE MOUTH

The mouth, or oral cavity, is bounded externally by the lips and is contiguous with the oropharynx posteriorly (Fig. 4-3).

- The tongue is attached to the symphysis of the mandible anteriorly and anterolaterally and the stylohyoid process and hyoid bone posterolaterally and posteriorly, respectively. The posterior limit of the tongue corresponds to the position of the hyoid bone (Fig. 4-1). The clinical importance of this relationship will become apparent when the 3-3-2 rule is described in Chapter 6.
- The potential spaces in the hollow of the mandible are collectively called the mandibular space, which is subdivided into three potential spaces on either side of the midline sublingual raphe: the submental, submandibular, and sublingual spaces. The tongue is a fluid-filled noncompressible structure. During conventional laryngoscopy the tongue is largely displaced into the mandibular space, permitting one to expose the larynx for intubation under direct

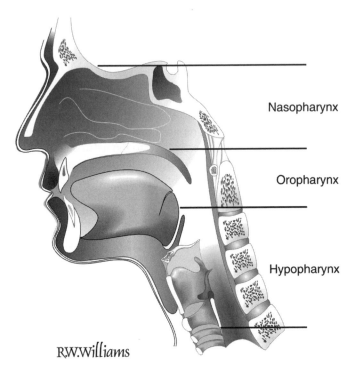

Nasopharynx

Oropharynx

Hypopharynx

R.W.Williams

FIG. 4-3. Pharynx divided into three segments: nasopharynx, oropharynx, and hypopharynx. (From Redden RJ. Anatomic considerations in anesthesia. In: Hagberg CA, ed. *Handbook of difficult airway management.* Philadelphia: Churchill Livingstone, 2000:7, with permission.)

vision. If the mandibular space is small relative to the size of the tongue (e.g., hypoplastic mandible, lingual edema in angioedema, lingual hematoma, etc.) the ability to visualize the larynx may be compromised. Infiltration of the mandibular space by infection (e.g., Ludwig's angina), hematoma, or other lesions may limit the ability to displace the tongue into this space and render orotracheal intubation difficult or impossible.

- Subtle geometric distortions of the oral cavity that limit working and viewing space, such as a high arched palate with a narrow oral cavity or buck teeth with an elongated oral cavity, may render orotracheal intubation difficult. Chapter 6 elaborates on these issues.

- Salivary glands continuously secrete saliva, which can defeat attempts at achieving sufficient topical anesthesia of the airway to undertake awake laryngoscopy or other active airway intervention maneuvers in the awake or lightly sedated patient—for example, laryngeal mask airway (LMA) insertion, lighted stylet intubation, etc.

- The condyles of the mandible articulate within the temperomandibular joint (TMJ) for the first 30 degrees of mouth opening. Beyond 30 degrees the condyles *translate* out of the TMJ anteriorly onto the zygomatic arches. Once translation has occurred it is possible to employ a jaw thrust maneuver to pull the mandible and tongue forward. This is the most effective method of opening the airway to alleviate obstruction or permit bag and mask ventilation. A jaw thrust to open the airway is not possible unless this translation has occurred.

THE PHARYNX

The pharynx is a U-shaped fibromuscular tube extending from the base of the skull to the lower border of the cricoid cartilage where, at the level of the sixth cervical vertebra, it is continuous with the esophagus. Posteriorly it rests against the fascia covering the prevertebral muscles and the cervical spine. Anteriorly it opens into the nasal cavity (the nasopharynx), the mouth (the oropharynx), and the larynx (the laryngo- or hypopharynx).

- The oropharyngeal musculature has a normal tone, like any other skeletal musculature, and this tone serves to keep the upper airway open during quiet respiration. Respiratory distress is associated with pharyngeal muscular activity that attempts to open the airway further. Benzodiazepines and other sedative hypnotic agents may attenuate some of this tone. This explains why sedation may lead to total airway obstruction in patients presenting with partial airway obstruction.

- An 'awake look' is advocated during the difficult airway algorithm (see Chapter 2). Being able to see the epiglottis or posterior glottic structures generally assures one that the same structures will be seen during intubation if neuromuscular blockade is used to secure the airway. In practice, the glottic view is usually better with neuromuscular blockade than with the awake look because of the increased muscle relaxation. Rarely, however, the loss of pharyngeal muscle tone caused by the neuromuscular blocking agent might actually hinder one's ability to expose the larynx. Although uncommon, this tends to occur more often in morbidly obese or late-term pregnancy patients, in whom there may be submucosal edema.

- The glossopharyngeal nerve supplies sensation to the posterior one-third of the tongue, the valleculae, the superior surface of the epiglottis, and most of the posterior pharynx. This nerve is accessible to blockade (topically or by injection) as it runs past the inferior portion of the palatopharyngeus muscle, also known as the posterior tonsillar pillar (Fig. 4-4).

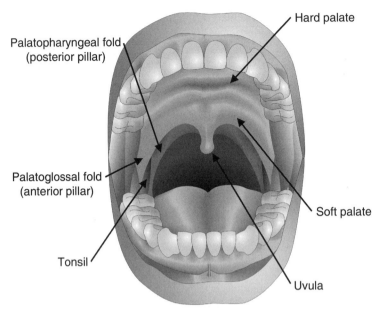

R.W.Williams

FIG. 4-4. The oral cavity: Note the position of the posterior pillar. The glossopharyngeal nerve runs at the base of this structure. (Redden RJ. Anatomic considerations in anesthesia. In: Hagberg CA, ed. *Handbook of difficult airway management.* Philadelphia: Churchill Livingstone, 2000:8.)

THE LARYNX

The larynx extends from its oblique entrance formed by the aryepiglottic folds, the tip of the epiglottis, and the posterior commissure between the arytenoid cartilages through the vocal apparatus to the cricoid ring (Fig. 4-5).

- The superior laryngeal branch of the vagus nerve supplies sensation to the undersurface of the epiglottis, all of the larynx to the level of the false vocal cords, and the pyriform recesses posterolateral to either side of the larynx (Fig. 4-5). The nerve enters the region by passing through the thyrohyoid membrane just below the inferior cornu of the hyoid bone (Fig. 4-6). It then divides into a superior and an inferior branch; the superior branch passes submucosly through the vallecula, where it is visible to the naked eye, on its way to the larynx; and the inferior branch runs along the medial aspects of the pyriform recesses (described below).
- The larynx is the most heavily innervated sensory structure in the body, followed closely by the carina. Stimulation of the unanesthetized larynx during intubation causes tremendous reflex sympathetic activation. Blood pressure and heart rate may increase by as much as 100%.
- The pyramidal arytenoid cartilages sit on the posterior aspect of the larynx (Fig. 4-5). The intrinsic laryngeal muscles cause them to swivel, opening and closing the vocal cords. An endotracheal tube (ETT) that is too large may, over time, compress these structures causing mucosal and cartilagenous ischemia and resultant permanent laryngeal damage. A traumatic intubation may dislocate these cartilages, and unless diagnosed early and relocated, may lead to permanent hoarseness.
- The larynx bulges posteriorly into the hypopharynx, leaving deep recesses on either side called the pyriform recesses or sinuses. Ingested material passes through the pyriform

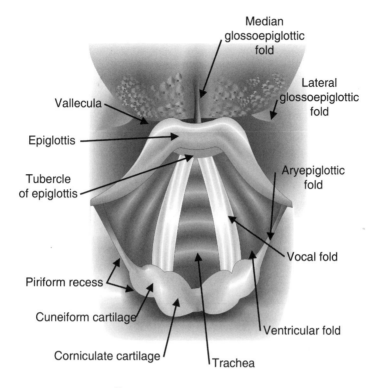

R.W.Williams

FIG. 4-5. Larynx visualized from the oropharynx. Note the median glossoepiglottic fold. It is pressure on this structure by the tip of a curved blade that flips the epiglottis forward, exposing the glottis during laryngoscopy. Note that the valleculae and the pyriform recesses are different structures, a fact often confused in the anesthesia literature. The cuneiform and corniculate cartilages are called the arytenoid cartilages. The ridge between them posteriorly is called the posterior commissure. (Redden RJ. Anatomic considerations in anesthesia. In: Hagberg CA, ed. *Handbook of difficult airway management.* Philadelphia: Churchill Livingstone, 2000:9.)

recesses into the esophagus when swallowed, and foreign bodies (e.g., fishbones) occasionally become lodged there.

- The cricothyroid membrane extends between the upper surface of the cricoid cartilage to the inferior border of the thyroid cartilage. Its height tends to be about the size of the tip of the index finger externally in both male and female adults. Locating the cricoid cartilage and the cricothyroid membrane quickly in an airway emergency is crucial. It is usually easily done in men, because of the obvious laryngeal prominence (Adam's apple). Locate the laryngeal prominence, then note the anterior surface of the thyroid cartilage immediately caudad, usually about one index finger's breadth in height. There is an obvious soft indentation caudad to this anterior surface with a very hard ridge immediately caudad to it. The soft indentation is the cricothyroid membrane and the ridge is the cricoid cartilage. Because of the lack of a distinct laryngeal prominence in women, locating the membrane can be much more difficult. In the woman, place your index finger in the sternal notch. Then drag it cephalad in the midline until the first, and ordinarily the biggest, transverse ridge is felt. This is the cricoid ring. Superior to the cricoid cartilage is the cricothyroid membrane, and superior to that, the anterior surface of the thyroid cartilage, then the thyrohyoid space and

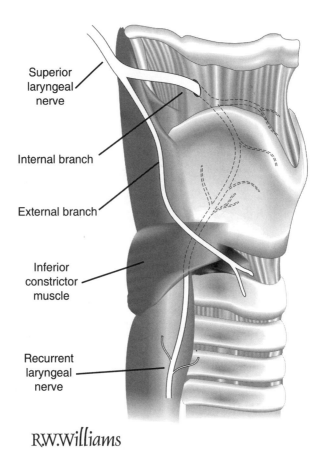

Superior
laryngeal
nerve

Internal branch

External branch

Inferior
constrictor
muscle

Recurrent
laryngeal
nerve

R.W.Williams

FIG. 4-6. Oblique view of the larynx. Note how the internal branch of the superior laryngeal nerve pierces the thyrohyoid membrane midway between the hyoid bone and the superior border of the thyroid cartilage. (Redden RJ. Anatomic considerations in anesthesia. In: Hagberg CA, ed. *Handbook of difficult airway management.* Philadelphia: Churchill Livingstone, 2000:11.)

thyroid cartilage. The cricothyroid membrane is higher in the neck in a woman than a man because the woman's thyroid cartilage is relatively smaller than the man's.

- The cricothyroid membrane measures 6 to 8 mm from top to bottom. If one pierces the membrane in its midportion to perform a retrograde intubation, the puncture point is a mere 3 to 5 mm below the vocal cords, which may not be far enough into the airway to retain the ETT when the wire is cut at the skin. The technique of passing the wire from the outside to the inside of the distal end of the ETT through the Murphy eye enables an additional 4 to 5 mm of insertion, generally minimizing this risk. The proximity of the cricothyroid membrane to the vocal cords is also the driving factor in using small tracheal hooks during surgical cricothyroidotomy to minimize any risk to the cords (see Chapter 15).

TRACHEA

The trachea begins at the inferior border of the cricoid ring. The sensory supply to the tracheal mucosa is derived from the recurrent laryngeal branch of the vagus nerve. The trachea is between 9 and 15 mm in diameter in the adult and 12 to 15 cm long. It may be somewhat larger in the elderly. The adult male trachea will generally easily accept an 8.5-mm inner diameter (ID) ETT, but a 7.5-mm ID ETT may be preferable in women. If the patient being intubated might require bronchoscopic pulmonary toilette after admission (e.g., chronic obstructive pulmonary disease, COPD; airway burns), consider increasing to a 9.0-mm ID tube for men and an 8.0 mm ID tube for women.

SUMMARY

Functional anatomy is important to expert airway management. Attention to the nuances and subtleties of anatomy in relation to technique will often spell the difference between success and failure in managing airways, particularly difficult airways. A clear understanding of the relevant anatomical structures, their blood supply, and their innervation will guide the choice of intubation and anesthesia techniques and will enhance understanding regarding the best approach to each patient.

EVIDENCE

1. General: The reviews by Morris (1) and Redden (2) provide excellent descriptions of the functional anatomy of the upper airway.

2. Nasotracheal intubation: Nasotracheal intubation has largely been supplanted by other methods of emergency airway management that have a higher success rate and fewer complications. Several authors have addressed the complications of nasotracheal intubation (3–10). Some are serious, such as severe epistaxis (1% to 10%), intracranial intubation (3), and bronchial obstruction (4). Others are potentially serious, such as retropharyngeal dissection (5,6) and sinusitis, particularly if the nasotracheal tube is left in place longer than 3 to 7 days (7,8). Most immediate complications of nasotracheal intubation are mild and self-limited (e.g., mild to moderate epistaxis) (2,11). Softening the ETT in warmed water or saline has been demonstrated to reduce the complication rate, particularly epistaxis (12).

3. Cocaine and coronary vasoconstriction: It is well known that recreational cocaine use is associated with coronary spasm leading to myocardial ischemia and infarction as well as sudden death (13). It is important to realize that medically administered cocaine to produce nasal vasoconstriction has produced similar complications (14,15,16).

REFERENCES

1. Morris IR. Functional anatomy of the upper airway. *Emerg Med Clin NA* 1988;6:639–669.
2. Redden RJ. Anatomic considerations in anesthesia. In: Hagberg CA, ed. *Handbook of difficult airway management*. Philadelphia: Churchill Livingstone, 2000:1–13.
3. Marlow TJ, Goltra DD Jr, Schabel SI. Intracranial placement of a nasotracheal tube after facial fracture: a rare complication. *J Emerg Med* 1997;15:187–191.
4. Skouteris CA, Mylonas AI, Galanaki EJ, et al. Acute bronchial obstruction after nasotracheal intubation: report of a case. *J Oral Maxillofac Surg* 2002;60:1188–1192.
5. Tintinalli JE, Claffey J. Complications of nasotracheal intubation. *Ann Emerg Med* 1981;10:142–144.
6. Landess WW. Retropharyngeal dissection: a rare complication of nasotracheal intubation revisited—a case report. *AANA J* 1994;62:273–277.
7. Holdgaard HO, Pedersen J, Schurizek BA, et al. Complications and late sequelae following nasotracheal intubation. *Acta Anaesthesiol Scand* 1993;37:475–480.
8. Bach A, Boehrer H, Schmidt H, et al. Nosocomial sinusitis in ventilated patients. Nasotracheal versus orotracheal intubation. *Anaesthesia* 1992;47:335–339.
9. Conetta R, Nierman DM. Pneumocephalus following nasotracheal intubation. *Ann Emerg Med* 1992;21:100–102.
10. Rhee KJ, Muntz CB, Donald PJ, et al. Does nasotracheal intubation increase complications in patients with skull base fractures? *Ann Emerg Med* 1993;22:1145–1147.

11. Rosen CL, Wolfe RE, Chew SE, et al. Blind nasotracheal intubation in the presence of facial trauma. *J Emerg Med* 1997;15:141–145.
12. Lu PP, Liu HP, Shyr MH, et al. Softened endotracheal tube reduces the incidence and severity of epistaxis following nasotracheal intubation. *Acta Anaesthesiol Sin* 1998;36:193–197.
13. Minor RL Jr, Scott BD, Brown DD, et al. Cocaine induced myocardial infarction in patients with normal coronary arteries. *Ann Intern Med* 1992;115:797–806.
14. Lange RA, Cigarroa RG, Yancy CW Jr, et al. Cocaine induced coronary artery vasoconstriction. *N Engl J Med* 1989;321:1557–1562.
15. Ross GS, Bell J. Myocardial infarction associated with inappropriate use of topical cocaine as treatment for epistaxis. *Am J Emerg Med* 1992;10:219–222.
16. Laffey JG, Neligan P, Ormonde G. Prolonged perioperative myocardial ischemia in a young male: due to topical intranasal cocaine? *J Clin Anesth* 1999;11:419–424.

5

Bag/Mask Ventilation and Endotracheal Intubation

Robert E. Schneider and Michael F. Murphy

> **Bag and mask ventilation is the cornerstone of airway management.**

Although all airway skills are important, perhaps the most important skill is the ability to use a bag and mask alone or with upper airway adjuncts to effectively oxygenate and ventilate a patient. This process is known as basic airway management. Substantial skill is required to establish and maintain an adequate mask seal, position the head, and ensure a patent airway with one hand while ventilating with the other. Once mastered, however, confident bag and mask ventilation reduces both the urgency to intubate and the anxiety that universally accompanies a failed attempt at laryngoscopy and intubation, especially if muscle relaxants have been used to facilitate intubation. Bag and mask ventilation is a reasonable airway management technique for a limited period of time, provided one takes steps to minimize the risks of gastric aspiration. In fact, competence with bag and mask ventilation is a prerequisite to using paralytic agents to secure the airway. A well-designed sequential approach to basic airway management is essential to the practice of emergency medicine and critical care.

SUPPLEMENTAL OXYGENATION

There is a stepwise progression that must be understood and followed in administering oxygen to nonintubated, spontaneously breathing patients who cannot maintain an acceptable oxygen saturation on room air. Many patients arrive in the emergency department with a nasal cannula connected to oxygen at 2 to 3 liters per minute flow rate. If ineffective at maintaining an adequate oxygen saturation, the nasal cannula should immediately be replaced with a nonrebreathing mask at 15 liters of flow, so named because of the inherent one-way valves designed to prevent the patient from entraining room air. There has been tremendous confusion in the past regarding the actual percentage of oxygen that can be successfully delivered through a nonrebreathing mask. For years, most physicians felt a nonrebreather was capable of delivering upwards of 95% oxygen. This belief was fueled by the original name of the mask, 100% nonrebreather mask, that is clearly misleading. Many well-conducted studies have subsequently shown that the *maximum* percentage of oxygen that can be delivered effectively is actually 70% to 75%, as the mask does not effectively seal and prevent the entrainment of room air and the reservoir is too small to provide sufficient oxygen to meet the large demand that occurs during inspiration. In common use, the nonrebreather probably provides oxygen at about 65%. A newly introduced nonrebreathing mask called the HiOx[80] uses a dual system of valves and is capable of delivering 90% oxygen at 8 or more liters of flow. Replacing the nasal cannula with a nonrebreathing mask and then observing changes in pulse oximetry readings over a 2- to 3-minute period allows one to quickly assess the efficacy of the nonrebreathing mask.

If expected improvement in oxygenation does not occur, the nonrebreather should be removed and replaced with any one of several specific resuscitation bags and masks (described later). Initially the patient must be reassured that a tight-fitting mask will be placed on his or her face and encouraged to continue breathing spontaneously without any assistance from the care provider. Utmost attention must be directed to ensuring a tight mask seal. After 3 or 4 minutes, the patient's oxygenation should be reassessed and if not improving, synchronous augmentation of the patient's inspiratory effort (500 to 700 cc tidal volume of oxygen with each spontaneous inspiration) should be undertaken. In a nontachypneic patient (less than 20 breaths/minute), this procedure is simply done. In a tachypneic patient (greater than 20 breaths/minute), synchronous augmentation will be quite difficult if not impossible. Continued attempts at augmenting each inspiratory effort may result in asynchronous bagging, leading to insufflation of the patient's stomach and increasing the risk of vomiting or regurgitation of gastric contents. To combat this, an appropriate cadence of bagging must be selected to allow effective enhancement of every third or fourth inspiratory effort. This is fairly easy to do and allows the care provider time to be certain a good seal is achieved and maintained. If synchronous assist fails, continuous positive airway pressure (CPAP) or bi-level positive airway pressure (BL-PAP) may be helpful (see Chapter 35) or endotracheal intubation will most likely be required.

BAG AND MASK VENTILATION

There is a paucity of literature that adequately describes effective techniques of bag and mask ventilation. It is not glamorous, most health care providers mistakenly think that they are proficient at it, and it is given little attention in most airway textbooks and courses. All of this makes bag and mask ventilation appear mundane within the spectrum of airway management. However, one quickly realizes its importance, given the fact that effective bag and mask oxygenation and ventilation buys time as one works through the array of potential solutions in managing a difficult or failed airway. Simply stated, the ability to effectively oxygenate and ventilate a patient with a bag and mask leaves three failed attempts at laryngoscopy and intubation as the only pathway to failed airway.

Successful bag and mask ventilation is dependent on two things: an adequate mask seal and a patent airway. Creating an adequate mask seal requires an understanding of the design features of the mask, the anatomy of the patient's face, and the interrelationship between the two. A patent airway permits the delivery of appropriate tidal volumes without insufflating the stomach. Techniques used in producing a patent airway often include head extension, chin lift, and jaw-thrust maneuvers.

The specific type of bag used in bag/mask ventilation is also important. Recent studies have demonstrated that bags that minimize dead space, incorporate unidirectional airflow valves (e.g., duckbill inspiratory valves), and use one-way expiratory valves to prevent the entrainment of room air during inspiration will deliver 90% to 97% oxygen to spontaneously breathing or ventilated patients. This result is in sharp distinction to improperly configured bags that provide high oxygen concentration during active bagging, but deliver only 30% oxygen during spontaneous patient breathing because of entrainment of room air.

A typical mask consists of three main parts:

- A round, protruding 15-mm male connector that fits a standard 22-mm female connector on the bag portion of the assembly
- The hard shell, or body of the mask, which most often is clear, providing continuous visualization of the patient's mouth and nose so that immediate intervention can be employed if the patient regurgitates
- The circumferential cushion, or inflatable collar, which, when properly filled, evenly distributes appropriately placed downward pressure onto the patient's face, promoting an effective mask seal

It is easier to establish an adequate mask seal if the mask is too large than if it is too small. In masks with inflatable collars, the collar must be inflated correctly to effect an adequate seal. If the seal is not adequate initially, air should be added to or removed from the mask empirically according to the operator's best judgment as to whether the mask was initially under- or overinflated.

Opening the Airway

Opening the airway should be accomplished before placing the mask on the face. Employ a jaw-thrust maneuver, then place an oral airway and one or two nasal airways depending on the clinical responsiveness of the patient. The jaw-thrust maneuver moves the tongue anteriorly with the mandible, minimizing its obstructing potential. An effective jaw thrust is achieved by forcibly and fully opening the mouth to 'translate' the condyles of the mandible out of the temperomandibular joint (TMJ), then pulling the mandible forward and maintaining a forward position with the help of the oral airway.

With the mandible pulled forward, the mask is placed on the face and sealed. The three facial landmarks that must be approximated by the mask are the bridge of the nose, the two malar eminences, and the mandibular alveolar ridge (Fig. 5-1). The mentum of the chin is not important in initial mask placement, but may become crucial if the patient is edentulous or if adjunctive chin-lift maneuvers are needed to ensure an effective seal. One must be cognizant at all times of the patient's orbits and resist any temptation to rest the ulnar surfaces of either wrist or the mask cushion on the orbits during bag and mask ventilation. This inadvertent compression may produce a profound vagal response and significantly reduce retinal blood flow.

Positioning the Mask

The mask should be placed on the patient's face detached from the bag. This is a simple point but often neglected. Leaving the bag and mask connected during initial placement makes the procedure awkward and clumsy. The nasal part of the mask should be opened and placed on the bridge of the nose (Fig. 5-2). The body of the mask is then levered down onto the patient's face (Fig. 5-3), covering the nose and mouth, and is adjusted cephalad (superior) or caudad (inferior) to allow optimum positioning.

Single-Hand Mask Hold

The operator's nondominant hand is placed on the mask. Many techniques have described how the hand should fit the mask. Ordinarily the distal pads of the thumb and the index finger are

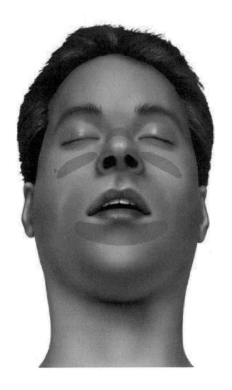

FIG. 5-1. Three facial landmarks that must be approximated by the mask cushion to achieve an effective mask seal: nasal bridge, two malar eminences, and the alveolar ridge.

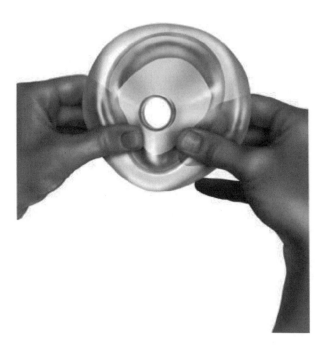

FIG. 5-2. Opening of the nasal portion of the mask facilitates initial placement onto the patient's nasal bridge.

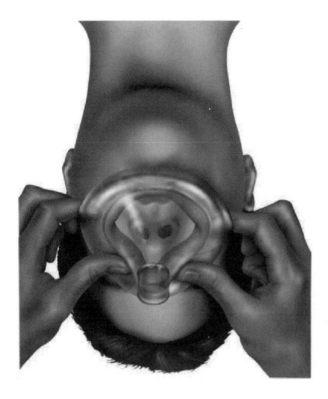

FIG. 5-3. After initial placement, the mask is positioned on the face to incorporate the nares and mouth inside the body of the mask.

used to hold the mask in place, rocking it gently from side to side to achieve the best seal. The remaining fingers are used to pull the mandible up into the mask, keeping the airway open. A common tendency, especially if any difficulty is encountered, is to pinch the body of the mask with the thumb and index finger pads. If this occurs, a mask leak may be produced or worsened if already present. If the operator's hand is large enough, the webspace between the thumb and index finger may appose the mask connector, allowing the rest of the hand to fall comfortably onto the body of the mask at a 45-degree angle (Fig. 5-4). This oblique angle allows even distribution of downward pressure as the mask is gently sealed onto the patient's face. The long, ring and little fingers should lie comfortably on the body of the mask as well. Their respective finger pads should approximate the mentum of the chin and body of the mandible and must be ready to pull the mandible into the mask (chin lift) if necessary (Fig. 5-5). It is important to be certain the volar pads stay off the soft tissues of the neck; otherwise relative airway obstruction may be produced. It may be necessary to gather the left cheek with the hypothenar eminence of the hand and compress it into the mask cushion while rocking the mask to the right to establish a more efficient mask seal. Several authors recommend placing the volar pad of the little finger posterior to the angle of the mandible to attempt a jaw-thrust maneuver. This method of producing a jaw-thrust maneuver is extremely difficult to perform and maintain for any length of time, especially with small hands.

Two-Hand Mask Hold

This is the most effective method of opening the airway and achieving an adequate mask seal and is the method of choice in an emergency situation when one-handed ventilation is not producing adequate ventilation. The two handed–two-person technique mandates that

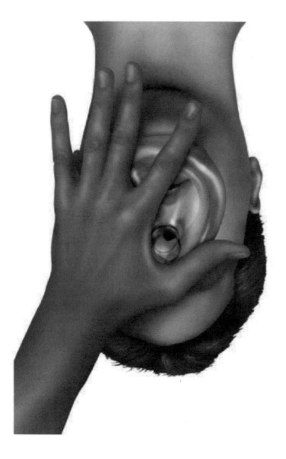

FIG. 5-4. The most effective single-handed mask seal is achieved by placing the thumb/index finger web space against the mask connector at 45 degrees and gently pushing the mask onto the face with the web space, not the palm of the hand.

the operator's sole responsibility is to ensure proper mask placement on the patient's face while simultaneously using both hands to open the airway and achieve an effective mask seal. An assistant is needed to squeeze the bag, but the most experienced airway manager should be handling the mask/face seal. The hands may be placed on the mask in one of two ways. One method capitalizes on placement of the index finger and thumb distal phalanges of both hands in apposition to one another along the inferior and superior ridges of the mask respectively (Fig. 5-6). The volar pads of the remaining three fingers (long, ring, little fingers) are fully abducted and used to capture the mandible and perform a simultaneous jaw-thrust and chin-lift maneuver, opening the airway and creating an optimum mask seal. Alternatively, both thenar eminences can be positioned parallel to one another with the thumbs pointing caudad (inferior) and the thumb meta-caupophalangeal (MCP) joints placed directly opposite the mask connector, executing gentle downward pressure pushing the mask into the face (Fig. 5-7). The thenar eminences are stronger and will fatigue much later than the index fingers. The remaining four fingers of both hands are placed along the mandible in the following locations: the volar pads of the index fingers lift the mentum of the chin and provide an effective chin-lift maneuver; the same pads of the little fingers should capture both angles of the mandible, unhinge it, and perform and maintain an effective jaw-thrust maneuver; the volar pads of the long and ring fingers should fall comfortably onto the body of the mandible and help lift the remainder of the mandible tightly into the mask. This latter technique is easier to perform and is more comfortable to sustain for any length of time. In desperate situations, a single care provider can achieve oxygenation and ventilation

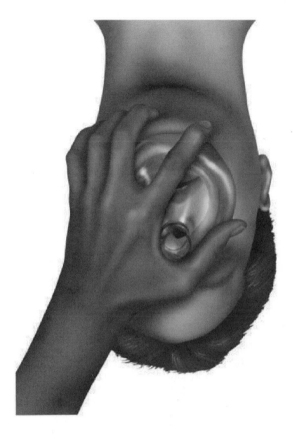

FIG. 5-5. The thumb and index finger lie passively on the mask. The long, ring, and little finger volar pads capture the body of the mandible and mentum and perform a chin lift maneuver.

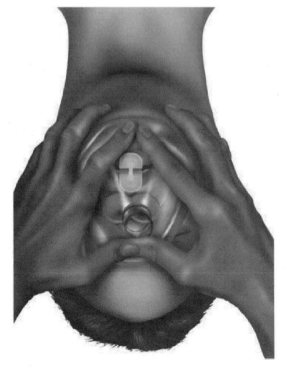

FIG. 5-6. Commonly taught method of effectively sealing the mask with two hands: thumbs cephalad (superiorly) and index fingers caudad (inferiorly). Leaves only three fingers to create and maintain jaw-thrust and chin-lift maneuver. Not a comfortable position to maintain for any length of time.

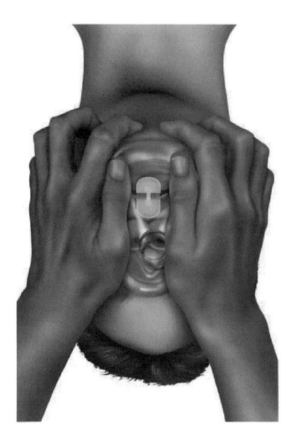

FIG. 5-7. Airway Course technique of effectively sealing the mask with two hands: MCP joints of both thumbs appose the mask connector, allowing four fingers to create and maintain jaw-thrust and chin-lift maneuver. Much more comfortable position for prolonged ventilation.

by squeezing the bag between his or her elbow and chest/lateral abdomen, or between his or her knees while using both hands to optimize the mask seal until help can be recruited.

Bagging the Patient

The resuscitation bag is then connected to the mask and the patient is ventilated. When fully inflated, the standard adult resuscitation bag contains 1500 cc of oxygen. This entire volume should not and cannot be delivered repeatedly without insufflating the stomach. The goal of effective oxygenation and ventilation is to deliver 16 to 24 reduced tidal volume breaths (500 cc) per minute without exceeding the proximal and distal esophageal sphincter opening pressures of approximately 25 cm of water. To be successful on both accounts, an appropriate cadence of bagging must be established and should be similar to "squeeze . . . release . . . release" cadence recommended by Advanced Cardiac Life Support (ACLS) but at a slightly faster pace (squeeze, release, release, squeeze, release, release). The goal is to deliver smaller tidal volumes with each breath at an increased rate to maintain an effective minute ventilation of 10 liters per minute. Application of Sellick's maneuver (Fig. 5-8) will minimize passage of air into the stomach of the unresponsive patient.

Bag and mask ventilation is a dynamic process. One must continually assess responses to changes that are made, while at the same time listening and feeling for any potential areas of mask leak. With the nondominant hand placed appropriately on the mask, a left-sided mask leak will be felt by the care provider's hypothenar eminence. An assistant may be required to

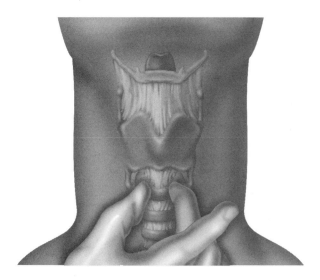

FIG. 5-8. Proper application of Sellick's maneuver (cricoid pressure) involves the thumb and long finger properly positioned on the cricoid cartilage and applying posterior pressure to occlude the esophagus against the anterior surface of the C-6 vertebral body.

evaluate the integrity of the seal on the right side of the mask and compress the right cheek into the mask cushion as needed. It may be necessary to rock the mask up or down or from side to side (pronation or supination) to achieve a better mask seal. While squeezing the bag and delivering effective tidal volumes, the care provider should simultaneously feel resistance in the bag and observe rise and fall of the chest, improvement in oxygen saturation, the appearance of an appropriate waveform on a capnograph, and color change from purple to yellow on an end-tidal carbon dioxide (CO_2) detector, provided the patient is generating CO_2.

When initial bag and mask ventilation fails to establish or maintain adequate oxygen saturation, better bag and mask techniques must be used. One should immediately employ a two-handed–two-person technique and focus on the following options:

1. Is the mask seal optimal? If not, how can this be improved: e.g., applying KY jelly to a beard; placing unfolded gauze 4×4s fluffed and compressed inside the mouth along the buccal pouches (cheeks) to create a more anatomically normal mask seal; reinserting the patient's false teeth; gathering both cheeks inside the body of the mask; ensuring that the entire mouth and all airway adjuncts are within the body of the mask, not on the seal (Fig. 5-9).
2. Are all upper airway adjuncts being properly used? The most common mistake observed in unsuccessful bag and mask ventilation is the omission of the oral airway. The unsupported tongue falls back, obstructs the glottic opening, and prevents one from being able to adequately oxygenate and ventilate the patient. An oral airway should always be used when an unresponsive patient is being ventilated with a bag and mask.
3. Does the jaw-thrust maneuver need to be redone to more effectively open the airway?
4. Does a more experienced person need to be recruited to help optimize bag and mask technique?

LARYNGOSCOPY AND OROTRACHEAL INTUBATION

Direct laryngoscopy is the centerpiece of orotracheal intubation. Laryngoscopy is a learned skill, and when it is performed properly, it provides optimal exposure of the glottic opening,

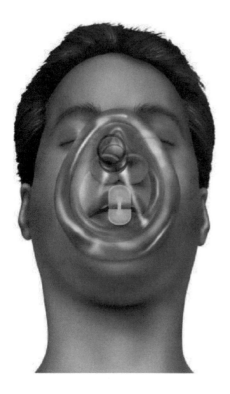

FIG. 5-9. Two nasal airways and an oral airway inserted and placed inside the body of the mask to ensure an effective mask seal.

facilitating endotracheal intubation. Laryngoscopy is a multifaceted procedure that requires both dexterity and creativity to align the oral, pharyngeal, and laryngeal axes of the airway so that the laryngoscopist will be provided the best possible view of the glottis.

Though there are many different types of laryngoscopic blades, they are essentially either straight or curved. Typically, the straight blades are intended to pick up the epiglottis to optimize visualization of the glottic opening. The curved blades, once placed in the vallecula, indirectly expose the glottis by compressing the hyoepiglottic ligament and dragging the epiglottis forward. Either blade can be used either way, though the best success rates are experienced when they are used as intended. Despite the many myths that have been perpetuated in airway management, the curved blade does not have to be placed in the vallecula. The curved blade technique (placement in the vallecula) is the one most frequently taught and used in clinical practice. However, the straight blade technique (picking up the epiglottis) is the one first described in the early 20th century when orotracheal intubation became commonplace. Airway managers need to be familiar with both techniques so that if one fails the other can be used.

Chapter 6 discusses difficult laryngoscopy and intubation. A *best attempt* at laryngoscopy has six components: (i) performance by a reasonably experienced endoscopist, (ii) no significant muscle tone (paralysis), (iii) the use of the optimal sniff position, (iv) the use of external laryngeal manipulation (OELM or BURP, discussed later in this chapter), (v) appropriate length of blade, and (vi) type of blade. With this definition and no other confounding considerations, the optimal attempt at laryngoscopy and intubation may be achieved on the first attempt and should take no more than three attempts. Because there are different techniques of laryngoscopy, the laryngoscopist needs to choose one method that works best and use or practice it often, though not to the exclusion of the others.

Anatomy of Intubation

To appreciate the intricacies of laryngoscopy, one must first understand the anatomy of the upper airway, how to handle the laryngoscope, how to select the best blade for the patient at hand, and how to maneuver the patient and his or her laryngeal anatomy into the optimum position to provide the best view of the vocal cords.

The anatomy of the upper airway, including the larynx, is described in Chapter 4. In the larynx, the vocal cords, which define the glottic opening, lie at the mid portion of the thyroid cartilage, inferior and posterior to the flexible epiglottis, which emanates from the hyoid bone and base of the tongue. During laryngoscopy, these constant relationships serve as very important anatomic landmarks. When in trouble, one *must* find the epiglottis, because it leads to the cords (unless the airway is transected). There will be occasions during routine or difficult laryngoscopy when the esophagus is exposed and mistaken for the vocal cords. Unless one has a landmark or consistent reference point to confirm the airway anatomically, esophageal intubation may ensue or intubation may be unsuccessful. Whenever one is uncertain whether the visualized opening is the glottis or the esophagus, the epiglottis must be found. Once identified, the tip of the epiglottis can usually be elevated with either the straight or curved blade exposing the cords and the arytenoid cartilages, allowing confident placement of the endotracheal tube (ETT) into the airway.

The single greatest obstacle to successful laryngoscopy is the tongue. To the laryngoscopist, the tongue is your enemy, and the epiglottis is your friend. Anatomically, the base of the tongue may block access to the glottic opening. When the tongue is large in relation to the oral cavity (Mallampati Class III or IV), it can inhibit adequate exposure of the glottic aperture. For this reason, preintubation assessment of the patient's airway is essential. In the mnemonic LEMON, discussed in Chapter 6, the *M* stands for Mallampati, serving as a reminder to examine the oral cavity to assess the relative size of the tongue in relationship to the oropharynx and the mandibular space. The laryngoscope blade is the tool that controls and maneuvers the tongue. In general, the larger the tongue, the wider the blade (i.e., no. 3 or no. 4) that should be selected. Fundamental to successful laryngoscopy is the selection of a blade, curved or straight, that will be wide and long enough to capture the tongue at the initiation of laryngoscopy and sweep it leftward out of the visual field and permit direct visualization of the airway.

Technique of Laryngoscopy

Overview of the Technique

In the emergent situation, it is important to have a laryngoscopic technique that is safe, quick, simple to perform, consistent, and most important, universally applicable to every clinical situation, (i.e., it can be used for curved- or straight-blade intubations in pediatric or adult patients). The most common errors associated with failed orotracheal intubation are listed in Box 5-1.

The Airway Course technique of laryngoscopy and intubation that will be described is traditionally associated with the use of a straight blade but can be used with any blade, curved or straight. In the first stage (nonvisual) of this technique, the laryngoscope blade is fully inserted blindly, but gently, into the esophagus. In the second stage (visual), the blade is slowly withdrawn from the esophagus under direct vision to initially expose the glottis, then the epiglottis (which can be picked up with the tip of either blade, providing maximum laryngeal exposure for successful intubation), and lastly the base of the tongue. The traditional technique of inserting a curved blade into the vallecula and then compressing it to flip the epiglottis

---

Box 5-1. Laryngoscopy: *Three things:*

- No tongue should be visible on the right side of the blade. If there is, remove the blade and reinsert it.
- Once the glottis is visualized using the left arm and hand, *keep it in view!* Don't relax the left hand/arm when you pick up the ETT with the right hand/arm
- Keep your wing up. Though it is more comfortable to rest your elbow on the pillow or stretcher, once you've done that, all that you can do with the laryngoscope is lever it, pushing the target up and away from you.

---

forward while lifting the tongue into the mandibular space has many technical subcomponents, requires more visual checkpoints, and may take more time to perform, especially in an emergency.

The intial stage of the Airway Course laryngoscopic technique is totally nonvisual. The laryngoscope blade is passed blindly and gently through the cervical esophagus into the upper body of the esophagus by feel and subconscious appreciation of the oral, pharyngeal, and esophageal anatomy. The second stage is totally visual. It may require transient forearm muscle power to further elevate the tongue into the mandibular space just before intubation to achieve maximum glottic exposure.

Handling the Laryngoscope

The laryngoscope should always be grasped in the left hand. Though laryngoscope manufacturers can supply devices for use with the right hand, they are very difficult to acquire and both left- and right-handed care providers are advised to learn to use the laryngoscope in their left hand. Most often it is grasped differently for each of the two stages of laryngoscopy. During the nonvisual stage of laryngoscopy, the laryngoscope is held by the volar pads of the fingers and thumb, not clenched in the palm of the hand ('death grip'). The handle of the laryngoscope should be grasped with the fingertips of the index through fifth fingers, while the volar pad of the thumb is positioned on the proximal end of the blade at the connection with the handle providing the push that accompanies simultaneous pronation of the hand in a lift and advance motion, permitting the atraumatic delivery of the blade into the proximal body of the esophagus. Holding the laryngoscope handle in the palm of the hand and applying constant, firm forearm muscle power (the death grip) throughout this initial stage of laryngoscopy is not recommended. The fidelity of tactile sensation is less with the palm of the hand than with the fingertips, and muscle fatigue is more likely to occur (Fig. 5-10). For the visual stage of laryngoscopy, the laryngoscope handle can be grasped using any familiar technique, including the death grip.

Positioning the Airway

Laryngoscopy will be more successful if the laryngoscopist assumes or creates a comfortable intubating position that allows in-line visualization of the anatomic field. This can be accomplished by either adjusting the patient's stretcher or the height of the intubator (stool, kneeling) to bring the airway into the laryngoscopist's central field of vision. Uncomfortable, contorted

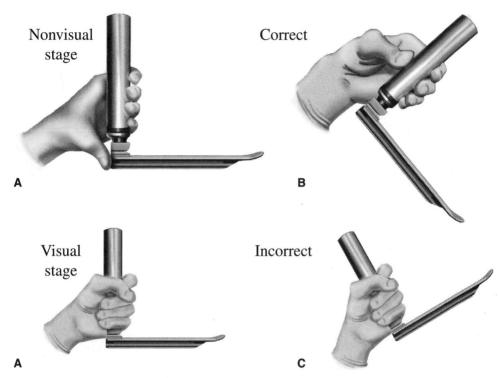

FIG. 5-10. Laryngoscopy. **A:** Recommended grip of the laryngoscope. **B:** Technique of achieving greater glottic exposure. Note how the end of the laryngoscope handle is directed at approximately 45 degrees and lift is applied longitudinally. **C:** Absence of the rocking motion will prevent dental injury and trauma.

body positions lead to bad decisions and unnecessarily complicate laryngoscopy. The laryngoscopist's right hand must remain free at all times and not succumb to the habit of wanting to hold the ETT when initiating laryngoscopy. Throughout laryngoscopy and intubation the free right hand will be used in a dynamic fashion to lift, flex, and extend the patient's head to produce the best view of the glottis; to employ a tonsil suction (Yankauer) to remove any secretions, blood, emesis, or other debris that might be obscuring the distal visual field; to apply the BURP maneuver to improve the view of the glottis (see later); and last, to insert the ETT when intubating the patient.

Before placing the laryngoscope into the patient's mouth, the sniffing position is created by placing a pillow, folded towel, or sheet under the patient's head to facilitate extension of the head on the neck and slight forward flexion of the lower cervical spine on the chest ('sniffing the morning air' or 'sipping English tea') (Fig. 5-11). Though there has been some controversy as to whether or not the sniffing position is best, it is generally accepted that this is the best *starting* position. Active positioning of the head on the neck with the laryngoscopist's free right hand should facilitate the parallel alignment of the oral, pharyngeal, and laryngeal axes. In the trauma victim, where in-line stabilization of the cervical spine is recommended, or in patients with decreased cervical spine mobility, flexion of the lower cervical spine onto the chest and extension of the head on the neck may be impossible or inappropriate, thus making laryngoscopy more difficult. Patients with advanced cervical arthritis may have markedly reduced neck motion, which may also confound laryngoscopy.

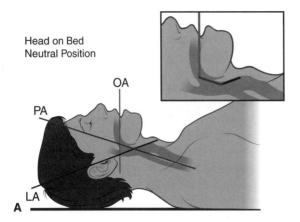

Head on Bed
Neutral Position

OA

PA

LA

A

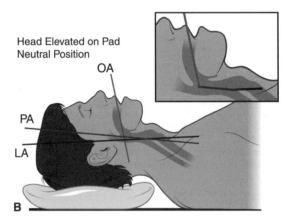

Head Elevated on Pad
Neutral Position

OA

PA

LA

B

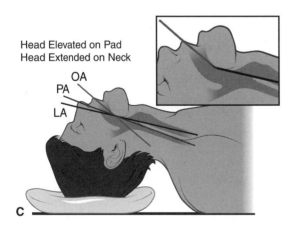

Head Elevated on Pad
Head Extended on Neck

OA
PA
LA

C

FIG. 5-11. A: Anatomic neutral position. The oral (OA), pharyngeal (PA), and laryngeal (LA) axes are at greater angles to one another. **B:** Head, still in neutral position, has been lifted by a pillow flexing the lower cervical spine and aligning the pharyngeal (PA) and laryngeal (LA) axes. **C:** The head has been extended on the cervical spine, aligning the oral axis (OA) with the pharyngeal (PA) and laryngeal (LA) axes, creating the optimum sniffing position for intubation.

Opening the Mouth

Once the optimal position for laryngoscopy has been achieved, the mouth is opened with the right hand to gain access to the oropharynx. It is a matter of personal preference whether one wishes to use the scissor technique of opening the mouth or simply tilt the head back to indirectly effect mouth opening or grasp the lower lip and mandible with the thumb, index, and long fingers of the right hand and open the mouth. The latter technique permits retraction of the lower lip, providing full exposure of the mandibular teeth and the entire oropharynx without any visual obstruction from the long finger on the maxillary teeth as might occur with the scissor technique.

Stage 1—Nonvisual Insertion of the Blade

Assuming the patient is totally paralyzed with maximum mandibular mobility, the laryngoscope blade is placed into the right side of the patient's mouth alongside the lingual surface of the right mandibular molar teeth (Fig. 5-12). This is an extremely important initial anatomic relationship in controlling the tongue. The laryngoscopist must be certain there is no tongue between the flanged surface of the blade and the lingual surface of the mandibular molar teeth before beginning laryngoscopy. If any tongue is seen, the laryngoscope should be removed and then replaced in the correct starting position. Failure to establish this starting position will compromise control of the tongue, potentially obstruct visualization of the glottic opening, and hinder passage of the ETT (Fig. 5-13). Blade insertion is generally much easier with the patient in the sniffing position rather than the neutral position. In the latter instance (most trauma patients), the laryngoscope blade must hug the anterior surface of the tongue as the blade compresses the tongue into the floor of the mouth and simultaneously opens the mandible and atraumatically advances through the oropharynx, posterior pharynx, and into the esophagus.

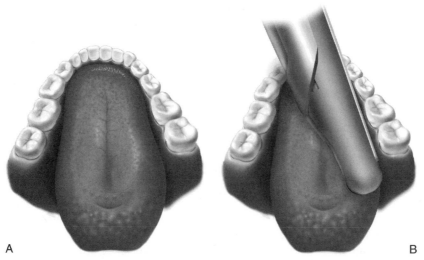

FIG. 5-12. A: Oral cavity. **B:** Initial anatomic relationship of the flange of the blade with the lingual surface of the molar teeth. Note there is no tongue between the flange of the blade and the teeth.

A   **B**   **C**
Incorrect   Incorrect   Correct

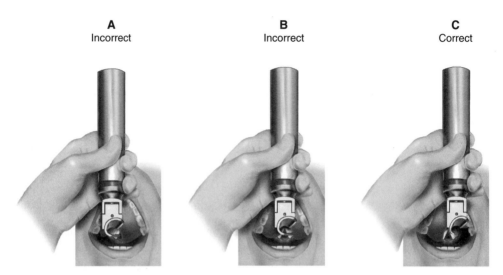

FIG. 5-13. Tongue control during laryngoscopy. **A** and **B** demonstrate poor visualization of the cords due to incorrect positioning of the blade. Note how the tongue folds over the blade and obscures the view. **C** demonstrates correct positioning of the blade to control and move the tongue to the left, providing an optimal view for intubation.

This procedure is gentle, but requires some muscle power. If more space is required to negotiate the posterior pharyngeal turn, it must be generated by further opening of the mandible.

Once the blade has been correctly positioned adjacent to the right mandibular molar teeth, its entire length is passed blindly and atraumatically into the patient's esophagus, traversing the base of the tongue, passing posterior to the epiglottis and cords, anterior to the posterior pharyngeal wall, and finally moving superiorly and anteriorly through the cervical esophagus into the proximal body of the esophagus. Active visualization of the posterior pharyngeal or laryngeal anatomy is neither possible nor required during this initial maneuver. As mentioned previously, the esophageal insertion is done completely by feel, with gentle pressure exerted by the volar pads of the fingers and thumb allowing the laryngoscopist to feel the advancing tip of the laryngoscopic blade. Any perception of resistance during this maneuver requires immediate cessation of advancement, slight withdrawal and realignment superiorly, then reinsertion. The tip of the advancing blade should move toward the midline during this insertion. The laryngoscopist can be assured that the application of cricoid pressure may need to be eased slightly to effect a complete atraumatic insertion.

How is esophageal placement of the blade beneficial to the laryngoscopist? With this initial position established, the cords will always be proximal to the tip of the laryngoscope blade, never distal (Fig. 5-14). In emergency laryngoscopy this is of paramount importance. If the visual stage of laryngoscopy is begun without passing the entire blade into the esophagus, the proximal position of the cords in relationship to the tip of the blade cannot be ensured, thus increasing the likelihood of not recognizing what is initially visualized and prompting the dreaded questions, "Where am I? Are the cords distal or more proximal? Do I need to go deeper or come out more?"... and the dance begins, frantically inserting and withdrawing the blade in search of the glottis, each time producing more laryngeal trauma and operator anxiety.

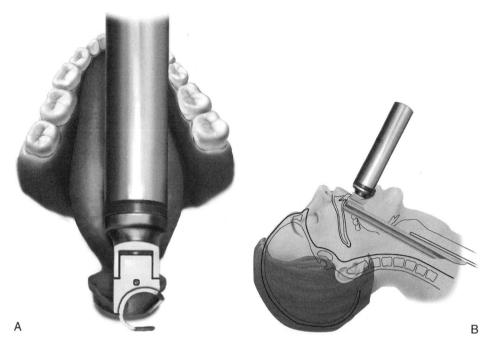

A   B

FIG. 5-14. A: The initial starting position for the visual phase of laryngoscopy. **B:** Note that the blade is in the esophagus and the blade/handle junction is at the patient's teeth. Note the position of the cords proximal to the tip of the blade.

Stage 2—Visual Laryngoscopy

Once fully inserted into the esophagus, the proximal end of the blade (connection of blade with handle) is swung to the midline of the mouth aligning with the midline positioned tip of the blade in the esophagus. Remaining in the midline throughout the visual phase of laryngoscopy is crucial to finding the glottis quickly. Under constant direct vision and in a comfortable intubating position that allows in-line visualization of the distal anatomic field, the laryngoscope and blade are slowly withdrawn in the same fashion as they were initially inserted. Gentle upward pressure rather than strong muscle power is maintained as the laryngoscope is withdrawn. The blade often contacts, but does not lever against, the upper incisors. There should not be any rocking motion of the handle or blade in attempts to find the airway as this withdrawal is accomplished. The withdrawal maneuver is simply a continuous, even-pressured removal of the laryngoscope until the cords are visualized, which almost always will be the first recognizable anatomic structure encountered. The cords will be seen sooner with a curved blade than with a straight blade because of the difference in blade length. The most common misperception that occurs during withdrawal of the straight blade is that the operator feels he or she has missed the airway when, in fact, the cords still lie proximal to the current visual field and will be exposed momentarily as the laryngoscope is withdrawn farther. When the cords are identified, the ETT is passed through the glottic opening, tube placement is confirmed, and the tube is secured in position.

If the vocal cords are missed or are not adequately visualized or simply not identified during initial laryngoscopic withdrawal, continued steady removal of the laryngoscope will next disclose the epiglottis as it comes free from the compressing surface of the blade and drops into view, similar to a trap door. Once the epiglottis has been found, the consistent anatomic relationship of the vocal cords to the epiglottis can be exploited. Under direct vision, the tip of the curved or straight blade is used to pick up and elevate the epiglottis, exposing the glottic aperture (Fig. 5-15).

Continued withdrawal of the laryngoscope will quickly disclose the base of the patient's tongue, a universally recognized structure. In this situation, gentle reinsertion of the blade under direct vision should identify the epiglottis and help locate the glottic aperture.

The BURP Maneuver

Cormack and Lehane quantified the extent to which one is able to visualize the larynx, epiglottis, and upper airway during laryngoscopy (Fig. 5-16). Grades 1 and 2 are usually associated with low laryngoscopic failure rates whereas grades 3 and 4 usually have higher failure rates. If the laryngoscopic view is less than adequate, firm backward, upward, and rightward pressure on the thyroid cartilage with the laryngoscopist's free right hand will most often improve the laryngeal view one full grade, producing maximum glottic exposure. This maneuver, which is distinct from cricoid pressure (Sellick's maneuver), is called the BURP maneuver (*B*ackward, *U*pward, *R*ightward *P*ressure) (Fig. 5-17). Once the vocal cords are exposed and positioned optimally, the assistant providing cricoid pressure with the right long finger and thumb can use the free right index finger to maintain this optimum view, and without releasing cricoid pressure, can perform a combined Sellick-BURP maneuver. This allows the laryngoscopist to reach down and pick up the ETT tube and intubate the trachea.

Intubating the Trachea

Once the airway has been identified, it is important that the laryngoscopist not lose sight of the target, the glottic aperture. The assistant, standing at the patient's right side applying Sellick's maneuver or Sellick-BURP with the right hand, should open the right side of the patient's mouth with the left index finger, providing generous access to the oropharynx and, most important, providing room for unimpeded passage of the ETT (Fig. 5-18). The ETT should be passed from the right side of the patient's mouth and must not be passed down the flange of the blade. The sole purpose of the flange is to capture the tongue, move it leftward out of the visual field, and maintain it in that location until the patient is intubated. If the ETT is mistakenly passed down the flange of the blade, it can become trapped, preventing advancement, or the cuff can be lacerated, necessitating reintubation over a tube exchanger once the patient is intubated. Entering from the right side of the patient's mouth prevents any obstruction or distraction of the laryngoscopist's central view of the cords. It is not possible to maintain one's central visual focus on two objects simultaneously. Ill-advised attempts to do so during laryngoscopy probably contribute to esophageal intubations.

As the ETT is initially passed into the right side of the patient's mouth, the bevel of the tube should lie in a horizontal position. The tube initially contacts the hard palate and then sweeps the soft palate as it is advanced toward the glottic opening occupying a position in the right peripheral field of vision. At the glottic opening the bevel should be simultaneously rotated counterclockwise 90 degrees from the horizontal (widest) to the vertical (narrowest) plane and moved into the midline to facilitate atraumatic passage through the cords (Fig. 5-19). Following passage through the cords, the laryngoscope and the stylet are removed and the balloon is inflated.

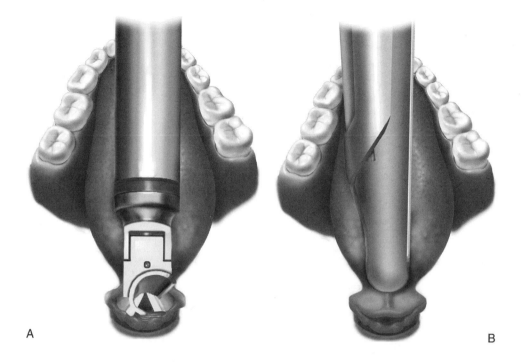

A

B

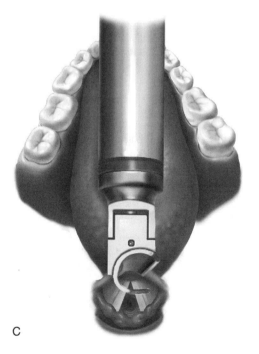

C

FIG. 5-15. Exposure of the cords. **A:** Initial withdrawal of the laryngoscope will usually expose the cords. If not, further withdrawal of the laryngoscope will disclose the epiglottis (**B**), which can be picked up and elevated (**C**), disclosing the glottic aperture.

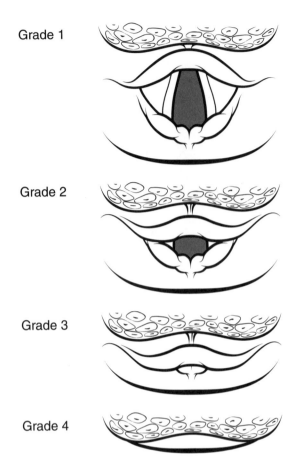

Grade 1

Grade 2

Grade 3

Grade 4

FIG. 5-16. Cormack-Lehane laryngoscopic grading system. Grade 1 is visualization of the entire glottic aperture. Grade 2 is visualization of just the arytenoid cartilages or the posterior portion of the glottic aperture. Grade 3 is visualization of only the epiglottis. Grade 4 is visualization of only the tongue or the tongue and soft palate.

USING AN INTUBATING STYLET

An intubating stylet is a device designed to facilitate a Seldinger type intubation of the trachea when a poor grade 2 or grade 3 view has prevented successful intubation despite traditional maneuvers such as 'hockey sticking' the distal end of the tube over a rigid stylet and attempting to fish the ETT anteriorly up into the trachea.

These stylets are made of plastic or gum-elastic and have a 1-cm, 30-degree deflection of the distal tip. The tip deflection enhances the anterior movement of the distal tip underneath the epiglottis, maximizing the chance it will pass into the glottis and hence the trachea. Once in the trachea, the tip can often transmit a click, click, click sensation generated by the tracheal rings as the stylet is moved gently in and out of the airway. Feeling this sensation enhances your confidence that the stylet is in the trachea; failing to sense it does not mean that you are not in the trachea. The tongue or other airway structures contacting the shaft of the stylet may insulate against the transmission of the corrugated vibrations.

Two types of stylets are recommended: the Eschmann (SIMS-Portex, Keene, NH) and the Frova (Cook Critical Care, Bloomington, IN). Other intubating stylets are available but design flaws prevent them from being recommended. The Frova has a hollow lumen and is supplied with both Luer lock and conventional 15-mm connectors to permit the insufflation of oxygen in the event of an intubation failure; the Eschmann is solid and has no lumen. The Frova

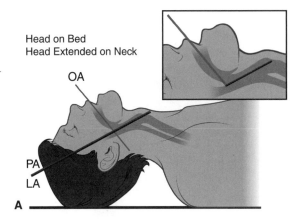

Head on Bed
Head Extended on Neck

OA

PA
LA

A

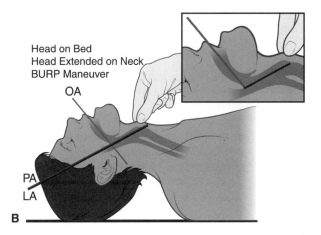

Head on Bed
Head Extended on Neck
BURP Maneuver

OA

PA
LA

B

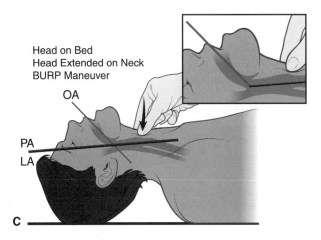

Head on Bed
Head Extended on Neck
BURP Maneuver

OA

PA
LA

C

FIG. 5-17. A: Relatively anteriorly placed larynx. **B:** BURP maneuver on the thyroid cartilage. **C:** BURP maneuver improves the laryngeal view for intubation.

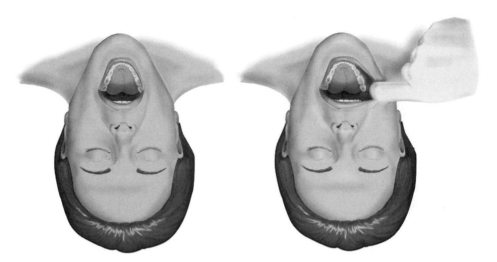

FIG. 5-18. Retraction of the corner of the mouth by an assistant's index finger will provide ample room for unobstructed passage of the ETT.

connectors will not tolerate much in the way of positive pressure before detaching from the end of the device. The theoretical advantage of luminal oxygenation is thus of marginal clinical import.

The stylets are labeled in centimeters, depicting the distance from the tip, and aligned on the same side of the bougie as the tip deflection. Positioning the inserted stylet at 25 cm at the patient's lip correlates with the tip of the bougie at midtrachea. It is important to keep the writing and hence the deflected tip up (anterior) as the ETT is passed over the stylet to minimize the chance of forcing the ETT posteriorly in the trachea, risking a posterior tracheal perforation.

Technique of Passing the Stylet

When using the intubating stylet, some laryngeal structure (epiglottis or better—grade 2 or 3) must be visible. *Under direct vision* an intubating stylet is inserted behind the epiglottis and an attempt is made to insert the tip through the glottis into the trachea. In a grade 2 view, the stylet

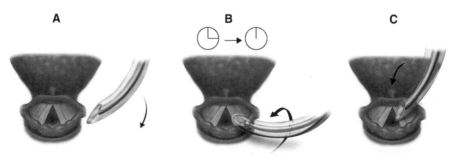

FIG. 5-19. The ETT is rotated 90 degrees counterclockwise (**B**) as it is passed through the cords, changing the initial horizontal (widest) axis of the bevel (**A**) to the vertical (narrowest) axis (**C**).

may be seen to enter the glottis. In a grade 3 view, the tip of the intubating stylet will not be seen to enter the glottis or trachea. In either case, if the intubator is confident that the stylet is in the trachea, an ETT is slid over the stylet into the trachea *while maintaining the best possible view with the laryngoscope*. The most common mistake is removing the laryngoscope. Keeping the laryngoscope in place minimizes the angle the tube/stylet combination must negotiate and enhances the chance of successfully intubating the trachea. Should passage of the ETT get hung up, rotate the tube through 180 degrees, first to the right and then to the left. The tip of the ETT may be caught on the posterior commissure of the glottis, the anterior commissure of the cords, either cord, or the cricoid cartilage, though it is impossible to know the exact location. A similar experience may occur when the intubating stylet is passed. The possibilities and remedies are identical. Once the ETT is in place, the intubating stylet is removed and tube position is confirmed.

Both the Eschmann and Frova can be coiled up and carried in your pocket to the patient. However, to prevent shipping damage the Frova is packaged with a rigid metal internal stylet that should be removed before use and to permit coiling for transport. The Eschmann is provided in both plastic and gum-elastic varieties. The gum-elastic has a more rounded tip, is potentially less traumatic, and softens when heated (a disadvantage). The plastic variety is sturdier. The Eschmann can be cleaned and reused, whereas the Frova is intended to be a single-use device.

CONFIRMING INTUBATION OF THE TRACHEA

Once the ETT has been placed, it is imperative to confirm that it is in the patient's trachea. Traditionally, the "gold standard" for this has been considered to be direct visualization of the endotracheal tube passing through the vocal cords, but this approach has proven fallible. The current standard is detection of end-tidal CO_2, most commonly using the colorimetric capnometer, which changes from purple to yellow in the presence of exhaled carbon dioxide, or capnography, where the presence of an appropriate waveform proves tracheal placement.

When using a colorimetric end-tidal carbon dioxide detector, the color will quickly change from *p*urple (poor) to *y*ellow (yes). This color change should occur within one or two breaths, but in certain circumstances may be delayed for up to six breaths. If the color change to yellow is not immediate, one has to be suspicious that the ETT is either in the esophagus or inflated above the cords, rather than being properly positioned in the trachea. A color change to tan rather than to bright yellow may also indicate a supraglottic or esophageal location of the ETT tip. In this circumstance, several options are available to confirm the anatomic location of the tube: The laryngoscopy may be repeated to confirm that the tube is indeed properly positioned through the cords; a new colorimetric device may be tried; or the patient may be extubated and reintubated. If any doubt remains, the tube should be assumed to be in the esophagus.

In those clinical circumstances where CO_2 is not produced (e.g., prolonged cardiac arrest), the colorimetric detectors are of limited value and esophageal detecting devices (EDD) may be used to confirm appropriate tube placement. There are two types of esophageal detecting devices: the piston syringe device and the self-inflating bulb device. Studies have shown that the sensitivity of the self-inflating bulb is greater than the piston syringe. The principle behind these devices relates to the anatomic differences between the trachea and the esophagus. The trachea is composed of anteriorly positioned cartilaginous rings that prevent the collapse of the airway into the ETT when the piston is aspirated or the compressed bulb is released and allowed to reinflate. Because the esophagus is a circumferentially muscular structure without any bony or cartilaginous support, placement of the ETT into the esophagus and aspiration of the syringe or release of the self-inflated bulb will invaginate the esophageal mucosa into the tube and prevent easy removal of the piston or rapid reinflation of the bulb. These devices are quite sensitive and specific, but again must be used in conjunction with other techniques to confirm proper placement of the ETT into the trachea.

Auscultation of the left supraclavicular area, left axilla, left chest, right chest, and epigastrium, respectively, are additive to end-tidal CO_2 and EDD confirmation techniques. The left side of the chest is preferentially auscultated first to confirm that a right mainstem intubation has not occurred. Fogging (condensation) of the ETT is a completely unreliable method of confirming tracheal intubation and should not be relied on. With the exception of bronchoscopic confirmation, none of these techniques taken alone guarantee proper placement of the ETT in the trachea. Thus, it is recommended that they all be done, especially in the arrested patient. Chest x-rays are used primarily to assess for mainstem intubation and to evaluate tube position within the trachea, not to determine whether the ETT is in the trachea.

FAILED LARYNGOSCOPY AND INTUBATION

When tracheal intubation is unsuccessful, the patient should be ventilated with a bag and mask and high-flow oxygen if the saturations are <90%. During this reoxygenation time, the laryngoscopist should systematically analyze the likely causes of the failure. It makes no sense to attempt a second laryngoscopy without changing something in the procedure to improve chances for success. The following questions should be addressed:

- Is the patient in the optimum sniffing position for laryngoscopy and intubation? Is there something additional in terms of positioning that would improve the view of the vocal cords? If the patient's head is lying flat on the stretcher, the placement of a pillow, sheet, or blanket under the patient's head might improve the glottic view. If the patient was placed in the sniffing position initially and the larynx still appeared quite anterior, reducing the degree of head extension could be helpful. Additionally, it may even help to elevate and *flex* the patient's head with the laryngoscopist's free right hand (actually flex both the head and neck) while performing laryngoscopy to create a better view of a true anterior airway.
- Would a different blade provide a better view? If the initial attempt at laryngoscopy was done with a curved blade, it may be advisable to change to a straight blade and vice versa. Alternatively, a different size blade of either type might be helpful.
- Is the patient adequately paralyzed? Laryngoscopy may have been attempted too soon after administering succinylcholine, or an inadequate dose of succinylcholine may have been administered. If the total time of paralysis has been such that the effect of succinylcholine is dissipating, then administration of a second full paralyzing dose of succinylcholine is advisable. Should this occur, atropine must be available to treat potential bradycardia that occasionally accompanies repeat dosing of succinylcholine. Appropriate paralysis will improve the view of laryngoscopy one full grade!
- Was everything possible done to optimize the view of the cords? Would the BURP maneuver be helpful? Most often, BURP improves the laryngeal view by one full grade.
- Is a more experienced laryngoscopist available? If so, a call for help may be in order.

EVIDENCE

1. Supplemental oxygen: Standard textbooks in respiratory therapy (1,2) and anesthesiology (3) describe oxygen delivery systems and the concentrations of oxygen that they characteristically deliver.

2. Bag and mask ventilation: Not all self-inflating ventilation bags deliver high concentrations of oxygen. Only those bags with duckbill inhalation valves, one way exhalation valves, and small dead space can be expected to deliver inhaled concentrations of oxygen greater than 90% (5,6). Duckbill valve bags without one-way exhalation valves have been shown to deliver less than 40% oxygen (6). The technique of squeezing the bag has been shown to affect the delivered tidal volume. The recommended tidal volume of 500 cc is best achieved by squeezing the bag with one hand rather than squeezing the bag against one's knee (7).

3. Positioning the airway: Cormack and Lehane have devised the most widely accepted system of categorizing the view of the larynx achieved with an orally placed laryngoscope (8). The sniffing position has been widely accepted as the optimum position for orotracheal intubation though Adnet et al. have recently challenged this dogma, suggesting that simple extension may be superior (9,10). In attempting to provide a framework or an approach to answering the question of optimum positioning of the head and neck, Levitan et al. devised a scoring system to quantitate the percentage of glottic opening (POGO) visible, though at the present time, this scale has yet to gain wide acceptance. The question has yet to be finally answered (11).

4. BURP: It has clearly been shown that optimum external laryngeal manipulation (OELM), also known as BURP (*b*ackward, *u*pward, *r*ightward *p*ressure) improves laryngeal view grade by one full grade, on average (12–14).

5. Intubating stylets: The literature clearly supports the use of intubating stylets to enhance success rates of intubation, particularly with grade 3 views (15–19). In one study the success rate improved from 66% to 96% after two attempts (18). Pathogenic bacteria may colonize both the device and its plastic container, emphasizing the importance of sterilizing the device after each use (20). Bronchial perforation has been reported with the device (21).

6. Laryngoscope blade selection and technique: It is generally felt that one's choice of a laryngoscope blade and the technique used to facilitate intubation is best guided by personal choice and experience (9,22,23). The literature suggests that straight blades improve laryngoscopic view (increased exposure of the vocal cords), whereas curved blades provide better intubating conditions (more room to maneuver) (23). The introduction of wider blades (e.g., Grandview) and use of intubating stylets improves intubation success rates with the straight-blade technique (18). The hinged laryngoscope (McCoy blade) has been shown to improve laryngeal view and intubating conditions and reduce cervical spine motion in some studies, though the findings remain controversial (24–28). Finally, use of the right paraglossal (or retromolar) approach initially described in the 1920s has been reevaluated by Henderson and advocated to improve laryngoscopic view, particularly in situations where visualization of laryngeal structures is difficult (29).

7. Confirmation of tracheal placement: Visualization of the ETT entering the larynx provides a reliable method of verifying correct position of the tube. Fiberoptic bronchoscopy remains the gold standard for verifying correct endotracheal tube placement in adults and pediatric patients by permitting the direct visualization of tracheal rings. This technique has also been used in the setting of emergency airway management (30–32). Auscultation of the chest for breath sounds and of the epigastrium for absence of air entry into the stomach and observation of chest motion during ventilation are common but notoriously inaccurate methods of ascertaining proper ETT placement. CO_2 detection and EDDs have become the standard of care to verify correct placement of the endotracheal tube in the trachea, though both techniques have shortcomings (33–52). As might be expected, CO_2 detection techniques tend to be less accurate in identifying correct placement of the ETT in patients with circulatory arrest, with reported false negative rates (CO_2 not detected, tube in the trachea) as high as 30% to 35% (37). In nonarrested patients CO_2 detection is highly reliable, indicating correct placement 99% to 100% of the time (33,35,38,48). Soft drinks in the stomach containing CO_2 may mimic the exhaled CO_2 from the lungs for a couple of breaths, the so-called Cola complication, though this confounding result ought not to persist beyond six breaths (53). The correct endotracheal placement of the tube can be evaluated by the 'esophageal detector device' that consists of a self-inflating suction bulb or syringe and an attached adapter to fit it to a standard ETT connector. The collapsed bulb or syringe rapidly fills with air if the ETT is in the trachea; it does not inflate if the tube is in the collapsed esophagus with a specificity of about 99% (41,54,55). Lighted stylets have also been used to verify tracheal placement (56).

REFERENCES

1. Shapiro BA, Kacmarek RM, Cane RD, et al. *Clinical application of respiratory care*, 4th ed. St Louis: Mosby, 1991.
2. Kacmarek RM, Stoller JK, eds. *Current respiratory care.* Toronto: BC Decker, 1988.
3. Vender JS, Clemency MV. Oxygen delivery systems, inhalation therapy and respiratory therapy. In: Benumof JL, ed. *Airway management: principles and practice.* St Louis: Mosby, 1996.
4. Barnes TA, Watson ME. Oxygen delivery performance of old and new designs of the Laerdal, Vitalograph and AMBU adult manual resuscitators. *Respir Care* 1983;28:1121.
5. Cullen P. Self-inflating ventilation bags. *Anaesth Intensive Care* 2001;29:203.
6. Nimmagadda U, Salem MR, Joseph NJ, et al. Efficacy of preoxygenation with tidal volume breathing. Comparison of breathing systems. *Anesthesiology* 2000;93:693–698.
7. Wolcke B, Schneider T, Mauer D, et al. Ventilation volumes with different self-inflating bags with reference to the ERC guidelines for airway management: comparison of two compression techniques. *Resuscitation* 2000;47:175–178.
8. Cormack RS, Lehane J. Difficult tracheal intubation in obstetrics. *Anaesthesia* 1984;39:1105.
9. Benumof JL. The ASA difficult airway algorithm: new thoughts and considerations. 51st annual refresher course lectures and clinical update program, #235. American Society of Anesthesiologists, 2000.
10. Adnet F, Baillard C, Borron SW, et al. Randomized study comparing the "sniffing position" with simple head extension for laryngoscopic view in elective surgery patients. *Anesthesiology* 2001;95:836–841.
11. Levitan RM, Ochroch AE, Hollander J, et al. Assessment of airway visualization: validation of the percent of glottic opening (POGO) scale. *Acad Emerg Med* 1998;5:919–923.
12. Knill RL. Difficult laryngoscopy made easy with a "BURP". *Can J Anaesth* 1993;40:279–282.
13. Benumof JL, Cooper SD. Quantitative improvement in laryngoscopic view by optimal external laryngeal manipulation. *J Clin Anesth* 1996;8:136–140.
14. Takahata O, Kubota M, Mamiya K, et al. The efficacy of the "BURP" maneuver during a difficult laryngoscopy. *Anesth Analg* 1997;84(Feb):419–421.
15. Green DW. Gum elastic bougie and simulated difficult intubation. *Anaesthesia* 2003;58:391–392.
16. Henderson JJ. Development of the 'gum-elastic bougie'. *Anaesthesia* 2003;58:103–104.
17. Toyoyama H, Hirose Y, Toyoda Y. When and by whom was the curved tip of a gum-elastic bougie first introduced. *Anaesthesia* 2002;57:932.
18. Gataure PS, Vaughan RS, Latto IP. Simulated difficult intubation. Comparison of the gum elastic bougie and the stylet. *Anaesthesia* 1996;51:935–938.
19. Kidd JF, Dyson A, Latto IP. Successful difficult intubation. Use of the gum elastic bougie. *Anaesthesia* 1988;43:437–438.
20. Cupitt JM. Microbial contamination of gum elastic bougies. *Anaesthesia* 2000;55:466–468.
21. Viswanathan S, Campbell C, Wood DG, et al. The Eschmann tracheal tube introducer (gum elastic bougie). *Anesthesiol Rev* 1992;19:29.
22. Practice guidelines for management of the difficult airway. An updated report by the American Society of Anesthesiologists task force on management of the difficult airway. *Anesthesiology* 2003;98:1269–1277.
23. Arino JJ, Velasco JM, Gasco C, et al. Straight blades improve visualization of the larynx while curved blades increase the ease of intubation: a comparison of the Macintosh, Miller, McCoy, Belscope and Lee-Fairview blades. *Can J Anaesth* 2003;50:501–506.
24. Yardeni IZ, Gefen A, Smolyarenko V, et al. Design evaluation of commonly used rigid and levering laryngoscope blades. *Acta Anaesthesiol Scand* 2002;46:1003–1009.
25. McCoy EP, Mirakhur RK. The levering laryngoscope. *Anaesthesia* 1993;48:516–519.
26. Cook TM, Tuckey JP. A comparison between the Macintosh and the McCoy laryngoscope blades. *Anaesthesia* 1996;51:977–980.
27. MacIntyre PA, McLeod AD, Hurley R, et al. Cervical spine movements during laryngoscopy. Comparison of the Macintosh and McCoy laryngoscope blades. *Anaesthesia* 1999;54:413–418.
28. Chisholm DG, Calder I. Experience with the McCoy laryngoscope in difficult laryngoscopy. *Anaesthesia* 1997;52:906–908.
29. Henderson JJ. The use of paraglossal straight blade laryngoscopy in difficult tracheal intubation. *Anaesthesia* 1997;52:552–560.

30. Nielsen LH, Kristensen J, Knudsen F, et al. Fibre-optic bronchoscopic evaluation of tracheal tube position. *Eur J Anaesthesiol* 1991;8:277–279.
31. Lee YS, Soong WJ, Jeng MJ, et al. Endotracheal tube position in pediatrics and neonates: comparison between flexible fiberoptic bronchoscopy and chest radiograph. *Zhonghua Yi Xue Za Zhi* (Taipei) 2002;65:341–344.
32. Hutton KC, Verdile VP, Yealy DM, et al. Prehospital and emergency department verification of endotracheal tube position using a portable, non-directable, fiberoptic bronchoscope. *Prehosp Disast Med* 1990;5:131–136.
33. Grmec S. Comparison of three different methods to confirm tracheal tube placement in emergency intubation. *Intensive Care Med* 2002;28:701–704.
34. Katz SH, Falk JL. Misplaced endotracheal tubes by paramedics in an urban emergency medical services system. *Ann Emerg Med* 2001;37:32–37.
35. Takeda T, Tanigawa K, Tanaka H, et al. The assessment of three methods to verify tracheal tube placement in the emergency setting. *Resuscitation* 2003;56:153–157.
36. Kelly JJ, Eynon CA, Kaplan JL, et al. Use of tube condensation as an indicator of endotracheal tube placement. *Ann Emerg Med* 1998;31:575–578.
37. MacLeod BA, Heller MB, Gerard J, et al. Verification of endotracheal tube placement with colorimetric end-tidal CO_2 detection. *Ann Emerg Med* 1991;20:267–270.
38. Ornato JP, Shipley JB, Racht EM, et al. Multicenter study of a portable, hand-size, colorimetric end-tidal carbon dioxide detection device. *Ann Emerg Med* 1992;21:518–523.
39. Zaleski L, Abello D, Gold MI. The esophageal detector device. Does it work? *Anesthesiology* 1993;79:244–247.
40. Hayden SR, Sciammarella J, Viccellio P, et al. Colorimetric end-tidal CO_2 detector for verification of endotracheal tube placement in out-of-hospital cardiac arrest. *Acad Emerg Med* 1995;2:499–502.
41. Bozeman WP, Hexter D, Liang HK, et al. Esophageal detector device versus detection of end-tidal carbon dioxide level in emergency intubation. *Ann Emerg Med* 1996;27:595–599.
42. Pelucio M, Halligan L, Dhindsa H. Out-of-hospital experience with the syringe esophageal detector device. *Acad Emerg Med* 1997;4:563–568.
43. Schaller RJ, Huff JS, Zahn A. Comparison of a colorimetric end-tidal CO_2 detector and an esophageal aspiration device for verifying endotracheal tube placement in the prehospital setting: a six-month experience. *Prehosp Disast Med* 1997;12:57–63.
44. Kasper CL, Deem S. The self-inflating bulb to detect esophageal intubation during emergency airway management. *Anesthesiology* 1998;88:898–902.
45. Cardoso MM, Banner MJ, Melker RJ, et al. Portable devices used to detect endotracheal intubation during emergency situations: a review. *Crit Care Med* 1998;26:957–964.
46. Falk JL, Falk Sayre MR. Confirmation of airway placement. *Prehosp Emerg Care* 1999;3:273–278.
47. Tanigawa K, Takeda T, Goto E, et al. Accuracy and reliability of the self-inflating bulb to verify tracheal intubation in out-of-hospital cardiac arrest patients. *Anesthesiology* 2000;93:1432–1436.
48. Li J. Capnography alone is imperfect for endotracheal tube placement confirmation during emergency intubation. *J Emerg Med* 2001;20:223–229.
49. Tanigawa K, Takeda T, Goto E, et al. The efficacy of esophageal detector devices in verifying tracheal tube placement: a randomized cross-over study of out-of-hospital cardiac arrest patients. *Anesth Analg* 2001;92:375–378.
50. Bhende MS, LaCovey DC. End-tidal carbon dioxide monitoring in the prehospital setting. *Prehosp Emerg Care* 2001;5:208–213.
51. Hendey GW, Shubert GS, Shalit M, et al. The esophageal detector bulb in the aeromedical setting. *J Emerg Med* 2002;23:51–55.
52. Tong YL, Sun M, Tang WH, et al. The tracheal detecting-bulb: a new device to distinguish tracheal from esophageal intubation. *Acta Anaesthesiol Sin* 2002;40:159–163.
53. Zbinden S, Schüpfer G. Detection of oesophageal intubation: the cola complication. *Anaesthesia* 1989;44:81.
54. Kapsner CE, Seaberg DC, Stengel C, et al. The esophageal detector device: accuracy and reliability in difficult airway settings. *Prehosp Disast Med* 1996;11:60–62.
55. Wee MY. The oesophageal detector device. Assessment of a new method to distinguish oesophageal from tracheal intubation. *Anaesthesia* 1998;43:27–29.
56. Stewart RD, LaRosee A, Stoy WA, et al. Use of a lighted stylet to confirm correct endotracheal tube placement. *Chest* 1987;92:900–903.

6

Identification of the Difficult and Failed Airway

Michael F. Murphy and Ron M. Walls

DEFINITIONS OF THE DIFFICULT AND FAILED AIRWAY

Although both difficult and failed airways are discussed in this chapter, the two concepts are distinct. A difficult airway is one for which a preintubation examination has identified attributes that are likely to make laryngoscopy, intubation, bag/mask ventilation, or surgical airway management more difficult than would be the case in an ordinary patient without those attributes. Identification of a difficult airway is a key component of the approach to airway management in the emergency department patient and becomes a key branch point on the main airway algorithm (see Chapter 2). If a difficult airway is identified, the difficult airway algorithm is used, and the approach is therefore different from that taken when the patient is not anticipated to have a difficult intubation. A failed airway situation occurs when a provider has embarked on a certain course of airway management (e.g., RSI) and has identified that intubation by that method is simply not going to succeed, requiring immediate initiation of a rescue sequence (the failed airway algorithm, Chapter 2). Certainly, in retrospect, a failed airway can be called a difficult airway, as it has proven to be impossible to intubate, but the terms "failed airway" and "difficult airway" must be kept distinct, for they represent different situations, require different approaches, and arise at different points in the airway management sequence.

> *"The difficult airway is something one anticipates; the failed airway is something one experiences."*
>
> *Walls, 2002*

Airways that are difficult to manage are fairly common in emergency practice with some estimates being as high as 20% of all emergency intubations. However, the incidence of intubation failure is quite low, being in the 0.5% to 2.5% range. Moreover, the disastrous situation of being able neither to intubate nor to ventilate rarely occurs (0.1% to 0.5%).

The use of neuromuscular blockade to facilitate oral endotracheal intubation followed the introduction of curare into anesthetic practice in the 1940s and succinylcholine in the early 1950s. Until that time orotracheal intubation was largely performed with the patient ventilating spontaneously under inhalational anesthesia (e.g., ether). The consequence of a failed intubation was mitigated by the fact that the patient continued to breathe spontaneously. The threat of failure to intubate in the face of neuromuscular blockade and apnea suddenly required anesthesia providers to evaluate the airway for difficulty before paralysis was induced. Thus the clinical use of neuromuscular blocking agents became inseparable from the requirement to perform an airway evaluation and from the ability to rescue the airway in the event of failure. Emergency medicine practitioners began to use neuromuscular blockade to facilitate orotracheal intubation in the late 1970s. By the late 1980s the use of neuromuscular blockade for this purpose was widely referred to as rapid sequence intubation (RSI), deliberately creating a distinction from the anesthesia term rapid sequence induction, which is also abbreviated RSI. By the mid to late 1990s most emergency practitioners were using neuromuscular blockade in some form, and most intubations were being done using neuromuscular blocking agents. It had become evident that neuromuscular blockade not only made the technical task of intubation easier and faster, but that the complication rates were lower and the success rates higher. However, for many practitioners the need to evaluate the airway for difficulty and the development of a systematic method of doing so lagged behind the clinical introduction of RSI. There was also the need to expand the rescue options beyond cricothyrotomy.

This chapter will explore the concepts of the failed and the difficult airway. The premise is that recognizing the difficult airway and dealing with it appropriately ought to minimize the likelihood that airway management will fail. Furthermore, recognizing the failed airway promptly will optimize the chances that failing techniques will be abandoned and an approach undertaken that is reasonably anticipated to succeed.

THE FAILED AIRWAY

A failed airway exists when either of the following conditions is met:

1. Failure to maintain acceptable oxygen saturations during or after one or more failed laryngoscopic attempts, or
2. Three failed attempts at orotracheal intubation by an experienced intubator, even when oxygen saturation can be maintained.

Clinically, the failed airway presents itself in two ways, depending on the urgency created by the situation:

1. There is not sufficient time to evaluate or attempt a series of rescue options, and the airway must be secured immediately because of an inability to maintain oxygen saturation by bag and mask ventilation. This is the can't intubate/can't oxygenate scenario. (defined by the previous number 1).
2. There is time to evaluate and execute various options because the patient is in a can't intubate/can oxygenate situation (defined by the previous number 2).

The most important way to avoid airway management failure is to identify in advance those patients who might be difficult to intubate, bag/mask ventilate, or perform a cricothyrotomy on, particularly if one is relying on the latter two techniques to rescue the airway in the event that oral intubation proves impossible.

In 2002, in characterizing the distinctions between the difficult and failed airway, Walls coined the expression: "The difficult airway is something one anticipates; the failed airway is something one experiences." In an ideal world this would be so, and we would be sufficiently adept at predicting difficulty that experiencing failure would never occur.

The adage in anesthesia with respect to neuromuscular blockade and the orotracheal intubation of a patient that has some effective spontaneous ventilation has always been: "Don't take anything away from the patient that you cannot replace," which can be truncated to: "Don't burn any bridges." Although such advice is certainly sound in terms of elective anesthesia, this rigid principle is not always consistent with the realities of emergency airway management, where intubation is often required emergently regardless of the patient's underlying physiological condition or difficult airway attributes, and the approach must be chosen that is most likely to result in success. Thus, many patients with identified difficult airways are best managed using RSI, but the approach is customized by the standardized consideration of options for the difficult airway (Chapter 2).

THE DIFFICULT AIRWAY

The universal airway algorithm was introduced in Chapter 2. When one is presented with a patient who requires intubation, the first decision is whether or not this is a crash airway. If it is not a crash airway, one must ask, "Is this a difficult airway?" Asking the question presumes that one has a framework with which to answer it.

In clinical practice, the difficult airway has four dimensions:

1. Difficult bag/mask ventilation (BMV)
2. Difficult laryngoscopy
3. Difficult intubation
4. Difficult cricothyrotomy

These four dimensions can be reduced to three technical operations:

1. Difficult bag/mask ventilation (BMV)
2. Difficult laryngoscopy and intubation
3. Difficult cricothyrotomy

Sakles has depicted the relationship among these technical operations as a triangle (Fig. 6-1). According to the main emergency airway management algorithm, RSI is the method of choice for airway management in the event airway management difficulty is not anticipated. This requires a reliable and reproducible method for identifying the difficult airway. This evaluation

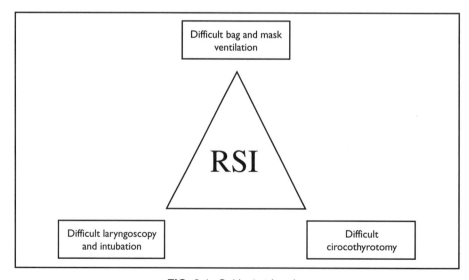

FIG. 6-1. Sakles's triangle.

must be expeditious, easy to remember, and complete. A distinct evaluation is required for difficult bag/mask ventilation, difficult laryngoscopy/intubation, and difficult surgical airway management.

Difficult Bag/Mask Ventilation: MOANS

Chapter 5 highlights the importance of bag/mask ventilation in airway management, particularly as a rescue maneuver when orotracheal intubation has failed. If the airway manager is uncertain that neuromuscular blockade-facilitated orotracheal intubation (RSI) will be successful, he or she must be confident that bag/mask ventilation is possible, or at the very least that a cricothyrotomy can rapidly be performed.

The validated indicators of difficult bag and mask ventilation can be easily recalled for rapid use in the emergency setting by using the mnemonic MOANS. Perhaps one can recall this mnemonic by picturing the obtunded, *moan*ing patient as in need of bag/mask ventilation, or conversely, the involuntary *moan* that might escape the lips of the provider when he or she is confronted by a patient on whom bag/mask ventilation is not possible.

M *Mask Seal*: Bushy beards, crusted blood on the face, or a disruption of lower facial continuity are the most common examples of conditions that may make an adequate mask seal difficult. Some experts recommend smearing a substance, such as KY jelly, on the beard as remedy to this problem, though this action may simply make a bad situation worse in that the entire face may become too slippery to hold the mask in place.

O *Obesity/Obstruction*: Patients who are obese (body mass index > 26 kg/m^2) are often difficult to ventilate adequately by bag and mask. Women in third-trimester gestation are a prototype for this problem, because the increased body mass and the resistance to diaphragmatic excursion by the gravid uterus create elevated resistance to bag/mask ventilation. Pregnant patients also desaturate more quickly, making the bag ventilation difficulty of even greater import (see Chapter 3). The difficulty bagging the obese patient is not caused solely by the weight of chest and abdominal walls and the resistance by the abdominal contents to diaphragmatic excursion. Obese patients also have redundant tissues, creating resistance to airflow in the supraglottic airway. Similarly, patients with angioedema, Ludwig's angina, upper airway abscesses (e.g., peritonsillar), epiglottitis, and others, ought to be considered at this juncture. There is a sense that edematous lesions (e.g., angioedema, croup, epiglottitis, etc.) are more amenable to bag and mask rescue should sudden obstruction occur or be induced, though not reliably. On the other hand, firm, immobile lesions such as hematomas, cancers, and foreign bodies are less amenable to rescue by bag and mask ventilation, so inciting total obstruction (airway manipulation, poor positioning, medications, etc.) in these patients is ill-advised, except as part of a carefully laid out plan.

A *Age*: Age greater than 55 is associated with a higher risk of difficult bag/mask ventilation, perhaps because of a loss of muscle and tissue tone in the upper airway as we age.

N *No teeth*: An adequate mask seal may be difficult in the edentulous patient as the face tends to cave in. An option is to leave dentures (if available) *in situ* for bag/mask ventilation and remove them for intubation. Alternatively, gauze flats may be inserted in the cheeks to puff them out in an attempt to improve the seal.

S *Stiff*: This refers to patients whose lungs are themselves resistant to ventilation and require high ventilation pressures. These patients are primarily those with reactive airways disease with medium and small airways obstruction (asthma; chronic obstructive pulmonary disease, COPD) and those with pulmonary edema, acute respiratory diseases (ARDS), advanced pneumonia, or any other condition that reduces pulmonary compliance to bag/mask ventilation. A separate but unrelated *S* that connotes difficult bag/mask ventilation is a history of snoring. This condition is not of practical value in the emergency department, however, as it is unlikely that it will be determined in the setting of an emergency intubation.

Difficult Laryngoscopy and Intubation: LEMON

Difficult laryngoscopy and intubation ordinarily implies that the operator had a poor view of the target, i.e., the glottis. Cormack and Lehane provided some clarity to the way we think of the difficult airway by parsing the act of intubation into its two subcomponents: laryngoscopy and intubation. They also introduced the most widely used system of categorizing the degree of visualization of the larynx during laryngoscopy, in which an ideal laryngoscopic view is designated grade 1 and the worst possible view grade 4. (Fig. 6-2) Cormack–Lehane view grades 3 (epiglottis only visible) and 4 (no glottic structures at all visible) are accepted to represent difficult laryngoscopy and are highly correlated with difficult intubation. View grades 1 (visualization of the entire laryngeal aperture) and 2 (visualization of some portion of the cords and arytenoids) are not typically associated with difficult intubation, though a patient with a grade 2 view in which only the arytenoids are visible is significantly more difficult to intubate than a patient with a grade 2 view in which any portion of the cords can be seen. Patients with a limited grade 2 view or a grade 3 view may greatly benefit by use of an intubating stylet, such as the Eschmann or Frova devices (see Chapter 5). The Cormack–Lehane grading system does not differentiate precisely the degree to which the laryngeal aperture is visible during laryngoscopy: A grade 2 view may reveal little of the vocal cords (or none at all if only the arytenoids are visible, a circumstance that has led some authors to propose a 2a/2b system, wherein a 2a shows any portion of the cords, a 2b only the arytenoids),

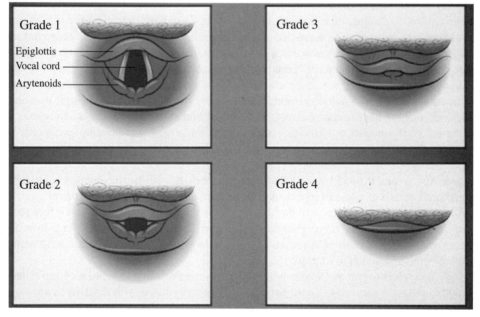

FIG. 6-2. Cormack–Lehane laryngeal view grade system.

whereas a grade 1 view reveals the entire glottis. The question is often asked: How much of the cords must be visible during direct laryngoscopy to ensure intubation success? How much is *enough*?

To put this grading system into context, one must first define *best attempt*. Benumof defines the six components of the best attempt as: (i) performance by a reasonably experienced endoscopist, (ii) no significant muscle tone, (iii) the use of the optimal sniff position, (iv) the use of external laryngeal manipulation (BURP), (v) length of the blade, and (vi) type of blade. With this definition and no other confounding considerations, the optimal attempt at laryngoscopy may be achieved on the first attempt and should take no more than three attempts. Most times the circumstances of an emergency intubation preclude the first attempt from being the best attempt. Should an orotracheal intubation attempt fail and an additional attempt be contemplated, it seems reasonable to change something on the subsequent attempt to enhance the chances of success. That something may be one, some, or all of these factors. This approach to the components of the optimum or best attempt provides the framework to address what to change.

Optimizing all six components may not be possible in an emergency. For example, in certain situations where difficulty is predicted, it may not be advisable to paralyze the patient. Additionally, in the event the cervical spine is immobilized, it may not be possible to place the patient in the sniff position. Most experts on airway management agree that positioning the head and neck is an important step in optimizing conventional laryngoscopy as a prelude to orotracheal intubation. Though there is some debate about the relative role of cervical extension versus the sniffing position (Chapter 5), in any case, optimal positioning of the patient for direct laryngoscopy improves laryngoscopic view.

The object of identifying difficult laryngoscopy and intubation preemptively is to minimize to the greatest extent possible the likelihood of encountering a failed airway. Benumof's six principles provide a framework for evaluating those elements that might be present in an individual case that might limit laryngoscopic success.

Many researchers over the years have addressed the ability to determine with precision those airways where laryngoscopy and intubation will succeed and those in which it will fail. None have been able to do so. Lists of anatomical features, radiologic findings and complex scoring systems have all been explored without success. In the absence of a proven and validated system that is capable of predicting intubation difficulty with 100% sensitivity and specificity, it is important to develop an approach that will enable a clinician to quickly and simply identify those patients who *might* be difficult to intubate, so that an appropriate plan can be made using the difficult airway algorithm. In other words, sensitivity (i.e., identifying all those who might be difficult) is more important than specificity (always being correct when identifying a patient as difficult) when we ask the question, Does this airway meet the threshold of being sufficiently difficult to warrant using the difficult airway algorithm, or is it appropriate and safe to proceed directly to RSI?

To identify as many of the risks as possible as quickly as possible to meet the demands of an emergency situation, the mnemonic LEMON is a useful guide. The elements of the mnemonic are assembled from an analysis of the difficult airway prediction instruments in the elective anesthesia literature and are the subject of a validation study (NEAR III) by the investigators of the multicenter National Emergency Airway Registry project. The LEMON mnemonic is recalled by the popular idiom that a defective product is a lemon, thus the difficult airway is a LEMON:

L *Look externally*: Although a gestalt of difficult intubation is not particularly sensitive (meaning that many difficult airways are not readily apparent externally), it is quite specific, meaning that if the airway looks difficult, it probably is. Most of the litany of physical features associated with difficult laryngoscopy and intubation (e.g., small mandible, large tongue, large teeth, short neck, etc.) are accounted for by the remaining elements of LEMON and so do not need to be specifically recalled as a list, which can be a difficult memory challenge in a critical situation. The external look specified here is for external evidence of lower facial disruption that might make both intubation and mask ventilation difficult. It is during this part of LEMON, i.e., the external look, that the MOANS evaluation for difficult bag/mask ventilation occurs (discussed earlier) along with the SHORT evaluation for difficult cricothyrotomy (discussed later).

E *Evaluate 3-3-2:* This step is an amalgamation of the much-studied geometric considerations that relate mouth opening and the size of the mandible to the position of the larynx in the neck in terms of likelihood of successful laryngoscopy and intubation. This relationship was first articulated by Patil in 1983 when he associated a thyromental distance of less than 6 cm with difficult intubation. The thyromental distance is the hypotenuse of a triangle, the axis being the length of the mandible and the abscissa being the distance between the base of the mandible and the top of the larynx. Mouth opening is also key to the need to visualize the glottis during laryngoscopy. A normal patient can open his or her mouth sufficiently to accommodate three of his or her own fingers between the incisors. The thyromental distance is represented by the patient's ability to accommodate three of his or her own fingers between the tip of the mentum and hyoid bone (Fig. 6-3a) and to fit two fingers between the hyoid bone and the thyroid notch (Fig. 6-3b). Thus in the 3-3-2 rule, the first 3 assesses the adequacy of oral access and the second 3 addresses the capacity of the mandibular space to accommodate the tongue on laryngoscopy. More than or less than three fingers are both associated with greater degrees of difficulty in visualizing the larynx at laryngoscopy: the former because the length of the oral axis is elongated; the latter because the mandibular space may be too small to accommodate the tongue, requiring it to remain in the oral cavity or move posterior, obscuring the view of the glottis. The final 2 identifies the location of the larynx in relation to the base of the tongue. If significantly more than two fingers are accommodated, meaning the larynx is distant from the base of the tongue, it may be difficult to visualize the glottis on laryngoscopy. Fewer than two fingers may mean that the larynx is tucked up under the base of the tongue and may be difficult to expose. This condition is often called anterior larynx.

M *Mallampati score:* Mallampati determined that the degree to which the posterior oropharyngeal structures are visible reflects the relationships among mouth opening, the size of the tongue, and the size of the oral pharynx that dictates access via the oral cavity for intubation, and that these relationships are loosely associated with intubation success. Mallampati's classic assessment required that patients sit on the side of the bed, open their mouths as widely as possible, and protrude their tongue as far as possible without phonating. Fig. 6-4 depicts how the scale is constructed. Though Class I and II patients are associated with low intubation failure rates, the importance with respect to the wisdom of using neuromuscular blockade rests with those in Classes III and IV, particularly Class IV where intubation failure rates may exceed 10%. By itself the scale is neither sensitive nor specific; however, it is easily performed in an emergency and may reveal important information about access to the oral cavity and the potential for difficult glottic visualization. Usually in the emergency situation, it is not possible to have the patient sit up and follow instructions. Therefore, a crude Mallampati measure is often all that can be acquired, by looking into the supine, obtunded patient's mouth with a tongue blade and light, or with a lighted laryngoscope blade to gain an appreciation of how much mouth opening is present (at least in the preparalyzed state) and how likely the tongue and oral pharynx are to conspire to prevent successful

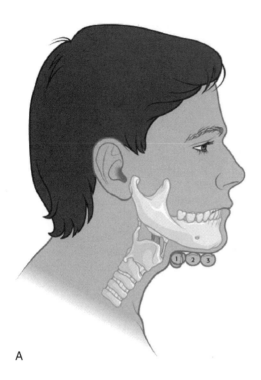

A

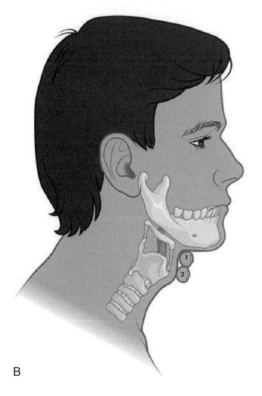

B

FIG. 6-3. A: The second 3 of the 3-3-2 rule.
B: The 2 of the 3-3-2 rule.

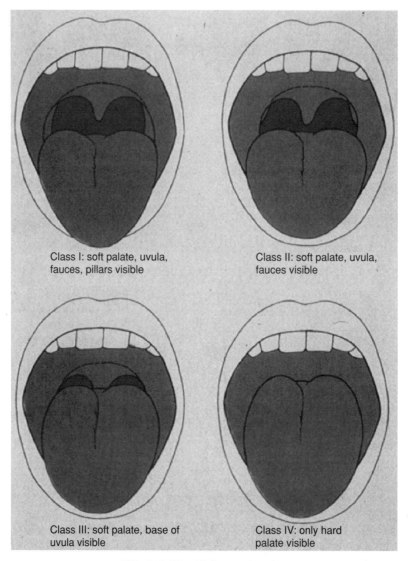

Class I: soft palate, uvula, fauces, pillars visible

Class II: soft palate, uvula, fauces visible

Class III: soft palate, base of uvula visible

Class IV: only hard palate visible

FIG. 6-4. The Mallampati scale.

laryngoscopy. Although not validated in the supine position using this approach, there is no reason to expect that the assessment would be any less reliable than the original method with the patient sitting and performing the maneuver actively.

O *Obstruction*: Upper airway obstruction should always be considered as a marker for a difficult airway. The three cardinal signs of upper airway obstruction are muffled voice (hot potato voice), difficulty swallowing secretions (because of either pain or obstruction), and stridor. The first two signs do not ordinarily herald imminent total upper airway obstruction in adults, but stridor is a particularly ominous sign. The presence of stridor is generally considered to indicate that the circumference of the airway has been reduced to roughly 10% of its normal caliber. Upper airway obstruction should always be considered a difficult airway and managed with extreme care. The administration of small doses of opioids and benzodiazepines to manage anxiety may induce total obstruction as the tone of the upper airway musculature stenting the airway open relaxes. Chapter 26 deals with this topic in detail, particularly in relation to the management of the patient with upper airway obstruction, the selection of rescue interventions, and the timing of those interventions.

N *Neck mobility:* The ability to position the head and neck is one of the six factors necessary to the achievement of the optimal laryngoscopic view of the larynx. Cervical spine immobilization in trauma, by itself, may not constitute a degree of difficulty that automatically leads one to defer RSI from consideration, pending application of the difficult airway algorithm. However, cervical spine immobilization will make intubation more difficult and will compound the effects of other identified difficult airway markers. In addition, intrinsic cervical spine immobility, such as in cases of ankylosing spondylitis or rheumatoid arthritis, can make intubation by direct laryngoscopy extremely difficult or impossible and should be considered as a much more serious issue than the ubiquitous cervical collar (that mandates in-line manual immobilization).

Difficult Cricothyrotomy: SHORT

There are no absolute contraindications to performing an emergency cricothyrotomy (see Chapter 15). However, some conditions may make it difficult or impossible to perform the procedure, making it imperative to identify those conditions in advance and allowing consideration of alternatives rather than simply relying on a rapidly performed cricothyrotomy as a rescue technique. The mnemonic SHORT is used to quickly assess the patient for features that may indicate that a cricothyrotomy might be difficult. The mnemonic can be recalled by remembering that a patient with a *short* neck is difficult to perform a surgical airway on, or that time is *short* when cricothyrotomy is indicated. The SHORT mnemonic is applied as follows:

S *Surgery (or other airway disruption):* The anatomy may be subtly or obviously distorted, making the airway difficult to find or impeding access to the anterior portion of it (e.g., halo device after spine surgery).

H *Hematoma (includes infection/abscess):* A hematoma (postoperative or traumatic) or an infective process in the pathway of the cricothyrotomy may make the procedure technically difficult, but should never be considered a contraindication in a life-threatening situation.

O *Obesity (includes any access problem):* Obesity should be considered a surrogate for any problem that makes percutaneous or open surgical access to the anterior neck problematic, such as a very short neck; large, descending pannus; subcutaneous emphysema.

R *Radiation distortion (and other deformity):* Past radiation therapy may distort tissues making the procedure difficult, or fixed flexion deformity of the spine may limit the working access to the anterior landmarks.

T *Tumor:* Tumor either in or around the airway may present difficulty, both from an access perspective as well as bleeding.

SUMMARY

• When intubation is indicated, the most important question is, "Is this airway difficult?" Considerations of pretreatment agents for RSI, for example, do not come into play until the patient has been thoroughly assessed for difficulty (MOANS, LEMON, and SHORT) and the appropriate issues addressed using the algorithms.

• MOANS is always crucially important. The ability to bag/mask ventilate a patient is what turns a potential can't intubate, can't oxygenate situation requiring urgent cricothyrotomy into a can't intubate, *can* oxygenate situation, in which many rescue options can be considered. The ability to prospectively identify and avoid situations in which bag ventilation will be difficult or impossible is critical to avoiding unnecessary emergency cricothyrotomy.

• When cricothyrotomy is necessary, virtually always the possibility will have been identified in advance, and application of SHORT will permit the operator to be mentally and physically prepared for the surgical airway.

• No single indicator, combination of indicators, or even weighted scoring system of indicators can be relied on to guarantee success or predict inevitable failure for oral intubation. Application of a systematic method to identify the difficult airway and then analysis of the situation to identify the best approach, given the anticipated degree of difficulty and the skill, experience, and judgment of the individual performing the intubation, will lead to the best decisions regarding how to manage the particular clinical situation.

EVIDENCE

1. Incidence of difficult and failed airway: In anesthesia practice the incidence of the failed airway has been identified as 1:2230 (0.05%) in surgical patients (1) and in approximately 1:280 (0.36%) of parturients for cesarian section under general anesthesia (2). The largest single-center series in the emergency medicine literature has demonstrated a failure rate for RSI of approximately 1% (3). Emerging numbers from the multicenter NEAR project show cricothyrotomy rates of approximately 0.5% in medical cases and 2.3% in trauma (4).

2. Predicting difficult intubation: Many studies have attempted not only to define the features that may predict difficulty, but also to precisely define those airways where failure will occur. The goal has been to attempt to precisely divide the population into those who can be safely anesthetized and paralyzed and those who ought to be intubated awake. The landmark publication in 1956 by Cass et al. identified those anatomical features that may predict difficult intubation (5). This work coincided with the introduction of paralytic agents into anesthetic practice in the late 1940s and early 1950s. Many subsequent investigators attempted to deliver tools that could accurately predict failure (6–13). Though all failed to craft a formula or identify a specific predictor for failure, Mallampati had a measure of success in that he identified oral access as a crucial feature of the assessment for difficulty (13). Langeron in particular contributed greatly to the scientific validation of those features predicting difficult bag/mask ventilation with his study published in 2000 (14,15).

3. Positioning of the airway: Cormack and Lehane have devised the most widely accepted system of categorizing the view of the larynx achieved with an orally placed laryngoscope (16). The sniffing position has been widely accepted as the optimum position for orotracheal intubation (17) though Adnet et al. have recently challenged this dogma, suggesting that simple extension may be sufficient or possibly even superior (18). In attempting to provide a framework or an approach to answering the question of optimum positioning of the head and neck, Levitan et al. devised a scoring system to quantify the percentage of glottic opening (POGO) visible during a best laryngoscopy, though at the present time, this scale has yet to gain widespread acceptance (19).

REFERENCES

1. Samsoon GLT, Young JRB: Difficult tracheal intubation: a retrospective study. *Anaesthesia* 1987;14:17–27.
2. Rocke DA, Murray WB, Rout CC, et al. Relative risk analysis of factors associated with difficult intubation in obstetric anesthesia. *Anaesthesiology* 1992;77:67.
3. Sakles JC, Laurin EG, Rantapaa AA, et al. Airway management in the emergency department: a one-year study of 610 tracheal intubations. *Ann Emerg Med* 1998;31(Mar):325–332.
4. Bair AE, Filbin MR, Kulkarni RG, et al. The failed intubation attempt in the emergency department: analysis of prevalence, rescue techniques, and personnel. *J Emerg Med* 2002;23(Aug):131–140.
5. Cass NM, James NR, Lines V. Difficult direct laryngoscopy complicating intubation in anaesthesia. *BMJ* 1956;1:488–490.
6. Bellhouse CP, Dore C. Criteria for estimating likelihood of difficulty of endotracheal intubation with the MacIntosh laryngoscope. *Anaesth Intensive Care* 1988;16:329.
7. Savva D. Prediction of difficult tracheal intubation. *Br J Anaesth* 1994;73:149.
8. Tse JC, Rimm EB, Hussain A. Predicting difficult endotracheal intubation in surgical patients scheduled for general anesthesia: a prospective blind study. *Anesth Analg* 1995;81:254.
9. El-Ganzouri AR, McCarthy RJ, Turman KJ, et al. Preoperative airway assessment: predictive value of a multivariate risk index. *Anesth Analg* 1996;82:1197.
10. Oates JD, MacLeod AD, Oates PD, et al. Comparison of two methods for predicting difficult intubation. *Br J Anaesth* 1991;66:305.
11. Rose DK, et al. The airway: problems and predictions in 18,500 patients. *Can J Anesth* 1994;41:372.
12. Mallampati SR. Clinical sign to predict difficult tracheal intubation (hypothesis). *Can Anesth Soc J* 1983;30:316.
13. Mallampati SR, Gatt SP, Gugino LD, et al: A clinical sign to predict difficult intubation: a prospective study. *Can Anesth Soc J* 1985;32:429.
14. Langeron O, et al. Prediction of difficult mask ventilation. *Anaesthesiology* 2000;92:1229.
15. Wilson ME, Spiegelhalter D, Robertson JA, et al. Predicting difficult intubation. *Br J Anaesth* 1988;61:211.
16. Cormack RS, Lehane J. Difficult tracheal intubation in obstetrics. *Anaesthesia* 1984;39:1105.
17. Benumof JL. The ASA difficult airway algorithm: new thoughts and considerations. 51st annual refresher course lectures and clinical update program, #235. American Society of Anesthesiologists, 2000.
18. Adnet F, Baillard C, Borron SW, et al. Randomized study comparing the "sniffing position" with simple head extension for laryngoscopic view in elective surgery patients. *Anesthesiology* 2001;95:836–841.
19. Levitan RM, Ochroch AE, Hollander J, et al. Assessment of airway visualization: validation of the percent of glottic opening (POGO) scale. *Acad Emerg Med* 1998;5:919–923.

7

Sedation and Anesthesia for Awake Intubation

Michael F. Murphy

DESCRIPTION

Human beings protect their airway at virtually all cost. To suggest that any method of intubation can be performed in a fully awake and aware patient is clearly ludicrous, unless, of course, several muscular individuals are involved and there is no regard for the integrity of airway structures. In fact, it is generally impossible even to get a glimpse of the glottis with a laryngoscope in a fully awake and aware patient. This is why the *"awake" methods of laryngoscopy referred to* in the difficult airway algorithm always enclose the term *awake* in quotation marks, meaning that though the patient may be nominally aware, his or her sensibilities are attenuated by local anesthesia, sedation, or both.

Ordinarily, local anesthesia and sedation are used concurrently for diagnostic or therapeutic upper airway interventions in patients. If the patient is uncooperative or when time is of the essence, systemic sedation dominates and less local anesthesia is used. Cooperative patients requiring nonemergent diagnostic maneuvers tend to receive more local anesthesia and less systemic sedation because there is sufficient time to dry the airway of secretions and perform the various local anesthesia techniques.

Awake laryngoscopy has two main roles, both of which apply to patients with anticipated difficult intubation:

1. To determine whether intubation will be feasible, thus facilitating a decision regarding the use of neuromuscular blocking agents, or
2. Actually performing the intubation, particularly in circumstances in which the patient's airway may be deteriorating, as in angioedema or upper airway burns or trauma.

An awake look intended to determine the feasibility of intubating the trachea nasally or orally can be accomplished in two ways:

- A flexible fiberoptic bronchoscope or nasopharyngoscope inserted through the nostril may be used to determine if nasal intubation is feasible or to locate the glottis in patients suffering from blunt or penetrating neck trauma to determine if orotracheal intubation will be possible. Topical nasal anesthesia and minimal, if any, sedation are usually all that is required.
- A laryngoscope blade is inserted into the mouth as for a direct laryngoscopy with the intention of confirming that glottic visualization (and thus, orotracheal intubation) is possible.

Substantial local anesthesia of the mouth, oropharynx, and hypopharynx or very deep sedation is usually required to get a decent look at the glottis using this technique. If the glottis is adequately visualized, the airway manager may elect to proceed immediately to an awake intubation or withdraw the laryngoscope and perform RSI. The approach will be dictated by the clinical circumstance. In general:

○ If the difficult airway is dynamic, i.e., evolving, and is the reason for the intubation, then it is usually advisable to intubate the patient during the awake direct laryngoscopy, because the airway may deteriorate significantly over time or as a result of the direct laryngoscopy. A good rule of thumb is, if the airway might change, intubate it when you have the chance.

○ If the difficult airway is chronic (e.g., cervical rheumatoid arthritis) and is not the reason for the airway crisis but simply a confounder to the intubation, then it is reasonable to withdraw the laryngoscope and perform a proper RSI, in the knowledge that the airway is not going to deteriorate further while the RSI is being done.

An awake intubation is more invasive and requires greater degrees of local anesthesia, sedation, and usually, both.

INDICATIONS AND CONTRAINDICATIONS

Awake intubation is indicated when the individual responsible for airway management is not confident that bag and mask ventilation, intubation, or both can be accomplished if the patient is rendered apneic, particularly if an awake laryngoscopy has confirmed that intubation will be challenging. Sedation, upper airway local anesthesia, or both may be indicated for the insertion of supraglottic rescue devices such as nasal and oral airways, LMAs and Combitubes.

Similarly, sedation or local anesthesia of the upper airway may be indicated to facilitate upper airway evaluation (e.g., endoscopy) to identify the location of foreign bodies and remove them, identify a cause of hoarseness, evaluate airway integrity in blunt and penetrating neck trauma, diagnose epiglottitis in a patient with throat pain out of keeping with the oropharyngeal examination, and others.

There are really no contraindications to the use of local anesthetic agents and systemic sedation to enable upper airway evaluation, particularly in an emergency. However, there are some precautions with respect to the choice of sedative agents and how they are used.

SEDATION TECHNIQUES

An awake look in an emergency airway situation relies *entirely* on the intravenous titration of systemically active sedation. There is not enough time to produce adequate local anesthesia of the oropharynx and the hypopharynx for a patient to tolerate awake look procedure without at least a moderate level of sedation. The level of sedation sought is similar to that used for painful procedures in the emergency department, such as reduction of a dislocated shoulder or drainage of a deep cutaneous abscess. A variety of sedating type medications may be used including midazolam, propofol, etomidate, ketamine, and others. Agent selection depends on the clinical situation, medication availability, and the familiarity of the sedating professional with the medication. In general, it is best to achieve sedation for airway examination by the same methods used for other procedures, so that the airway manager is using those agents with which he or she is most familiar and in similar doses.

All agents classified as sedative hypnotics (e.g., benzodiazepines, barbiturates, ethanol, propofol, chloral hydrate, and to some extent etomidate) cause respiratory depression in a dose-dependent fashion. So do the opioids such as fentanyl, morphine, and meperidine, particularly when use in conjunction with sedative hypnotic agents. Patients with borderline ventilatory drive or barely compensated respiratory failure may be rendered apnoeic by relatively small doses of these agents. They also produce some degree of muscle relaxation. Patients with upper airway obstruction may become totally obstructed if these agents cause any loss of upper airway muscle tone, and the operator should always be prepared to proceed directly to a surgical airway when sedation and local anesthesia are undertaken on a patient with partial or impending airway obstruction (see Chapter 6).

Levels of sedation lighter than deep general anesthesia are associated with increased intubation difficulty and failure rates. In addition, deep general anesthesia defeats the fundamental purposes of an awake approach: i.e., the maintenance of spontaneous ventilation and active airway protection while one explores alternatives to induction and paralysis.

Ketamine is a dissociative agent and in doses exceeding 1 mg/kg IV has respiratory and cardiovascular depressant properties. It may also sensitize the larynx to laryngospasm in the face of laryngeal inflammatory disorders. However, in low to moderate doses it stimulates respiration, causes mild elevation in heart rate and blood pressure, and maintains muscle tone. Thus, on balance, in the setting of an airway emergency it may be the best agent to choose to enable the patient to tolerate the evaluation and to continue breathing. The method is to titrate the ketamine in 10 to 20 mg aliquots intravenously until the patient will tolerate an awake look. The patient may be dissociated, but ordinarily will continue to breathe spontaneously and maintain patency of the airway. Some authors have advocated a combination of ketamine and propofol drawn up in the same syringe to make a concentration of 5 mg/mL (5 mL of 10 mg/mL ketamine plus 5 mL of 10 mg/mL of propofol in a 10-mL syringe) titrated 1 to 2 mL at a time. Although this method administers two agents in a fixed combination, it appears to be effective and safe. Alternatives include balanced use of a benzodiazepine (such as midazolam) and an opioid (such as fentanyl), intravenously titrated etomidate, or other agents used for painful, stimulating procedures. All agents require continuous vigilance with respect to airway patency and adequacy of ventilation.

LOCAL ANESTHESIA TECHNIQUES

Local anesthesia of the airway may be produced topically, by injection, or by combining these two techniques. The selection of a local anesthetic agent will depend on the properties of the agent and how it is supplied (concentration and preparation—aqueous, gel, or ointment). Although the provision of profound local anesthesia in a highly cooperative patient may enable the airway to be visualized and the trachea to be intubated even without sedation, almost always in the emergency setting significant systemic sedation will be necessary.

The Nose

Topical anesthesia with vasoconstriction is the technique of choice for the nose.

- Using bayonet nasal forceps, place an *agent-soaked* cotton ball along the floor of the nose toward the back of the inferior turbinate (see Fig. 4-1) Place a second ball just anterior to that, another up against the front of the middle turbinate, and a final one in the vestibule of the nose. It is advisable to place a suture through the cotton balls to retrieve them, though

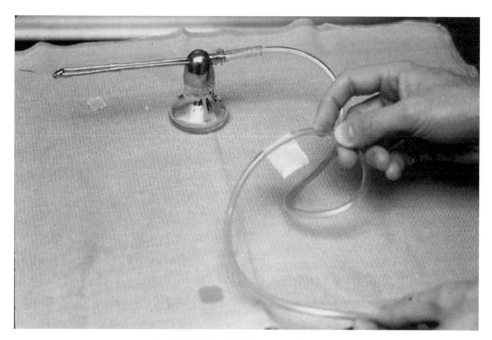

FIG. 7-1. DeVilbiss atomizer.

the author has yet to lose one into the airway. Alternatively, surgical patties (strings already attached) or nasal tampons can be used. Some prefer to place a dry nasal Zomed merocel wick along the floor of the nose and then inject the agent through a plastic IV cannula along the length of the wick. Leave the soaked wick in place for 10 minutes.

- Adequate topical anesthesia of the *dried* upper airway can often be achieved by nebulizing a mixture of 4 cc of 4% lidocaine with 1 cc of 1% phenylephrine. This procedure typically takes 10 to 15 minutes, though, and may still require some augmentation by topical spray during the procedure. Note that this approach will administer 160 mg of lidocaine topically, so must be dose adjusted for small adults and children (toxic dose of lidocaine is 4 mg/ kg.)
- Alternatively, one may elect to use a DeVilbiss atomizer (Fig. 7-1) or a Mucosal Atomization Device to atomize the agent into the nostril while asking the patient to sniff. Atomization produces larger droplets than nebulization. The result is that more of the medication rains out in the upper airway with atomizers than nebulizers, producing a denser block.
- Vasoconstriction is crucial. Not only does it enlarge nasal passageways, it also reduces the risk of mucosal damage and bleeding and enhances the effectiveness of the topical block (Chapter 4). One-fourth percent phenylephrine (Neosynephrine) or oxymetazoline (Afrin) sprayed and sniffed into the nostrils 2 to 3 minutes before the local anesthetic agent is applied is effective. Alternatively, one can prepare tetracaine 0.45% with epinephrine 1:25,000 (40 mcg/mL) or use 4% cocaine (40 mg/mL) applied by either of the previous methods. The maximum safe dose of tetracaine is 50 to 80 mg; for cocaine, 1 to 3 mg/kg, though toxic reactions have been reported with as little as 20 to 30 mg.
- Virtually all of the local anesthetic agents are effective when used topically in the nose. However, a cocaine 4% and tetracaine 0.45% are particularly effective because of their ability

to deeply penetrate tissues and eliminate the deep pressure type pain commonly associated with inserting devices through the nose. Lidocaine is effective, particularly the 4% aqueous solution (discussed earlier), though it tends to cause an intense burning dysesthesia when applied and produces less deep anesthesia, and at 40 mg/mL, toxicity is a real risk as the volume increases. Most consider 3 to 4 mg/kg applied to a mucosal surface to be a safe maximum dose for lidocaine.

The Mouth

The only reason to achieve topical anesthesia of the oral cavity is to reduce the discomfort generated by grasping the tongue with a gauze and pulling it forward to control it and draw the epiglottis forward during a procedure such as bronchoscopic intubation. Secretion of saliva can be eliminated by using an antimuscarinic agent such as glycopyrrolate (Robinul) (0.01 mg/kg IM or IV; usual adult dose 0.8 mg). This approach will enhance the block of the oral cavity, the tongue, the oropharynx, and the hypopharynx by permitting superior penetration of the local anesthetic agent. If there is sufficient time (20 minutes is required for this medication to effectively dry the oropharyngeal secretions), it is always advisable to administer glycopyrrolate as part of the local anesthesia of the upper airway.

- The mouth is best anesthetized topically by having the patient gargle and swish with a 4% aqueous solution of lidocaine. The gargling augments the anesthesia of the oro- and hypopharynx.
- An atomizer can also be used to spray the structures of the oral cavity.

The Oropharynx and Hypopharynx

Begin by having the patient gargle, swish, then spit out 30 mL of 4% lidocaine. For the most part the sensory supply of the oro- and hypopharyngeal areas is via the glossopharyngeal nerve (Chapter 4). The best way to achieve local anesthesia of these areas that is sufficiently dense to permit laryngoscopy or awake intubation is to use a technique that blocks this nerve at the base of the palatopharyngeal arch (posterior tonsillar pillar; see Fig. 4-4). Two techniques are commonly used:

- A 23-gauge angled tonsillar needle with 1 cm of exposed needle tip is inserted 0.5 cm behind the midpoint of the posterior tonsillar pillar and directed laterally and slightly posteriorly (Fig. 7-2). Two cc of 2% lidocaine is then deposited following a negative aspiration test. Although this block can be effective, it is not widely used because of the proximity of the carotid artery. A risk of carotid injection up to 5% has been noted.
- A safer way is to use a topical technique. The oral cavity and the pharynx must be thoroughly dry for any topical technique to work. Put 2 mL of 20% benzocaine ointment on the end of a tongue depressor. Have the patient sitting erect and pull the tongue out using a gauze as described previously. Apply the benzocaine ointment as far back on the base of the tongue as possible using the tongue depressor. Put the tongue back in the mouth and wait 15 minutes. The ointment will liquefy as it warms and will run into the area at the base of the palatopharyngeal arch, penetrating the mucosa to reach the glossopharyngeal nerve. It will also run into the valleculae and pyriform recesses to block the superior branch of the internal laryngeal nerve, producing laryngeal anesthesia.

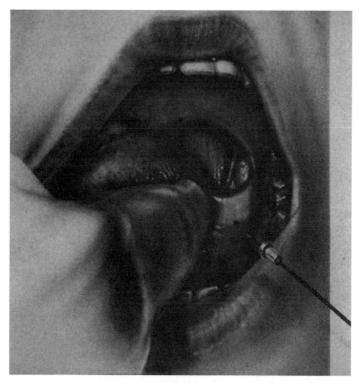

FIG. 7-2. Glossopharyngeal nerve block: insertion point for a 23-gauge angled tonsillar needle.

The Larynx

The drying imperative does not apply to the larynx. Topical local anesthesia of this structure can be provided by spraying using a manual spray device, an atomizer, or a nebulizer using 4 to 6 mL of 4% lidocaine aqueous. (See also the earlier description of nebulized lidocaine and phenylephrine) Alternatively, one can block the superior laryngeal branch of the vagus nerve (see Fig. 4-6):

- The internal branch of the superior laryngeal nerve can be blocked as it runs just deep to the mucosa in the pyriform recess using Jackson forceps to hold a cotton pledget soaked in 4% lidocaine against the mucosa for about one minute (Fig. 7-3).
- This block can also be performed using an external approach to the nerve as it perforates the thyrohyoid membrane just below the greater cornu of the hyoid bone. A 21 to 25-gauge needle is passed medially through skin to contact the hyoid bone as posteriorly as possible. The needle is then walked caudad off the hyoid. Resistance may be appreciated as the thyrohyoid membrane is perforated. Following aspiration to rule out entry into the pharyngeal lumen or a vessel, 3 cc 2% lidocaine can be injected. If the hyoid cannot be palpated or if palpation produces undue patient discomfort, the thyroid cartilage can be used as a landmark. The needle is then walked cephalad from a point on the thyroid cartilage about one-third of the distance from the midline to the greater cornu. Complications again include intraarterial injection, hematoma, and airway distortion.

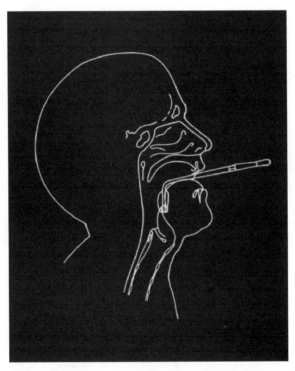

FIG. 7-3. Use of Jackson crossover forceps to perform a transmucosal superior laryngeal nerve block: A cotton pledget, soaked in 4% lidocaine, is held against the mucosa for about one minute.

The Trachea

The trachea is best anesthetized topically. Again, drying beforehand is unnecessary. Local anesthetic agent can be sprayed into the trachea using a handheld spraying device, an atomizer, a fiberoptic scope with a working channel, or a nebulizer.

- Tracheal and laryngeal anesthesia can be produced by puncturing the cricothyroid membrane and injecting local anesthetic agent directly into the trachea. A 5-mL syringe containing 3 mL of 4% lidocaine aqueous is attached to a 20-gauge IV catheter over a needle device. It may be helpful to cut the plastic cannula to about 1.5 cm in length to minimize tracheal stimulation and coughing. A small area of skin is anesthetized over the cricothyroid membrane using a 25 to 27-gauge needle TB or insulin syringe to create a wheal. The needle/IV cannula/syringe combination is then inserted into the trachea through the wheal, aspirating for air during insertion. Once the air column is entered, the cut plastic cannula is threaded in over the needle and the needle is discarded. The lidocaine is injected at end exhalation with the subsequent inspiration and cough facilitating downward and upward spread of the anesthetic, reaching the cords in 95% of cases.

SUMMARY

- Topical anesthesia of the mouth, oropharynx, and hypopharynx will not be successful unless the mucous membranes are first dried by administration of glycopyrrolate.

- An awake look in the context of a difficult airway is primarily accomplished by using intravenous agents, supplemented by local anesthetic agents. Titrate ketamine or other appropriate sedation agents as for sedation/analgesia for a painful procedure.
- Use benzodiazepines, propofol, and opioids with extreme caution in patients with impending airway obstruction.

EVIDENCE

1. Choice of sedative agents: The combination of ketamine and propofol for procedural sedation is a relatively new idea. References 1–3 are drawn from the anesthesia literature and describe how this combination is used.

2. Pharmacodynamics of local anesthetic agents: The physicochemical characteristics of the local anesthetic agents define their clinical behavior, such as their onset time, potency, and duration of action. References 4–7 provide detailed descriptions these agents and their properties.

3. Cocaine and coronary vasoconstriction: It is well known that recreational cocaine use is associated with coronary spasm leading to myocardial ischemia and infarction as well as sudden death (8). It is important to realize that medically administered cocaine to produce nasal vasoconstriction has produced similar complications (9–11).

4. Caution with injection glossopharyngeal block: Reference 12 describes the inadvertent intracarotid injection of a local anesthetic agent during an attempted glossopharyngeal block followed by an immediate seizure.

REFERENCES

1. Mortero RF, Clark LD, Tolan MM, et al. The effects of small dose ketamine on propofol sedation: respiration, postoperative mood, perception, cognition and pain. *Anesth Analg* 2001;92:1465–1469.
2. Badrinath S, Avrramov MN, Shadrick M, et al. The use of a ketamine-propofol combination during monitored anesthesia care. *Anesth Analg* 2000;90:858–862.
3. Frey K, Sukhani R, Pawlowski J, et al. Propofol versus propofol-ketamine sedation for retrobulbar nerve block: comparison of sedation quality, intraocular pressure changes, and recovery profiles. *Anesth Analg* 1999;89:317–321.
4. Cathrall W, Mackie K. Local Anesthetics. In: Hardman JC, Linbird LE, Molinoff PS, et al., eds. *Goodman and Gilman's the pharmacological basis of therapeutics,* 9th ed. New York: McGraw-Hill, 1996:331–347.
5. Ritchie JM, Greene NM. Local Anesthetics. In: Gilman AG, Goodman LS, Gilman A, eds. *Goodman and Gilman's the pharmacological basis of theraputics,* 6th ed. New York: Macmillan, 1980:300–320.
6. Lewin NA, Goldfrank LR, Weisman RS. Cocaine. In: Goldfrank LR, Weisman RS, Flomenbaum NE, et al., eds. *Goldfrank's toxicologic emergencies,* 3rd ed. Norwalk, CT: Appleton-Century-Crofts, 1986:477–485.
7. Morris IR. Pharmacologic aids to intubation and the rapid sequence induction. *Emerg Med Clin North Am* 1988;6:753–768.
8. Minor RL Jr, Scott BD, Brown DD, et al. Cocaine induced myocardial infarction in patients with normal coronary arteries. *Ann Intern Med* 1992;115:797–806.
9. Lange RA, Cigarroa RG, Yancy CW Jr, et al. Cocaine induced coronary artery vasoconstriction. *N Engl J Med* 1989;321:1557–1562.
10. Ross GS, Bell J. Myocardial infarction associated with inappropriate use of topical cocaine as treatment for epistaxis. *Am J Emerg Med* 1992;10:219–222.
11. Laffey JG, Neligan P, Ormonde G. Prolonged perioperative myocardial ischemia in a young male: due to topical intranasal cocaine? *J Clin Anesth* 1999;11:419–424.
12. Mongan PD, Culling RD. Rapid oral anesthesia for awake intubation. *J Clin Anesth* 1992;4:101–105.

8

Blind Intubation Techniques

Steven A. Godwin

Blind intubation techniques are those methods of airway management that do not provide direct visualization of the larynx during the intubation process. Both blind nasotracheal intubation (NTI) and digital tracheal intubation (DTI) use indirect indicators of airway identification in lieu of direct-vision laryngoscopy. NTI relies on listening to and feeling air movement, whereas DTI depends on the provider's ability to use tactile senses to distinguish airway anatomy as the tube is inserted. Other methods of airway management that do not require direct visualization of the glottis but require specialized equipment, such as lighted stylets and gum-elastic bougies, are discussed in other chapters.

I. Blind nasal intubation

Although NTI was very widely used in emergency departments in the past, it is rapidly being supplanted by superior techniques of oral intubation with neuromuscular blockade, even in the prehospital setting. In general, NTI has a number of very serious drawbacks and very few advantages when compared with the other techniques that are now commonly used for emergency airway management. NTI has largely fallen out of favor in the emergency department because it takes longer, has a higher failure rate, has a higher complication rate, and requires smaller tube sizes than rapid sequence oral intubation. However, despite these inherent problems, NTI is still considered an important skill, as it may be useful in certain difficult airway situations, particularly in departments without fiberoptic capability.

A. Indications and contraindications

As clinicians become more facile and comfortable with neuromuscular blockade and a variety of other approaches, the one remaining indication for NTI may be the spontaneously breathing patient with an identified difficult airway, for whom rapid sequence intubation is judged to be inadvisable (Chapters 2 and 6). NTI is achieved by listening to the patient's spontaneous respirations through the tube and therefore should not be attempted in the apneic patient. It is contraindicated in combative patients; in those with anatomically disturbed airways (e.g., neck hematoma or upper airway tumor); in cases of increased intracranial pressure; in the context of severe facial trauma with suspected basal skull fracture; in upper airway infection, obstruction, or abscess; and in the presence of coagulopathy. NTI should be performed with great reservation on any patient who needs rapid intubation, because, despite optimistic claims to the contrary, intubation usually requires several minutes to complete using this technique and significant oxygen desaturation can occur. Therefore it is a poor choice for patients with respiratory failure, such as the asthmatic patient *in extremis,* who cannot be oxygenated during the protracted intubation attempt. In addition, one of the primary indications for NTI in the past, the multiply injured patient with potential cervical spine injury, has been discarded, and oral rapid sequence intubation (RSI) with in-line stabilization is now the recommended route (see Chapter 23).

B. Technique

1. Preoxygenate the patient with 100% oxygen as for RSI (see Chapter 3) if possible. Try to avoid bagging with positive pressure if spontaneous ventilation is adequate.

2. Choose the nostril to be used. Inspect the interior of the naris, with particular reference to the septum and turbinates. It may help to occlude each nostril in turn and listen to the flow of air through the orifices. If there appears no clear favorite, the right naris should be selected, as it better facilitates passage of the tube with the bevel out.

3. Instill two or three drops of neosynephrine or oxymetazoline nasal solution into each nostril. This will vasoconstrict the nasal mucosa and makes tube passage easier. The incidence of epistaxis may also be reduced. It may also be helpful to soak two or three cotton-tipped applicators in the vasoconstrictor solution and place them gently fully into the naris until the tip touches the nasopharynx. This provides vasoconstriction at the area that is often most difficult to negotiate blindly with the endotracheal tube (ETT). Nasal topical anesthesia may then be placed as time permits. Insertion of a 4% cocaine pack or instillation of 2% lidocaine jelly will provide anesthesia for the nose. The oral cavity can be sprayed with 4% lidocaine or a similar spray, and, if desired, the pharynx may be anesthetized similarly. An alternative is to nebulize a solution of 4 mL of 4% lidocaine with 1 mL of 0.5% neosynephrine in a gas-powered nebulizer, as one would do with albuterol. This takes approximately 5 to 10 minutes but provides excellent anesthesia, and is well tolerated. Still another suggested method involves insertion of an absorbent nasal tampon (as is used for epistaxis) and application of several milliliters of 2% lidocaine with 1:100,000 epinephrine. Cricothyroid puncture with instillation of 5 to 10 mL of 1% to 2% lidocaine is often advocated. This technique is reasonably simple and effective but usually produces coughing, perhaps an undesirable result. Importantly, complete anesthesia of the glottis may not be desirable in all cases. Advancing the tube during a cough sometimes allows immediate intubation of an otherwise elusive trachea. If the patient is awake, explain the procedure. This is a crucial step that is often neglected. If the patient becomes combative during the intubation, the attempt must cease, as epistaxis, turbinate damage, or even pharyngeal perforation may ensue. A brief, reassuring explanation of the procedure, its necessity, and anticipated discomfort may avert this undesirable situation.

4. Lubricate the tube and the nostril. The use of 2% lidocaine jelly has been advocated, but is not in contact with the nasal mucosa long enough to result in anesthesia. However, the jelly is an adequate lubricant and is not harmful, so it is a reasonable choice.

5. Select the appropriate size of ETT. In general, the tube should be the largest one that will fit through the nostril without inducing significant trauma. In most patients, a tube with an internal diameter (ID) of 6.0 to 7.5 cm will suffice. A smaller tube will fit through a difficult or tight space better than a larger tube. Test the ETT cuff for leaks.

6. It is probably easiest for a right-handed person to intubate from the patient's left side. This allows the right hand to be used for the intubation, while the left hand

applies cricoid pressure and provides feedback to the right hand. By leaning slightly forward between the two hands, the operator can listen to the breath sounds and guide the tube into place. Alternatively, a position immediately above the patient's head may be chosen. The patient may be placed in any comfortable position. The sitting position may be better, as it keeps the tongue forward. Positioning the head as for oral intubation is worthwhile, however. The so-called sniffing position, with the neck flexed on the body and the head extended on the neck, optimizes the alignment of the mouth and pharynx with the vocal cords and trachea. Care must be taken to avoid overextending the neck, which causes the tube to pass anteriorly to the epiglottis. A small towel may be placed behind the patient's occiput to help maintain this relationship.

7. Gently insert the tube into the nostril with the leading edge carefully avoiding the rich vascular area of the anterior septum. For consistency, the remainder of this discussion will assume a right naris intubation by a right-handed operator. The tube should be turned so that the leading edge of the bevel is "out" (i.e., away from the septum). This will minimize the chances of septum injury and epistaxis. This also positions the tube with the natural curve upward, which facilitates the slightly upward direction of the distal tip of the tube to clear the lower turbinate. The major nasal airway is located below the inferior turbinates, and placement of the ETT should follow the floor of the nose backwards. Once the tip of the tube is past the inferior turbinate, it should be directed caudad at approximately a 10-degree angle to follow the gently downsloping floor of the nose (see Chapter 4). This entire process should be done very slowly and with meticulous care. Once the nose is successfully intubated, further induction of epistaxis is unlikely. When the tip of the tube approaches the posterior pharynx, resistance will often be felt. At this point, rotate the proximal end of the tube approximately one-fourth of a turn toward the left nostril. This will place the short side of the bevel in the superior position and will facilitate "turning the corner" from the nose into the nasopharynx. Once the nasopharynx is successfully entered, restore the tube to the neutral (sagittal) position and proceed.

8. The tube should now be advanced until the breath sounds are best heard through it (usually approximately 3 to 5 cm). At this point, the distal tip of the tube is positioned immediately above the vocal cords. This process may be facilitated by occluding the opposite naris and closing the mouth.

9. Simultaneous with an inspiratory effort by the patient, advance the tube gently but firmly 3 to 4 cm while applying laryngeal pressure with the left hand. The vocal cords abduct during inspiration and are most widely separated at this time.

10. When the tube is advanced, one of three things will happen. If the trachea is entered, a series of long, wheezy coughs will usually emanate from the patient. Inflation of the cuff and a few ventilations with an end-tidal carbon dioxide (CO_2) detector will confirm intratracheal placement. If the trachea is not entered, the tube either will slide easily down the esophagus or will come to an abrupt halt as it tries to pass anterior to the vocal cords or abuts against the anterior wall of the larynx. In the former case, the patient will not cough and ventilation through the tube will be better heard over the stomach than over the lungs. End-tidal CO_2 will not be detected. If the tube has passed down the esophagus, it is necessary to bring the distal tip of the tube further anteriorly. Withdraw the tube until the breath sounds are well heard again. Then extend the patient's head slightly and try again. If the intubation is being

performed on a patient with possible cervical spine trauma, movement is impossible and the intubation should be reattempted without any change in patient position.

11. Inflate the cuff and confirm position with an end-tidal CO_2 detection device. *Do not administer neuromuscular blocking agents to a patient who has undergone NTI unless tracheal tube placement has been confirmed by end-tidal CO_2 detection.* Breath sounds are never reliable as an indicator of tracheal placement, but this is particularly true in the spontaneously breathing patient who has undergone nasoesophageal intubation, whose own breath sounds will continue to be heard over the lungs, even when the ETT is being bag ventilated. A chest radiograph should also be obtained. If the presence of the tube or inflation of the cuff leads to prolonged coughing by the patient, administer 2 mL of 2% lidocaine solution through the ETT during an inspiration. This will often dramatically improve tube tolerance in seconds.

12. Only 60% to 70% of intubations will succeed on the first attempt. The blind nature of the procedure requires adjustment and attention to feedback. If the intubation is proving extremely difficult, consider the various options in Box 8-1.

II. Digital tracheal intubation

Digital intubation is a tactile intubation technique in which the intubator uses his or her fingers to direct an ETT into the larynx. The technique has gained limited usefulness in clinical practice. It is not easy to perform, especially if the intubator has small hands or short fingers. Nor is it aesthetically pleasing. However, in certain failed airway circumstances in an austere environment, DTI may be an option.

A. Indications and contraindications

Digital intubation may be indicated:

1. In situations with poor lighting, difficult patient position, disrupted airway anatomy, or potential cervical spine instability. Many of these situations are more likely in the prehospital setting (e.g., a patient trapped in an automobile)
2. If laryngoscopy equipment is unavailable or not working
3. When visualization of the larynx is impossible (e.g., blood secretions) and no alternative devices or techniques are possible
4. In failed intubation in an austere environment without rescue airway devices

   The patients must be sufficiently obtunded to prevent a biting injury to the intubator. Generally, this technique should only be considered in a patient who is frankly comatose or who has arrested.

B. The technique of tactile DTI is as follows:

1. Have an assistant use a gauze sponge to gently but firmly retract the tongue.
2. Insert a stylet in the ETT and bend the ETT/stylet at a 90-degree angle just proximal to the cuff, as for a lighted stylet intubation (Chapter 11).
3. Slide the index and long fingers of the nondominant hand palm down along the tongue.
4. Identify the tip of the epiglottis with the tip of the long finger and direct it anteriorly.
5. Insert the ETT/stylet in the mouth and use the index finger to direct it gently into the glottic opening.

C. Success rates and complications

Perhaps the most substantial limitation in performing this technique successfully is the length of the intubator's fingers relative to the patient's oropharyngeal dimensions. Biting injuries or unintentional dental injuries to the hand with the risk of infectious disease transmission may occur. The technique has only infrequently been used in

Box 8-1. Options to Enhance Success in Difficult Blind Nasal Intubation

- The Endotrol tube, which has a ringlike apparatus connected to the distal end to allow anterior deflection of the tip of the tube, may be extremely helpful in such cases.
- If the tube has met with a dead end, it is anterior to the cords or abutted against the anterior wall of the trachea. It may be possible to ascertain by palpation with the left hand whether the tube is off to the left, off to the right, or anterior in the midline. If the tube is truly anterior, slight withdrawal of the tube until breath sounds are well heard followed by slight flexion of the head should facilitate passage. This is a common pitfall. When a first attempt fails, the operator often continues to further extend the neck in an attempt to succeed, each extension making the situation anatomically more impossible. If it is felt that the tube is off to the left or right in addition to being anterior, withdraw the tube, flex the head slightly (if possible), and turn the head slightly in the direction to which the distal tip of the tube was off the midline. For example, if the distal end of the tube was off to the right, turning the head to the right will cause the distal end of the tube to swing to the left (i.e., toward the midline), the desired corrective direction. Alternatively, if it is desirable to keep the patient's head in the midline, the proximal end of the ETT may be rotated to the side where the distal end was detected to achieve this effect.
- Inflation of the cuff as the tube lies in the oropharynx may aid in alignment of the ETT with the glottic opening. The tube is then advanced until it meets resistance at the cords; the cuff is then deflated before being pushed through the cords during inspiration. Inflation of the cuff is felt to lift the end of the tube away from the esophagus and into alignment with the vocal cords.
- Use of a guide such as a nasogastric tube or endotracheal tube changer in combination with the just-described inflated-cuff technique may improve success rates. With this method, after the ETT has been advanced with the cuff inflated to meet resistance at the laryngeal opening, the nasogastric tube is inserted through the ETT. The inflated cuff allows for alignment of the outlet of the ETT with the vocal cords, and the nasogastric tube will slide through the outlet, through the glottis, and into the trachea. As the nasogastric tube slides through the glottis coughing may occur, suggesting proper placement. The cuff can then be deflated and guided into the trachea over the nasogastric tube, which is then withdrawn from the ETT.
- Passing a fiberoptic laryngoscope or bronchoscope through the tube into the trachea (Chapter 12)
- Passing a lighted stylet through the tube to assist in locating the glottis (Chapter 11)
- Changing to a new tube, perhaps one that is 0.5 to 1.0 mm ID smaller. The tube often becomes warm and soft during the intubation attempt and is no longer capable of being appropriately manipulated.
- Using a laryngoscope and Magill forceps. This may require conditions that are not present (i.e., the ability to insert a laryngoscope into the mouth and visualize the vocal cords).
- Grasping the tongue with a piece of gauze and pulling it forward or sitting the patient up (if possible). This may improve the angle at the back of the tongue.
- Abandoning the attempt. Prolonged attempts are associated with hypoxemia and glottic edema caused by local trauma. Either of these situations can worsen the situation substantially. Repeated attempts are not significantly more successful than the first. In 10% to 20% of cases, NTI will simply not be possible.
- In an unconscious patient, the nasal passage may be dilated with a nasopharyngeal airway or a gloved small finger if problems are encountered trying to get the tube through the naris. Again, a smaller tube may be advisable.

the emergency department, and most authors agree that some degree of experience is needed to perform this skill in an efficient and effective manner.

The two major tips for performing this technique are to have an assistant retract the tongue, thereby allowing the intubator the best access to the epiglottis, and to ensure that the patient is sufficiently obtunded to tolerate airway manipulation.

EVIDENCE

1. Although historically recommended as the primary method for difficult airway man-agement, nasotracheal intubation (NTI) is an infrequently performed procedure for patients requiring emergent airway management and is now less commonly selected as a rescue method: Since RSI has become the method of choice for intubation of emergency patients, fewer physicians routinely perform NTI. In a recent review of 610 intubations performed in a large emergency department with a Level I trauma center, Sakles et al. (1) reported only 8 (1.3%) NTIs. Of these patients, two attempts were unsuccessful. A review of emergency department intubations from 30 hospitals as part of the National Emergency Airway Registry (NEAR) databank project, identified 207 of 7,712 (2.7%) patients who required the use of rescue techniques and/or additional personnel. Rescue RSI was performed after failure of an alternative technique in 102 of 207 (49%) patients, whereas NTI was used as a rescue in 36 of 207 (17%) of patients. Although there was a greater number of rescue intubations with NTI than with fiberoptic devices (10 of 207, 4.8%), the authors emphasize the rapid growth in the use of fiberoptics over other methods for both primary and rescue airway management. (2) Although still an important backup skill to maintain, NTI has a diminished role in emergency airway management.

2. When no other alternatives are available, NTI may be performed safely in facial trauma but clinicians should be aware of rare, yet devastating, possible complications: Historically, facial trauma was felt to be an absolute contraindication for NTI because of the perceived associated risk of intracranial placement in the presence of cribiform plate disruption. There have been two reported cases of intracranial placement of a nasotracheal tube after facial trauma. (3,4) These case reports have been criticized for demonstrating the outcome of poor technique rather than the presence of facial trauma as the cause of these injuries. (5) At least one study has been published evaluating the risk of NTI in the presence of facial trauma. This retrospective review of 311 patients with intubation in the presence of facial fractures found that 82 patients underwent NTI. (6) The authors found no episodes of intracranial placement, significant epistaxis requiring nasal packing, esophageal intubation, or osteomyelitis. Although there is no evidence that facial trauma is a contraindication for NTI, in the modern era of RSI and the availability of multiple alternative airway devices, the indications for NTI in the emergency department setting are limited.

3. Cuff inflation provides an increase in success rates for NTI in both normal and difficult airways: Over time a number of improvements to the technique for passage of the nasotracheal tube through the oropharynx and into the glottis have been suggested. The most studied and successful aid to NTI appears to be the addition of cuff inflation during passage of the tube through the oropharynx until the outlet abuts the glottic opening. A prospective randomized trial evaluating successful NTI with the cuff inflated versus deflated technique demonstrated the inflated cuff technique to be superior. The results showed that 19 of 20 (95%) patients were intubated with the cuff inflated. In contrast, only 9 of 20 (45%) patients were intubated with the cuff deflated. (7) A separate study compared success rates for NTI and fiberoptic bronchoscope in patients with an immobilized cervical spine with ASA I and II status airways while undergoing elective surgery. The authors reported that there was no significant difference in success rates between the groups. (8) The study concluded that ETT cuff inflation could be used as an alternative to fiberoptic bronchoscopy in patients with an immobilized cervical spine, but this conclusion is not warranted by this small study, and both techniques are highly operator dependent. In the immobilized trauma patient without other identified difficult airway attributes (Chapter 6), RSI is still considered the primary method of airway management. In the context of specific difficult airway attributes that argue against administering a paralytic agent, either fiberoptic intubation or NTI, performed with the patient spontaneously breathing, may be appropriate (Chapters 2 and 6).

REFERENCES

1. Sakles JC, Lauren EG, Rantapaa AA, et al. Airway management in the emergency department: a one year study of 610 tracheal intubations. *Ann Emerg Med* 1998;31(Mar):325–332.
2. Bair AE, Filbin MR, Kulkarni RG, et al. The failed intubation attempt in the emergency department: analysis of prevalence, rescue techniques, and personnel. *J Emerg Med* 2002;23(Aug):131–140.
3. Horellou MF, Mathe D, Feiss P. A hazard of naso-tracheal intubation. *Anaesthesia* 1978;33:78.
4. Marlow FJ, Goltra DQ Jr, Schabel SI. Intracranial placement of a nasotracheal tube after facial fracture: a rare complication. *J Emerg Med* 1997;15:187–191.
5. Walls RM. Blind nasotracheal intubation in the presence of facial trauma—Is it safe? *J Emerg Med* 1997;15:243–244.
6. Rosen CL, Wolfe RE, Chew SE, et al. Blind nasotracheal intubation in the presence of facial trauma. *J Emerg Med* 1997;15:141–145.
7. Van Elstraete AC, Pennant JH, Gajraj NM, et al. Tracheal tube cuff inflation as an aid to bind nasotracheal intubation. *Brit J Anaesth* 1993;70:691–693.
8. Van Elstraete AC, Mamie JC, Mehdaoni H. Nasotracheal intubation in patients with immobilized cervical spine: A comparison of tracheal tube cuff inflation and fiberoptic bronchoscopy. *Anesth Analg* 1998;87:400–402.

9

Laryngeal Mask Airways

Michael F. Murphy

DESCRIPTION

The laryngeal mask airway (LMA) was designed by the British anesthesiologist Archie Brain and has been referred to as the Brain airway. The original LMA (LMA Classic, LMA North America, San Diego, CA) looks like an endotracheal tube (ETT) at the proximal end that is equipped with an inflatable, elliptical, silicone rubber collar (laryngeal mask) at the distal end. The device is designed to surround and cover the supraglottic area, providing upper-airway continuity. Two rubber bars cross the tube opening at the mask end to prevent herniation of the epiglottis into the tube portion of the LMA. The LMA Classic is a multiuse device. The disposable and much less expensive variety of this device is called the LMA Unique. The LMA-Flexible incorporates a nonkinkable design in the tube portion of the device to prevent kinking as the device warms. It is not useful in the management of the emergency airway. The LMA-ProSeal incorporates a tunnel through which one can pass a suction catheter into the esophagus or stomach to aspirate regurgitant material, but cannot be intubated through. It also has a higher sealing pressure than the LMA Classic, so theoretically should be better for ventilating patients with higher airway pressures, but the difference may not be clinically significant. At this time the LMA-ProSeal does not have a place in emergency airway management.

The LMA-Fastrach, also called the ILMA or intubating LMA is the most important version of the LMA for emergency airway management because it combines the high insertion and ventilation success rate of the other LMAs with specially designed features to facilitate blind intubation. The LMA-Fastrach has incorporated an epiglottic elevating bar and a guide channel that directs an ETT anteriorly into the larynx, enhancing the success rate of blind intubation. The LMA-Fastrach device is a substantial advance in airway management, particularly as a rapidly attempted rescue device in the can't intubate, can't oxygenate situation while preparations for cricothyrotomy are under way.

The devices are easy to use, produce little in the way of adverse cardiovascular responses on insertion, and have a significant potential role in emergency airway management. Ventilation success rates near 100% have been reported in operating room series, but patients with difficult airways were excluded, so the emergency airway ventilation success rate is probably somewhat lower. Intubation success rates through the ILMA are consistently in the 95% range, though closer to 80% through the standard LMA. Placement of an LMA does not constitute *definitive airway management,* defined as a protected airway (i.e., cuffed ETT in the trachea) unless one is successful at passing an ETT through the device into the trachea. Although they do not reliably prevent the regurgitation and aspiration of gastric contents, they have been demonstrated to protect the airway from aspiration of blood and saliva from the mouth and pharynx.

The patient must have a high level of local anesthesia of the airway or be significantly obtunded (e.g., by RSI medications) to tolerate insertion of these devices. The LMA Classic and the LMA-Fastrach are fairly expensive but can be autoclaved and reused. The LMA Unique is less expensive and disposable, but is not available in the intubating configuration.

INDICATIONS AND CONTRAINDICATIONS

The standard LMA is now widely used in anesthetic practice instead of mask anesthesia and the intubating LMA is becoming incorporated into difficult airway management.

However, for the patient to tolerate insertion of the LMA and certainly for subsequent passage of the ETT, the patient's airway must be anesthetized or the patient must be deeply sedated. Ketamine titration offers the advantage of deep sedation, or dissociation, while ventilation is maintained (see Chapter 7).

In emergency airway management the standard or intubating LMA is used as a rescue device in a can't intubate, *can* ventilate situation, or it may be tried as a first line can't intubate, can't ventilate rescue device in certain cases, simultaneous with preparations for a cricothyrotomy (see Chapter 2). In such cases, it is critical that the attempt to rescue the patient's airway with the ILMA does not delay initiation of the cricothyrotomy. The advantage of the ILMA is that, if it is readily at hand, it can be inserted, inflated, and manipulated to determine whether ventilation will be successful in a matter of seconds. Thus, if one operator (or an assistant) is opening the cricothyrotomy tray, the principal airway manager can be placing the ILMA without risk of delay to the patient and additional hypoxia time. If the ILMA is to be used as a rescue device for a can't intubate, can't ventilate airway, there must be some certainty that laryngeal pathology is not the reason bag/mask ventilation and intubation have been unsuccessful. Although both the LMA (and ILMA) and the Combitube can be rapidly inserted with minimal training and high ventilation success rates, the ILMA has the clear advantage of then facilitating intubation. These devices have been used successfully in pediatrics, by novice intubators, during cardiopulmonary resuscitation, and in emergency medical services (EMS).

TECHNIQUE

LMA Fastrach

The LMA-Fastrach comes in three sizes: no. 3, no. 4, and no. 5. The no. 3 will fit in a normal-sized 10 to 12 year old and small adults and is recommended for persons weighing approximately 30 to 50 kg. Most ordinary-sized women will require a no. 3. Larger women and smaller men will take a no. 4, recommended for patients weighing 50 to 70 kg, and large men will generally require a no. 5, recommended for those weighing greater than 70 kg. For patients on the borderline between one mask size and another, it is generally preferable to err by selecting the larger mask, which usually provides a better mask seal. The intention is to rescue a patent airway initially with the LMA-Fastrach and recover the oxygen saturations by ventilating through the LMA-Fastrach device. Once the saturations are adequate, endotracheal intubation through the mask using the silicone-tipped ETT that comes with the device can be accomplished. This can be done blindly or using either a fiberoptic scope or a lighted stylet. When using the Trach-light (Chapter 7), it is helpful to remove the semirigid metal stylet and and to then mount the silicone-tipped LMA-Fastrach ETT on the light-tipped wand. The result is instantaneous verification of successful tracheal intubation, using the transillumination attribute of the Trachlight.

Select the appropriate-sized LMA-Fastrach. Deflate the cuff of the mask and apply a water-soluble lubricant to the anterior and posterior surfaces. Inflating the mask, then deflating it while it is pressed down firmly against a flat surface produces a smoother leading surface for insertion. Hold the device in the dominant hand by the metal handle and open the airway with the other hand. Ensure that the curved silicone coated metal tube portion of the device is in contact with the chin and the mask tip is flat against the palate before rotation (Fig. 9-1A).

1. Rotate the mask into place with a circular motion, maintaining firm pressure against the palate and posterior pharynx (Fig. 9-1A, B, C). Insert the device until resistance is felt and only the metal end of the silicone-coated tube protrudes from the airway.
2. Inflate the cuff of the LMA-Fastrach and hold the metal handle firmly in the dominant hand, using a "frying pan" grip. Ventilate the patient with a ventilation bag, attached to the LMA-Fastrach using the other hand. While ventilating, manipulate the mask with the dominant hand by lifting slightly as if to pull the mask toward the ceiling over the patient's feet. This will provide a good mask seal and will ensure that the mask is correctly positioned for intubation. Correct mask positioning will be identified by essentially noiseless ventilation, almost as if the patient is being ventilated through a cuffed ETT.
3. Visually inspect and inflate the silicone-tipped ETT that is supplied with the LMA-Fastrach to verify cuff integrity and symmetry. Fully deflate cuff, lubricate the ETT liberally, and pass it through the LMA-Fastrach. With the black vertical line on the ETT facing the operator (indicates that the bevel will be oriented with the narrowest part advancing through the cords), insert the ETT to the 15-cm depth marker, which corresponds to the transverse black line on the silicone-tipped ETT. This indicates that the silicone tip of the tube is about to emerge from the LMA-Fastrach, pushing the epiglottic elevating bar up to lift the epiglottis. Use the handle to gently lift the LMA-Fastrach as just described as the ETT is advanced (Fig. 9-2). Carefully advance until intubation is complete. Do not use force. Inflate the ETT cuff and confirm intubation. Then deflate the cuff on the LMA-Fastrach.
4. Most of the time in the emergency situation, the LMA-Fastrach and ETT are left *in situ* together. However, the LMA-Fastrach can be removed fairly easily, leaving just the ETT in place. The key to successful removal of the mask is to remember that one is attempting to keep the ETT precisely in place and to remove the mask over it. First remove the 15 mm bag connector from the ETT. Then immobilize the ETT with one hand and gently ease the deflated LMA-Fastrach out over the ETT until the proximal end of the mask channel reaches the proximal end of the ETT. Use a stabilizer rod to hold the ETT in position as the LMA-Fastrach is withdrawn over the tube (Fig. 9-3). Remove the stabilizer rod from the LMA-Fastrach and grasp the ETT at the level of the incisors (Fig. 9-4). The stabilizer bar must be removed to allow the pilot balloon of the ETT to pass through the LMA-Fastrach. Failure to do so may result in the pilot balloon being avulsed from the ETT, rendering the balloon incompetent and necessitating reintubation, preferably over an ETT changer (Fig. 9-5).

LMA Classic and Unique

Although the LMA Classic and LMA Unique can be rapidly inserted to rescue a failed airway with ventilation success rates comparable to that of the LMA-Fastrach, they are not as effective

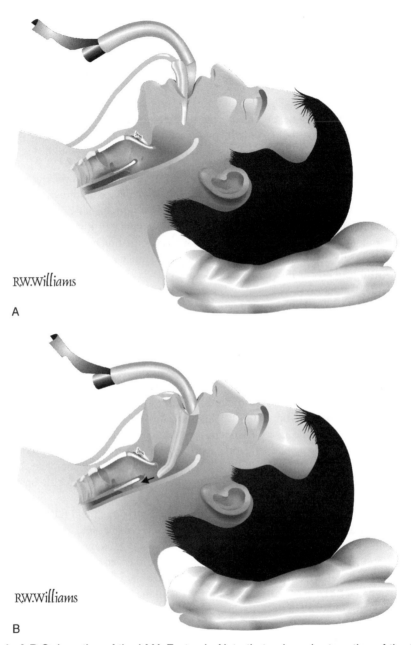

R.W.Williams

A

R.W.Williams

B

FIG. 9-1. A,B,C: Insertion of the LMA-Fastrach. Note that only a short portion of the tubular portion of the device extends beyond the lips. This metal tube accepts a bag/mask device fitting to enable bag/mask ventilation.   (continued)

as the LMA-Fastrach for facilitating intubation, and the LMA-Fastrach is often easier to insert because of the handle and guide channel, which serves as an introducer. The LMA Classic and LMA Unique should be considered as rescue ventilation devices only, even though modest success with intubation through them is reported. Select the appropriate size of LMA as described previously for the LMA-Fastrach. Unlike the LMA-Fastrach, the LMA Classic

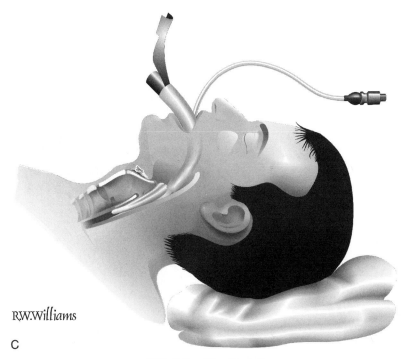

R.W.Williams

C

FIG. 9-1. *(Continued)*

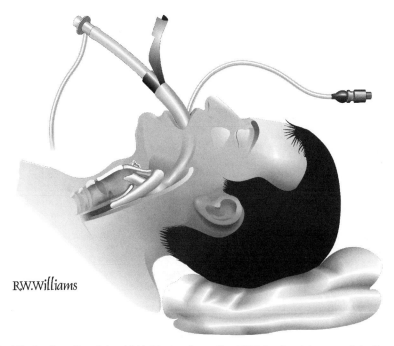

R.W.Williams

FIG. 9-2. Lift the handle of the LMA-Fastrach as the ETT is about to pass into the larynx to improve the success rate of intubation. This is called the Vergese maneuver after Dr. Brain's associate Dr. Chandy Vergese.

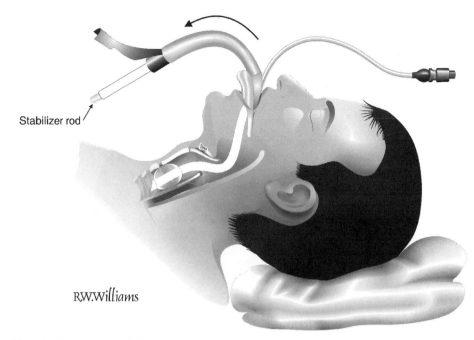

FIG. 9-3. Use of the stabilizer rod to ensure the ETT is not inadvertently dragged out of the trachea as the LMA-Fastrach is removed.

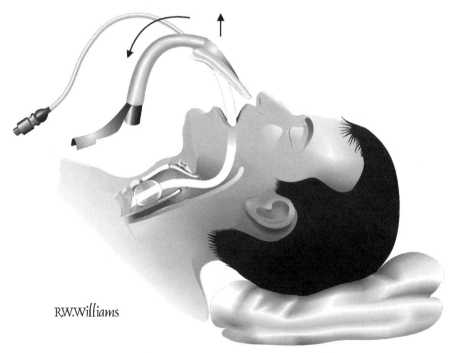

FIG. 9-4. The stabilizer rod is removed from the LMA-Fastrach to permit the pilot balloon of the ETT to go through the LMA-Fastrach and prevent it from being avulsed from the ETT.

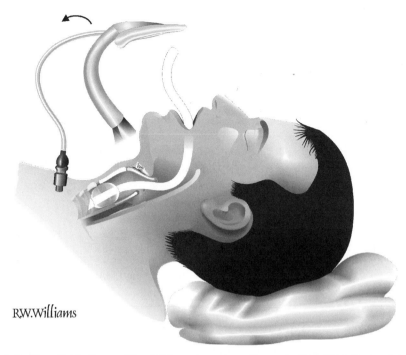

R.W.Williams

FIG. 9-5. The pilot balloon of the ETT emerges from the end of the LMA-Fastrach intact.

and the LMA Unique have smaller sizes (1, 1.5, 2, and 2.5) available for use in infants and children.

1. Place the device so that the collar is on a flat surface and inflate, then deflate the mask by aspirating the pilot balloon (Fig. 9-6). Completely deflate the cuff and ensure that it is not folded. The collar is designed to flip backwards so that the epiglottis is not trapped between the collar and the glottic opening. Lubricate both sides of the LMA with water-soluble lubricant to facilitate insertion.
2. Open the airway by using a head tilt as one would in basic airway management, if possible.
3. Insert the LMA into the mouth with the laryngeal surface directed caudally and your index or long finger placed along the tube with the tip resting against the cuff-tube junction (Fig. 9-7). Press the device onto the hard palate (Fig. 9-8) and advance it over the back of the tongue as far as the length of your index or long finger will allow (Fig. 9-9). Then use your other hand to push the device to its final seated position (Fig. 9-10). Allow the curve of the device to follow the natural curve of the oro- and hypopharynx to facilitate its falling into position over the larynx. The dimensions and design of the device allow it to wedge into the esophagus with gentle caudad pressure and to stop in the appropriate position over the larynx.
4. Inflate the collar with air—20 mL no. 3; 30 mL no. 4; 40 mL no. 5, or until there is no leak with bag ventilation (Fig. 9-11). If a leak persists, ensure that the tube of the LMA emerges from the mouth in the midline, flex the neck slightly, or as a last resort replace the device or go to the next larger size.

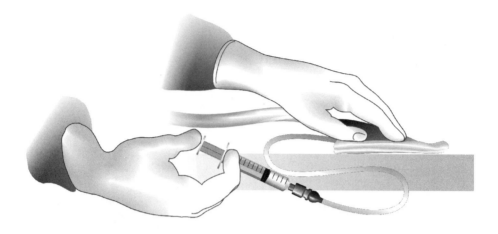

R.W.Williams

FIG. 9-6. Correct method of deflating the LMA cuff.

COMPLICATIONS AND LIMITATIONS

Getting the LMA to seal sufficiently to enable bag to LMA ventilation may at times be difficult. Keeping the tube portion of the device in the midline and altering the position of the head in neck from flexion (more usual) to extension may be of help. Overall, ventilation success rates are very high with any of the LMA devices, and optimal positioning improves ventilatory effectiveness, and facilitate intubation in the case of the LMA-Fastrach.

The LMA does not prevent the aspiration of gastric contents, serving to emphasize its role as a temporizing measure only. This limits its usefulness in prehospital and emergency airway

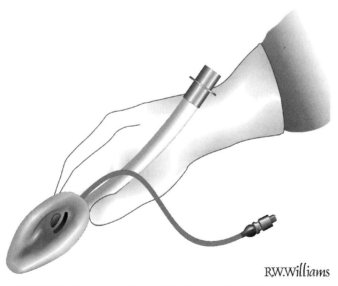

R.W.Williams

FIG. 9-7. Correct position of the fingers for LMA insertion.

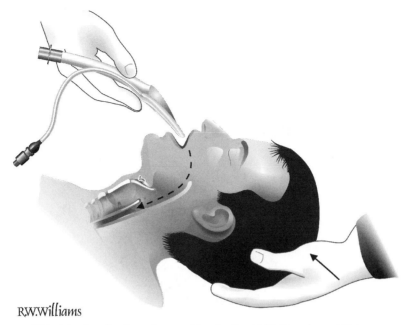

R.W.Williams

FIG. 9-8. Starting insertion position for the LMA Classic and Unique.

care beyond that of a temporizing measure, except when the LMA-Fastrach is used to achieve intubation. Cricoid pressure has variously been reported to hinder and aid in getting the LMA seated properly.

Negative pressure pulmonary edema, also known as post obstructive pulmonary edema (POPE), has been reported when a patient occludes an LMA Classic by biting down on the

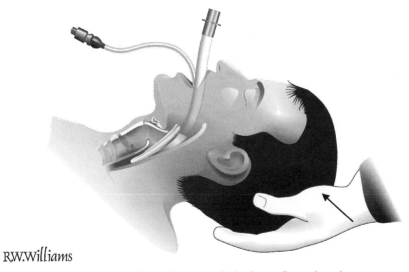

R.W.Williams

FIG. 9-9. Insert the LMA to the limit of your finger length.

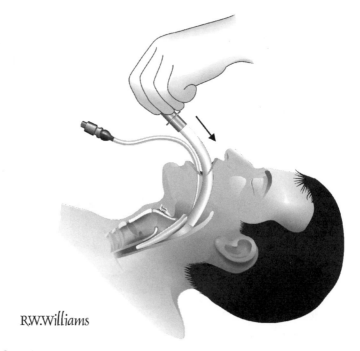

R.W.Williams

FIG. 9-10. Complete the insertion by pushing it in the remainder of the way with your other hand.

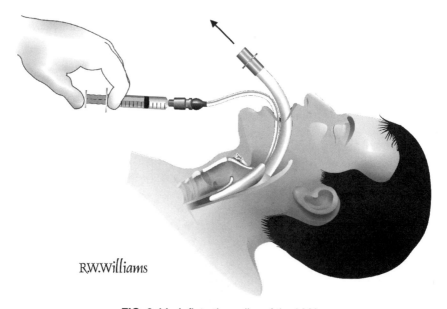

R.W.Williams

FIG. 9-11. Inflate the collar of the LMA.

flexible tube portion. It may be wise to place rolled-up gauze flats between the molars on each side of the LMA to prevent this complication. Alternatively any sort of bite block may work.

EVIDENCE

1. Difficult and Failed Airway Management: There is ample evidence that LMAs are useful in emergency airway management, both for the management of the difficult airway (1–12) and rescue of the failed airway (13–17), provided one is concurrently preparing to undertake a surgical airway.

2. Intubating through the Fastrack LMA: Success rates for blind intubation through the Fastrack range from 70% to 95% (18–20) and coupling the device with a Trachlight produces success rates of 100% (18–20). Some studies have described the technique of coupling the fastrack or Classic LMA with a fiberscope to ensure intubation success in both infants and adults (21,22).

3. LMAs and pediatrics: There is ample evidence that the LMA is appropriate and widely accepted as a rescue device in children (23–26). Some authors have described guidelines for selecting the appropriate size in children (23), and the manufacturer provides a pocket card to guide clinicians.

4. Ease of insertion: A variety of authors have described successful insertion and use of the device in basic rescuer nonmedical personnel (27,28), paramedics, nurses and respiratory therapists (29–31), and other naïve airway managers (29). Some of the EMS literature has questioned the ease of use of the device as a primary method of airway management in EMS (32), though analysis has shown that training is key to successful use of the devices (32–37).

5. The LMA in CPR: Numerous studies have demonstrated that the LMA (and Combitube) is at least as effective as other methods of airway management for patients requiring cardiopulmonary resuscitation (31,38).

6. LMA failure and complications: The LMA may fail to provide a seal sufficient to permit adequate ventilation, often attributed to the sensitivity of the seal to head and neck position (39–41). The head and neck should be neutral to slightly flexed, the tube of the LMA in the midline, and the natural anterior curve of the device maintained during ventilation. (42) Insufflation of the stomach may occur (43). Although the LMA may not offer total protection from the aspiration of regurgitated gastric contents (44–49), it does offer protection from the aspiration of material produced above the device (50). This same material accumulates above the cuff of an ETT and is suspected to be a major cause of ventilator-associated pneumonia in ventilated ICU patients. Cricoid pressure may or may not interfere with proper functioning of an LMA (51,52), though in practice each case is evaluated individually. Negative pressure pulmonary edema (POPE, mentioned earlier) is caused by a patient sucking hard to inspire against an obstruction. Fluid is sucked into the alveolar spaces. This complication has been reported with patients biting down on the LMA (53) and can be prevented by placing folded gauze flats between the molar teeth on either side. This also serves to keep the device in the midline, enhancing the seal.

7. Reviews: Comprehensive reviews of the use of the LMA in emergency medicine and rescue airway management are available (54–55).

REFERENCES

1. Foley LJ, Ochroch EA. Bridges to establish an emergency airway and alternate intubating techniques. *Crit Care Clin* 2000;16:429–444.
2. Cooper JR Jr. Use of a LMA and a sequential technique for unanticipated difficult intubations. *Anesthesiology* 2002;97:1326.

3. Fukutome T, Amaha K, Nakazawa K, et al. Tracheal intubation through the intubating laryngeal mask airway (LMA-Fastrach) in patients with difficult airways. *Anaesth Intensive Care* 1998;26:387–391.
4. McQuibban GA. LMA-FasTrach. *Can J Anaesth* 1998;45:95–96.
5. Fukutome T, Amaha K, Nakazawa K, et al. Tracheal intubation through the intubating laryngeal mask airway (LMA-Fastrach) in patients with difficult airways. *Anaesth Intensive Care* 1998;26:387–391.
6. Parmet JL, Colonna-Romano P, Horrow JC, et al. The laryngeal mask airway reliably provides rescue ventilation in cases of unanticipated difficult tracheal intubation along with difficult mask ventilation. *Anesth Analg* 1998;87:661–665.
7. Jones JR. Laryngeal mask airway: an alternative for the difficult airway. *AANA J* 1995;63:444–449.
8. Brimacombe J, Berry A, Van Duren P. Use of a size 2 LMA to relieve life-threatening hypoxia in an adult with quinsy. *Anaesth Intensive Care* 1993;21:475–476.
9. King CJ, Davey AJ, Chandradeva K. Emergency use of the laryngeal mask airway in severe upper airway obstruction caused by supraglottic oedema. *Br J Anaesth* 1995;75:785–786.
10. Defalque RJ, Hyder ML. Laryngeal mask airway in severe cervical ankylosis. *Can J Anaesth* 1997;44:305–307.
11. Brain AI. Use of the LMA in the unstable cervical spine. *Singapore Med J* 2001;Suppl 1:046–048.
12. Lee CM, Yang HS. Case of difficult intubation overcome by the laryngeal mask airway. *J Korean Med Sci* 1993;8:290–292.
13. DeMello WF, Kocan M. The laryngeal mask in failed intubation. *Anaesthesia* 1990;45:689.
14. Asai T, Appadurai I. LMA for failed intubation. *Can J Anaesth* 1993;40:802.
15. Levy DM. LMA for failed intubation. *Can J Anaesth* 1993;40:801–802.
16. Brimacombe J, Berry A. LMA for failed intubation. *Can J Anaesth* 1993;40:802–803.
17. Rosenblatt WH, Murphy M. The intubating laryngeal mask: use of a new ventilating-intubating device in the emergency department. *Ann Emerg Med* 1999;33:234–238.
18. Agro F, Hung OR, Cataldo R, et al. Lightwand intubation using the Trachlight: a brief review of current knowledge. *Can J Anaesth* 2001;48:592–599.
19. Agro F, Brimacombe J, Carassiti M, et al. Lighted stylet as an aid to blind tracheal intubation via the LMA. *J Clin Anesth* 1998;1:263–264.
20. Agro F, Brimacombe J, Carassiti M, et al. Use of a lighted stylet for intubation via the laryngeal mask airway. *Can J Anaesth* 1998;45:556–560.
21. Kannan S, Chestnutt N, McBride G. Intubating LMA guided awake fibreoptic intubation in severe maxillo-facial injury. *Can J Anaesth* 2000;47:989–991.
22. Bandla HP, Smith DE, Kiernan MP. Laryngeal mask airway facilitated fibreoptic bronchoscopy in infants. *Can J Anaesth* 1997;44:1242–1247.
23. Loke GP, Tan SM, Ng AS. Appropriate size of laryngeal mask airway for children. *Anaesth Intensive Care* 2002;30:771–774.
24. Park C, Bahk JH, Ahn WS, et al. The laryngeal mask airway in infants and children. *Can J Anaesth* 2001;48:413–417.
25. Tobias JD. The laryngeal mask airway: a review for the emergency physician. *Pediatr Emerg Care* 1996;12:370–373.
26. Paterson SJ, Byrne PJ, Molesky MG, et al. Neonatal resuscitation using the laryngeal mask airway. *Anesthesiology* 1994;80:1248–1253.
27. Levitan RM, Ochroch EA, Stuart S, et al. Use of the intubating laryngeal mask airway by medical and nonmedical personnel. *Am J Emerg Med* 2000;18:12–16.
28. Burgoyne L, Cyna A. Laryngeal mask vs intubating laryngeal mask: insertion and ventilation by inexperienced resuscitators. *Anaesth Intensive Care* 2001;29:604–608.
29. Choyce A, Avidan MS, Patel C, et al. Comparison of laryngeal mask and intubating laryngeal mask insertion by the naive intubator. *Br J Anaesth* 2000;84:103–105.
30. Davies PR, Tighe SQ, Greenslade GL, et al. Laryngeal mask airway and tracheal tube insertion by unskilled personnel. *Lancet* 1990;336:977–979.
31. Grayling M, Wilson IH, Thomas B. The use of the laryngeal mask airway and Combitube in cardiopulmonary resuscitation; a national survey. *Resuscitation* 2002;52:183–186.
32. Rumball CJ, MacDonald D. The PTL, Combitube, laryngeal mask, and oral airway: a randomized prehospital comparative study of ventilatory device effectiveness and cost-effectiveness in 470 cases of cardiorespiratory arrest. *Prehosp Emerg Care* 1997;1:1–10.
33. Miller GT. LMA fastrach. EMS discovers the intubating laryngeal mask airway. *J Emerg Med Serv* 2002;27:68–74.
34. Dries D, Frascone R, Molinari P, et al. Does the ILMA make sense in HEMS? *Air Med J* 2000;20:35–37.
35. Martin SE, Ochsner MG, Jarman RH, et al. Use of the laryngeal mask airway in air transport when intubation fails. *J Trauma* 1999;47:352–357.
36. Sasada MP, Gabbott DA. The role of the laryngeal mask airway in pre-hospital care. *Resuscitation* 1994;28:97–102.
37. Pennant JH, Walker MB. Comparison of the endotracheal tube and laryngeal mask in airway management by paramedical personnel. *Anesth Analg* 1992;74:531–534.
38. Samarkandi AH, Seraj MA, el Dawlatly A, et al. The role of laryngeal mask airway in cardiopulmonary resuscitation. *Resuscitation* 1994;28:103–106.

39. Zavattaro M, LMA failure. *Anaesth Intensive Care* 1996;24:119.
40. Okuda K, Inagawa G, Miwa T, et al. Influence of head and neck position on cuff position and oropharyngeal sealing pressure with the laryngeal mask airway in children. *Br J Anaesth* 2001;86:122–124.
41. Keller C, Brimacombe J. The influence of head and neck position on oropharyngeal leak pressure and cuff position with the flexible and the standard laryngeal mask airway. *Anesth Analg* 1999;88:913–916.
42. Brimacombe J, Berry A. Leak reduction with the LMA. *Can J Anaesth* 1996;43:537.
43. Latorre F, Eberle B, Weiler N, et al. Laryngeal mask airway position and the risk of gastric insufflation. *Anesth Analg* 1998;86:867–871.
44. Cassinello F, Rodrigo FJ, Munoz-Alameda L, et al. Postoperative pulmonary aspiration of gastric contents in an infant after general anesthesia with laryngeal mask airway (LMA). *Anesth Analg* 2000;90:1457.
45. Brimacombe JR, Berry A. The incidence of aspiration associated with the laryngeal mask airway: a meta-analysis of published literature. *J Clin Anesth* 1995;7:297–305.
46. Ismail-Zade IA, Vanner RG. Regurgitation and aspiration of gastric contents in a child during general anaesthesia using the laryngeal mask airway. *Paediatr Anaesth* 1996;6:325–328.
47. Brimacombe J, Berry A. LMA-related aspiration in children. *Anaesth Intensive Care* 1994;22:313–314.
48. Asai T. Aspiration and the LMA. *Can J Anaesth* 1992;39:746.
49. Barker P, Langton JA, Murphy PJ, et al. Regurgitation of gastric contents during general anaesthesia using the laryngeal mask airway. *Br J Anaesth* 1992;69:314–315.
50. Rosenblatt W. Personal communication.
51. Aoyama K, Takenaka I, Sata T, et al. Cricoid pressure impedes positioning and ventilation through the laryngeal mask airway. *Can J Anaesth* 1996;43:1035–1040.
52. Brimacombe J, White A, Berry A. Effect of cricoid pressure on ease of insertion of the laryngeal mask airway. *Br J Anaesth* 1993;71:800–802.
53. Bhavani-Shankar K, Hart NS, Mushlin PS. Negative pressure induced airway and pulmonary injury. *Can J Anaesth* 1997;44:78–81.
54. Pollack CV Jr. The laryngeal mask airway: a comprehensive review for the Emergency Physician. *J Emerg Med* 2001;20:53–63.
55. Berry AM, Brimacombe JR, Verghese C. The laryngeal mask airway in emergency medicine, neonatal resuscitation, and intensive care medicine. *Int Anesthesiol Clin* 1998;36:91–109.

10

Supraglottic Devices

Michael F. Murphy and Robert E. Schneider

COMBITUBE

Description

The Combitube is a dual-lumen, dual-cuff airway invented by Michael Frass, an Austrian intensivist. The goal of insertion is to place the device blindly into the esophagus, though it can be accommodated by the trachea should it inadvertently be placed there; it will function adequately in the short term as an endotracheal tube. One balloon seals the esophagus and the other the oropharynx, trapping the larynx between the two. It has two lumens, allowing ventilation whether placed into the esophagus or the trachea (Fig. 10-1).

The Combitube, in the context of emergency department airway management, is a rescue airway device. It is a dramatic improvement over the esophageal obturator airway (EOA), which has no place in modern emergency airway management. In addition, unlike its predecessors the EOA and the esophageal gastric tube airway (EGTA), an adequate mask seal is unnecessary to effect adequate ventilation.

The Combitube is supplied in two sizes: 37F SA (small adult), to be used in patients 4 to 5.5 feet tall, and 41F, which is for use in patients more than 5.5 feet tall. Combitubes suitable for use in children less than 4 feet tall are unavailable.

Indications and Contraindications

The indications for the use of the Combitube in emergency airway management include the following:

- Failed intubation, particularly the can't intubate, can't ventilate situation in which the etiology is felt *not* to be due to upper-airway obstruction at the level of the larynx, while preparations are being made to perform a cricothyrotomy. This is the same indication as mentioned for the LMA-Fastrach (see Chapter 9).
- Upper gastrointestinal or airway hemorrhage that threatens airway and tracheal patency.
- Primary airway management for cardiopulmonary arrest when endotracheal intubation is not permitted or impossible (e.g., prehospital care).
- The Combitube has been used in a case of severe facial burns, and may be of use in those rescue situations where mouth opening is too limited to admit an LMA or other device.

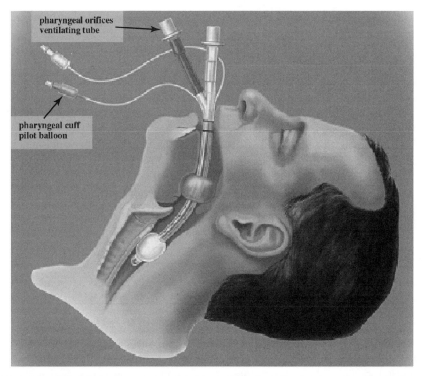

FIG. 10-1. The Combitube inserted and seated. Note how the laryngeal aperture is trapped between the two balloons.

Contraindications to the use of a Combitube include the following:

- Responsive patients with intact airway-protective reflexes. It is important to note that the Combitube is not indicated in managing the difficult airway (see Chapter 2), though there is one case report of Combitube use in the difficult airway.
- Patients with known esophageal disease
- Caustic ingestions
- Upper-airway obstruction due to laryngeal foreign bodies or pathology

Technique

Insertion of the Combitube is a blind technique, though a laryngoscope may be used, permitting insertion under direct vision.

1. With the patient supine (insertion is possible in any position) and the head and neck in a neutral position, lift the tongue and jaw upward with the nondominant hand.
2. Insert the device in the midline, allowing the curve of the device to follow the natural curve of the airway, and advance the device until the alveolar ridge is between the imprinted black bands on the device. Moderate force is required to enable the device to pass through the pharyngeal constrictor muscles into the esophagus. Substantial resistance should prompt the operator to withdraw and readvance. Inflate the proximal large oropharyngeal balloon with

approximately 100 mL of air (Combitube 37F: 85 mL) via the blue pilot balloon labeled #1.

3. Inflate the white distal balloon with 5 to 15 mL of air (Combitube 37F: 5 to 12 mL) via the white pilot balloon labeled #2.

4. Begin ventilation using the longer blue connecting tube. The presence of air entry into the lung and the absence of gastric insufflation by auscultation indicate that the Combitube is in the esophagus, which occurs virtually every time. The incidence of inadvertent tracheal intubation is less than 5%. Aspiration of gastric contents and gastric decompression is possible by passing the provided suction tube through the clear connecting tube into the stomach.

5. The absence of breath sounds in the chest and presence of gastric insufflation by auscultation indicates that the Combitube is in the trachea (a distinctly rare event), and ventilation should be performed through the shorter clear connection tube.

6. The absence of any sounds on auscultation may indicate that the device has been inserted too far and should be repositioned after the proximal balloon is deflated.

7. End-tidal carbon dioxide verification should be used to ensure pulmonary gas exchange.

Complications

The Combitube has been shown to be an effective airway management device. It is not difficult to position properly. The Combitube appears in one study to be superior to the LMA-Classic in the prehospital setting, and it has been shown to be a useful airway rescue device in the event of a failed intubation. However, like the LMA, it does not provide optimum protection against aspiration (although aspiration has never been reported), and its merit relative to the LMA-Fastrach is unknown. Complications are rare and mostly related to upper airway hematomas, pyriform perforation, and perforation of the esophagus.

Increasing cuff volumes are required at times to achieve a sufficient seal to permit adequate ventilation. As cuff volume is increased, the pressure transmitted to the mucosa is increased to the point where mucosal perfusion is compromised, particularly where the cuff is adjacent to rigid anatomic structures such as the cervical spine (pharyngeal balloon) and the larynx (esophageal balloon). Over time, this may lead to ischemic mucosal injury. A high rate of success with few complications has been reported in prehospital use for cardiac arrest.

OTHER SUPRALARYNGEAL DEVICES

The Cuffed Oropharyngeal Airway (COPA, Mallinkrodt Medical, St. Louis, MO) is an inexpensive disposable device that combines a Guedel airway with an inflatable distal high-volume, low-pressure cuff and a 15-mm proximal adapter (Fig. 10-2). The device is inserted like an oral airway and the cuff subsequently inflated to create an oropharyngeal seal and permit positive pressure ventilation (Fig. 10-3).

The Laryngeal Tube Airway (King LT Airway, King Systems Corp, Noblesville, IN) is a newly developed multiuse, latex-free, single-lumen silicon tube with oropharyngeal and esophageal low-pressure cuffs, a ventilation outlet between the two cuffs, and a blind distal tip (Fig. 10-4). It is inserted similarly to the Combitube, though there is substantially less resistance on insertion. When seated, it works in a fashion that is very similar to that of the

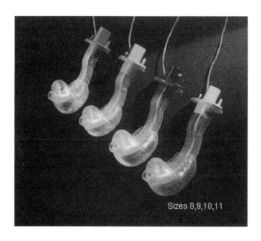

FIG. 10-2. Four sizes of COPAs. Note the cuffs on the distal ends of the airways.

Combitube (Fig. 10-5). Ventilation and oxygenation capabilities are similar to the LMA and Combitube.

Of the four supralaryngeal devices discussed in this section, the King LT Airway seems to have the most promise as an emergency failed airway rescue device in the opinion of the author (MM).

The Pharyngeal Airway Xpress (PAX, Vital Signs Inc., Totowa, NJ) is a sterile, latex-free, single-use airway device intended for use during routine anesthesia procedures. The PAX, with just one size, can accommodate all adults over 90 pounds. It is a curved tube designed with an anatomically shaped gilled tip at its distal end, a large oropharyngeal cuff, and an open hooded window that allows ventilation (Fig. 10-6). It is placed blindly, without the aid of any instrument, and when positioned correctly should provide an effective

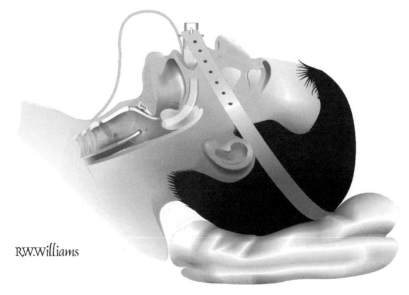

FIG. 10-3. The COPA seated and inflated. A head strap holds the device in place.

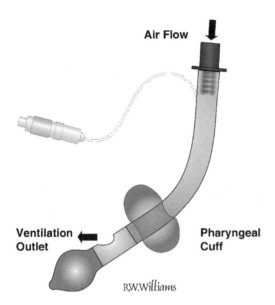

Air Flow

**Ventilation
Outlet**

**Pharyngeal
Cuff**

R.W.Williams

FIG. 10-4. The King LT Airway. Note that there is only one pilot balloon to inflate both balloons.

seal. There is insufficient published information at this time to support a recommendation to use this device in emergency airway management.

   The Glottic Aperture Seal Airway (GO$_2$ Airway, Augustine Medical, Eden Prairie, MN) is a newly developed, disposable, single-lumen airway that can achieve a highly effective seal against and within the laryngeal inlet (Fig. 10-7). It is inserted with the aide of a stainless steel insertion instrument (blade) (Figs. 10-8 and 10-9). Thus far two adult sizes have been developed, and pediatric sizes are under consideration.

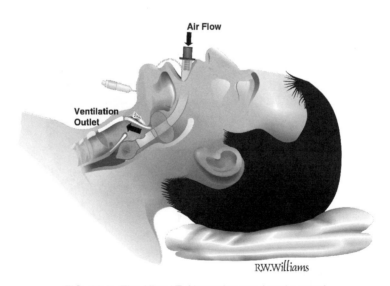

Air Flow

**Ventilation
Outlet**

R.W.Williams

FIG. 10-5. The King LT Airway inserted and seated.

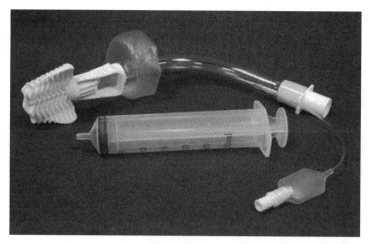

FIG. 10-6. The Pharyngeal Airway Express (PAX). The gilled tip seals the esophagus and is probably responsible for the superficial mucosal injuries seen with the device.

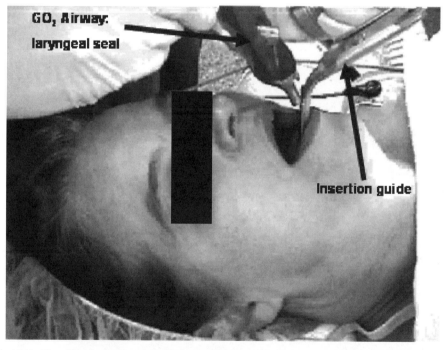

FIG. 10-7. The Glottic Aperture Seal Airway (GO$_2$ Airway). The insertion guide has been inserted into the mouth and over the back of the tongue using a tongue depressor. The GO$_2$ Airway is then inserted onto the guide and advanced into the airway, stopping when it can go no farther, rather like an LMA-Classic. Once seated and the laryngeal collar is inflated, the insertion guide is removed.

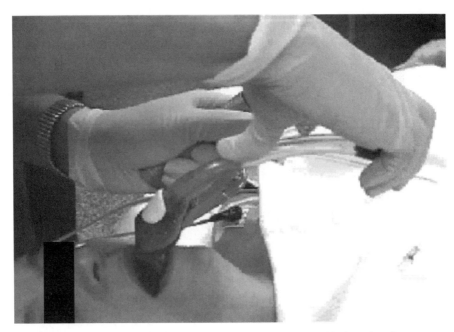

FIG. 10-8. The GO$_2$ Airway is slid down the insertion guide into the airway.

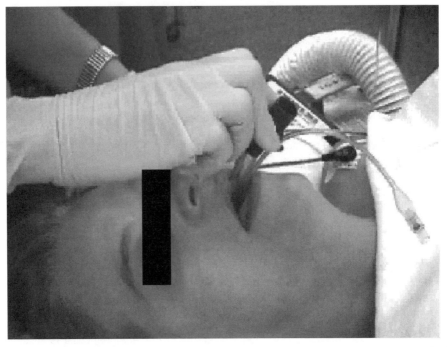

FIG. 10-9. The ventilating end of the GO$_2$ Airway that connects to the ventilating bag looks like an endotracheal tube or LMA.

EVIDENCE

1. The Combitube: The Combitube has been identified as a rescue airway device for the failed airway by authoritative bodies in the United States and Canada (1,2). Its use is well described in the anesthesia, resuscitation, emergency medicine, and emergency medical services literature both as a first-line device and in the face of a difficult and failed airway (3–9). Several authors have identified the Combitube as a valuable adjunct in cardiopulmonary resuscitation (10–12), performing as well as or better than the LMA and bag/mask ventilation. Success rates of 98 to 100% are regularly reported in these studies. The ease of insertion (13–17) and adequacy of ventilation by physicians and nonphysician providers is well established (17–20). The device has been demonstrated to be useful in the management of the difficult airway (21,22) and in rescuing a failed airway (23,24) while one prepares to undertake a cricothyrotomy. It has been demonstrated to protect the airway, control bleeding, and permit ventilation in a case of craniofacial trauma associated with severe bleeding (25) and to secure an airway in a case of severe facial burns preventing intubation (26). It is unclear whether or not the Combitube provides protection against the aspiration of gastric contents (27). The downside of the Combitube is reports of potentially serious complications related to the use of the Combitube, particularly pyriform sinus perforation (28–32) and esophageal perforation (33–37). A word of caution: Mucosal pressures exerted by the inflated balloons may exceed mucosal perfusion pressure, leading to mucosal ischemia (7).

2. Cuffed Oropharyngeal Airway: This device has limited evidence to support its use, and it has virtually disappeared from clinical use (38,39). It is designed to create an effective airway without stimulating the larynx and can be used during resuscitation (40) when face mask ventilation has proved difficult (41) and as an adjunct to fiberoptic intubation (42). Lingual and glossopharyngeal palsies have been reported after use of the device (43,44). There is no body of literature to support its use in emergency difficult or failed airways.

3. Laryngeal Tube Airway: Simple handling, possible aspiration protection, and availability in newborn to adult sizes are considered to be advantages of this airway device (45–48). As with the Combitube, mucosal compression by the inflated balloons may lead to mucosal ischemic injury (49).

4. Pharyngeal Airway Xpress: What little literature is available suggests a substantial incidence of superficial pharyngeal mucosal injury (50,51).

5. Glottic Aperture Seal Airway: There is virtually no literature at this time regarding this device to support a recommendation regarding emergency airway management (52).

REFERENCES

Combitube

1. Crosby ET, Cooper RM, Douglas MJ, et al. The unanticipated difficult airway with recommendations for management. *Can J Anaesth* 1998;45:757–776.
2. Practice guidelines for management of the difficult airway. An updated report by the American Society of Anesthesiologists task force on management of the difficult airway. *Anesthesiology* 2003;98:1269–1277.
3. Mercer M. The role of the Combitube in airway management. *Anaesthesia* 2000;55:394–395.
4. Gaitini LA, Vaida SJ, Agro F. The Esophageal-Tracheal Combitube. *Anesthesiol Clin North Am* 2002;20:893–906.
5. Idris AH, Gabrielli A. Advances in airway management. *Emerg Med Clin North Am* 2002;20:843–857.
6. Agro F, Frass M, Benumof JL, et al. Current status of the Combitube: a review of the literature. *J Clin Anesth* 2002;14:307–314.
7. Keller C, Brimacombe J, Boehler M, et al. The influence of cuff volume and anatomic location on pharyngeal, esophageal, and tracheal mucosal pressures with the esophageal tracheal combitube. *Anesthesiology* 2002;96:1074–1077.
8. Shuster M, Nolan J, Barnes TA. Airway and ventilation management. *Cardiol Clin* 2002;20:23–35.

9. Agro F, Frass M, Benumof J, et al. The esophageal tracheal combitube as a non-invasive alternative to endotracheal intubation. A review. *Minerva Anestesiol* 2001;67:863–874.
10. Grayling M, Wilson IH, Thomas B. The use of the laryngeal mask airway and Combitube in cardiopulmonary resuscitation; a national survey. *Resuscitation* 2002;52:183–186.
11. Gabrielli A, Layon AJ, Wenzel V, et al. Alternative ventilation strategies in cardiopulmonary resuscitation. *Curr Opin Crit Care* 2002;8:199–211.
12. Frass M, Staudinger T, Losert H, et al. Airway management during cardiopulmonary resuscitation—a comparative study of bag-valve-mask, laryngeal mask airway and Combitube in a bench model. *Resuscitation* 1999;43:80–81.
13. Levitan RM, Kush S, Hollander JE. Devices for difficult airway management in academic emergency departments: results of a national survey. *Ann Emerg Med* 1999;33:694–698.
14. Lefrancois DP, Dufour DG. Use of the esophageal tracheal combitube by basic emergency medical technicians. *Resuscitation* 2002;52:77–83.
15. Ochs M, Vilke GM, Chan TC, et al. Successful prehospital airway management by EMT-Ds using the combitube. *Prehosp Emerg Care* 2000;4:333–337.
16. Tanigawa K, Shigematsu A. Choice of airway devices for 12,020 cases of nontraumatic cardiac arrest in Japan. *Prehosp Emerg Care* 1998;2:96–100.
17. Rumball CJ, MacDonald D. The PTL, Combitube, laryngeal mask, and oral airway: a randomized prehospital comparative study of ventilatory device effectiveness and cost-effectiveness in 470 cases of cardiorespiratory arrest. *Prehosp Emerg Care* 1997;1:1–10.
18. Calkins MD, Robinson TD. Combat trauma airway management: endotracheal intubation versus laryngeal mask airway versus combitube use by Navy SEAL and Reconnaissance combat corpsmen. *J Trauma* 1999;46:927–932.
19. Yardy N, Hancox D, Strang T. A comparison of two airway aids for emergency use by unskilled personnel. The Combitube and laryngeal mask. *Anaesthesia* 1999;54:181–183.
20. Dorges V, Ocker H, Wenzel V, et al. Emergency airway management by non-anaesthesia house officers—a comparison of three strategies. *Emerg Med J* 2001;18:90–94.
21. Staudinger T, Tesinsky P, Klappacher G, et al. Emergency intubation with the Combitube in two cases of difficult airway management. *Eur J Anaesthesiol* 1995;12:189–193.
22. Blostein PA, Koestner AJ, Hoak S. Failed rapid sequence intubation in trauma patients: esophageal tracheal combitube is a useful adjunct. *J Trauma* 1998;44:534–537.
23. Enlund M, Miregard M, Wennmalm K. The Combitube for failed intubation—instructions for use. *Acta Anaesthesiol Scand* 2001;45:127–128.
24. Della Puppa A, Pittoni G, Frass M. Tracheal esophageal combitube: a useful airway for morbidly obese patients who cannot intubate or ventilate. *Acta Anaesthesiol Scand* 2002;46:911–913.
25. Morimoto F, Yoshioka T, Ikeuchi H, et al. Use of esophageal tracheal combitube to control severe oronasal bleeding associated with craniofacial injury: case report. *J Trauma* 2001;51:168–169.
26. Wagner A, Roeggla M, Roeggla G, et al. Emergency intubation with the combitube in a case of severe facial burn. *Am J Emerg Med* 1995;13:681–683.
27. Mercer MH. An assessment of protection of the airway from aspiration of oropharyngeal contents using the Combitube airway. *Resuscitation* 2001;51:135–138.
28. Urtubia RM, Gazmuri RR. Is the combitube traumatic? *Anesthesiology* 2003;98:1021–1022.
29. Urtubia RM, Carcamo CR, Montes JM. Complications following the use of the Combitube, tracheal tube and laryngeal mask airway. *Anaesthesia* 2000;55:597–599.
30. Oczenski W, Krenn H, Dahaba AA, et al. Complications following the use of the Combitube, tracheal tube and laryngeal mask airway. *Anaesthesia* 1999;54:1161–1165.
31. Moser MS. Piriform sinus perforation during esophageal-tracheal combitube placement. *J Emerg Med* 1999;17:129.
32. Richards CF. Piriform sinus perforation during esophageal-tracheal Combitube placement. *J Emerg Med* 1998;16:37–39.
33. Krafft P, Nikolic A, Frass M. Esophageal rupture associated with the use of the Combitube. *Anesth Analg* 1998;87:1457.
34. Krafft P, Frass M, Reed AP. Complications with the Combitube. *Can J Anaesth* 1998;45:823–824.
35. Walz R, Bund M, Meier PN, et al. Esophageal rupture associated with the use of the Combitube. *Anesth Analg* 1998;87:228.
36. Vezina D, Lessard MR, Bussieres J, et al. Complications associated with the use of the esophageal-tracheal Combitube. *Can J Anaesth* 1998;45:76–80.
37. Klein H, Williamson M, Sue-Ling HM, et al. Esophageal rupture associated with the use of the Combitube. *Anesth Analg* 1997;85:937–939.

Cuffed Oropharyngeal Airway (COPA)

38. Dravid RM, Popat MT. The cuffed oropharyngeal airway. *Anaesthesia* 1999;54:402–403.
39. Garcia-Guasch R, Ferra M, Benito P, et al. Ease of ventilation through the cuffed oropharyngeal airway (COPA), the laryngeal mask airway and the face mask in a cardiopulmonary resuscitation training manikin. *Resuscitation* 2001;50:173–177.

40. Rees SG. The cuffed oropharyngeal airway in resuscitation. *Anaesthesiol Reanim* 2001;26:18–20.
41. Asai T, Koga K, Stacey MR. Use of the cuffed oropharyngeal airway after difficult ventilation through a facemask. *Anaesthesia* 1997;52:1236–1237.
42. Greenberg RS, Kay N. Cuffed oropharyngeal airway aid to fiberoptic intubation. *Br J Anaesth* 1999;82:395–398.
43. Laffon M, Ferrandiere M, Mercier C, et al. Transient lingual and glossopharyngeal nerve injury: a complication of cuffed oropharyngeal airway. *Anesthesiology* 2001;94:719–720.
44. Kadry MA, Popat MT. Lingual nerve injury after use of a cuffed oropharyngeal airway. *Eur J Anaesthesiol* 2001;18:264–266.

Laryngeal Tube Airway (King LT Airway)

45. Dorges V, Ocker H, Wenzel V, et al. The Laryngeal Tube S: a modified simple airway device. *Anesth Analg* 2003;96:618–621.
46. Genzwuerker HV, Hilker T, Hohner E, et al. The laryngeal tube: a new adjunct for airway management. *Prehosp Emerg Care* 2000;4:168–172.
47. Dorges V, Ocker H, Wenzel V, et al. The laryngeal tube: a new simple airway device. *Anesth Analg* 2000;90:1220–1222.
48. Agro F, Cataldo R, Alfano A, et al. A new prototype for airway management in an emergency: the Laryngeal Tube. *Resuscitation* 1999;41:284–286.
49. Keller C, Brimacombe J, Kleinsasser A, et al. Pharyngeal mucosal pressures with the laryngeal tube airway versus Proseal laryngeal mask airway. *Anasthesiol Intensivmed Notfallmed Schmerzther* 2003;38:393–396.

Pharyngeal Airway Express (PAX)

50. Dimitriou V, Voyagis GS, Iatrou C, et al. A comparison of the PAxpress and face mask plus Guedel airway by inexperienced personnel after mannequin-only training. *Anesth Analg* 2003;96:1214–1217.
51. Cook TM, Rudd P, McCormick B, et al. An evaluation of the PAxpress pharyngeal airway. *Anaesthesia* 2003;58:191.

Glottic Aperture Seal Airway (GO$_2$ Airway)

52. Benumof JL. The glottic aperture seal airway: a new ventilatory device. *Anesthesiology* 1998;88:1219–1226.

11

Lighted Stylet Intubation

Michael F. Murphy and Orlando R. Hung

DESCRIPTION

Although direct-vision laryngoscopy and intubation has been proven over the years to be reliable and relatively easy, the accurate and prompt placement of an endotracheal tube (ETT) remains a major challenge in some patients, even in the hands of experienced laryngoscopists. It has been estimated that between 1% and 3% of patients present with difficult airways, leading to difficult endotracheal intubation under direct vision using a laryngoscope (see Chapter 6). In fact, it is impossible to intubate some patients using this technique, emphasizing the key role of cricothyrotomy in emergency airway management.

ETTs can be guided into place nonsurgically in the following ways:

- Under direct vision (via a laryngoscope, bronchoscope, etc.)
- With an indirect indicator, such as listening to and feeling air movement in nasal intubation, transillumination of light in the neck with lighted stylets and bronchoscopes and tactile digital intubation
- With a guide, such as an intubating laryngeal mask airway
- Blindly, without an indicator

Lighted stylet intubation is of use in those situations where conventional laryngoscopy has failed to provide visualization of the larynx sufficient to allow direct-vision intubation. In general, there must be adequate ventilation and oxygenation to allow time for the use of the lighted stylet (i.e., cannot intubate, *can* oxygenate).

The light-guided intubation technique relies on the transillumination of the soft tissues of the neck to indicate intratracheal tube placement. It was first used in 1959 by Yamamura and colleagues in Japan for blind nasal intubation. This technique takes advantage of the anterior location of the trachea, relative to the esophagus. With the light bulb of a lighted stylet placed at the tip of the ETT, a well-defined, circumscribed glow can readily be seen in the anterior neck area when the tip of the tube enters the trachea through the glottic opening. However, if the tip of the tube is in the esophagus, the light glow is diffuse and not easily seen.

Although the light-guided intubation technique had shown some promise, it was not widely used until the 1970s, following the introduction of the Flexilum (Concept Corporation, Clearwater, FL). The Tubestat (Concept Corporation, Clearwater, FL) was developed in the early 1980s, following minor refinements of the original Flexilum design. Despite these improvements, difficulties persisted with the use of these devices, mostly related to the degree of transillumination that could be achieved. A lighted stylet device from Vital Signs (Vital Light)

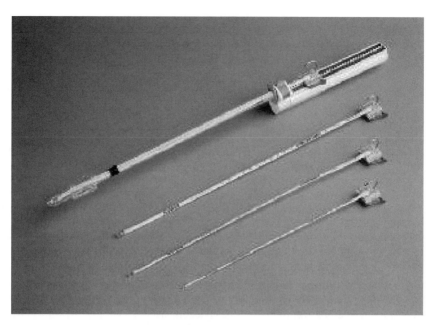

FIG. 11-1. Laerdal Trachlight handle and three sizes of wands: adult, pediatric, and infant. The wand and rigid internal stylet combination has been attached to the handle and an endotracheal tube loaded onto the wand. Note the point of connection of the endotracheal tube to the handle.

has the advantage of low cost, but is lacking some desirable features. Any fiberoptic device (rigid or flexible) with distal light emission can be used to intubate using this principle. The Shikani Optical Stylet (SOS) is an example and will be discussed in Chapter 13. The Trachlight (Laerdal Medical Corp., Wappinger Falls, NY) lighted stylet has incorporated many modifications to improve the transillumination features of the light, and has the flexibility to allow oral and nasal intubation (Fig. 11-1). Although there are several acceptable and approved lighted stylets available, the Trachlight seems to be superior, based on its features and adaptability. The remainder of the discussion will refer to the Trachlight.

INDICATIONS AND CONTRAINDICATIONS

The can't intubate, can't oxygenate situation is a relative contraindication to Trachlight intubation because of the time required, unless the operator has considerable skill and experience with the device and the intubation attempt can be made in parallel with preparations for cricothyrotomy. As with conventional intubation techniques, this technique requires moderate to substantial sedation and/or local anesthesia of the airway; it has been successfully used both for primary intubations during RSI and as a rescue device.

As with all procedures, practice in a controlled setting is important to develop facility with the device to allow predictable success rates. It has been demonstrated that this technique is easier to teach and the skill is easier to maintain than is true with conventional laryngoscopy. The Trachlight also appears to produce less airway trauma and physiological disturbance than conventional laryngoscopy. For the foreseeable future the majority of emergency physicians will undoubtedly continue to prefer the laryngoscope to the Trachlight. However, this device will serve as a valuable rescue device in the can't intubate, *can* ventilate situation. The

Trachlight ought to be considered a primary device when orotracheal intubation by other techniques is judged to be difficult or impossible (e.g., limited mouth opening or cervical spine mobility) because of inability to visualize the glottis, particularly if a fiberoptic device is not available. The device can be used to facilitate nasotracheal as well as orotracheal intubation. If the Trachlight is used to attempt nasotracheal intubation, transillumination replaces the use of audible breath sounds to guide the nasotracheal tube into place, making the technique possible in apnoeic patients.

This technique is contraindicated when there is reasonable suspicion that the anatomy of the airway is abnormal or shifted from the midline. Laryngeal pathology generally mandates intubation by direct visualization, so is also a contraindication to this technique.

TECHNIQUE

The Trachlight device consists of two parts: a reusable handle and a disposable, malleable lighted stylet, recommended by the manufacturer to be limited to ten uses (Fig. 11-1). The power control circuitry and batteries are within the handle. The Trachlight requires three AAA standard alkaline batteries, which are easily changed by opening the cover on the handle. A female connector with a locking lever located on the front of the handle accepts and secures the standard 15-mm male connector of ETTs. The stylet consists of a durable, flexible plastic tube with a bright light bulb at one end. The light bulb is sufficiently bright to permit transillumination and intubation under ambient light in most cases and offers 360-degree illumination at its tip. The light begins to blink after 30 seconds to prevent the bulb from overheating. Within the plastic sheath is a removable, malleable, metal stylet, and affixed to the end of the stylet opposite the light is a rigid plastic connector with a release arm, which attaches the stylet assembly to the handle (Fig. 11-2). This connector can be adjusted and slides along the handle to accommodate ETTs of different lengths. During intubation, the ETT and the wand become pliable when the rigid stylet is retracted. This design facilitates the advancement of the tube into the trachea.

1. ***Preparation.*** To ensure easy retraction during intubation, the internal rigid stylet of the wand should be well lubricated, preferably with a silicone fluid (Endoscopic Instrument Lubricant, ACMI), though any water soluble lubricant such as KY Jelly will suffice. Similarly, the external wall of the wand should be lubricated with a water-soluble lubricant. Cut the ETT to 26 cm for orotracheal intubation by removing, then reattaching, the ETT connector. This step makes the device easier to maneuver into the airway. Insert the wand into the ETT with the light just protruding from the end of the ETT so that it can be felt as you palpate the opening at the distal end of the ETT. Some recommend aligning the centimeter numbers of the wand with those in the ETT, but the transillumination is better with the light just emerging from the distal end of the tube. For most patients, the ETT–Trachlight (ETT–TL) combination should be bent just proximal to the ETT cuff where the words 'bend here' are located on the wand. In very large or very small patients, the bend may have to be more proximal or more distal respectively. The correct length for this distal limb of the ETT–TL combination is the distance from the base of the tongue to the cricothyroid membrane. This length corresponds externally to the distance from the angle of the mandible to the cricothyroid membrane, and the bend in the ETT–TL combination can easily be compared externally with these landmarks. The bend should be a sharp right angle, mimicking the shape of a field hockey stick. For a nasotracheal intubation, the length of the distal limb ought to correspond to the distance from the back of the nasopharynx to the cricothyroid membrane, externally

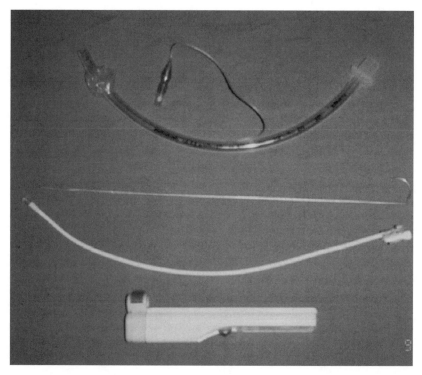

FIG. 11-2. Trachlight handle, flexible lighted wand and rigid internal stylet disassembled with an endotracheal tube.

represented by the distance from the tragus of the ear to the cricothyroid membrane. The bend is a more gentle sweep and slightly greater than 90 degrees to bring the tip sufficiently anterior to enter the glottis when the ETT is introduced nasally. For nasal intubation, some authors advocate leaving the rigid stylet in place; others recommend removing it entirely. Removing the stylet reduces the control one has over the distal end of the tube, and if this practice is followed, the use of an Endotrol control tip nasotracheal tube is recommended. Whether oral or nasal intubation is planned, the tip of the ETT should also be lubricated with a water-soluble lubricant.

2. *Positioning.* With the intubator standing at the head of the patient, the neck is bared to allow maximal visualization of the anterior neck of the patient during intubation. The technique can also be performed from the side of the patient. Usually, the patient's head and neck are placed in a *neutral* position, though it may be necessary to extend the head slightly to optimize visualization (Fig. 11-3). In obese patients or patients with an extremely short neck, placing a pillow under the shoulder and neck may be helpful, if possible, but the problems presented by these anatomical variations can also often be overcome by changing the angle of the tube bend or the length of the distal (bent portion) ETT.

3. *Ambient lighting.* In general, patients can be intubated easily under ambient lighting conditions. Dimming the light or shading the neck to optimize visualization of the transilluminated glow may be necessary in those with generous subcutaneous tissue or darkly pigmented skin.

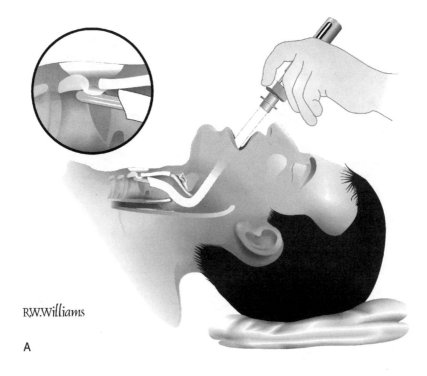

R.W.Williams

A

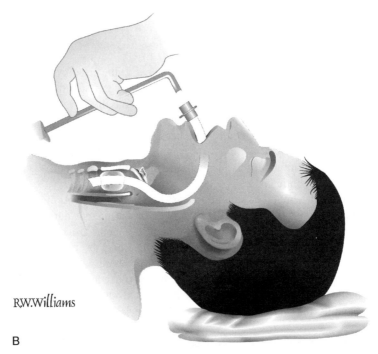

R.W.Williams

B

FIG. 11-3. Trachlight intubation. **A:** The operator is holding the device by the handle rather than holding the ETT–TL, a technical detail that most prefer. In this figure the head is rather more extended than ordinarily recommended. A neutral position is preferred. **B:** Once the ETT–TL have been placed in the trachea, the TL is removed.

Technique of Intubation

With the patient lying supine, the lower alveolar ridge and mentum are grasped and lifted upward using the intubator's nondominant hand. This lifts the tongue and epiglottis upward to facilitate the intubation. Alternatively, the thumb of the nondominant hand can be placed in the mouth along the patient's tongue to lift the tongue upward and forward as the interphalangeal joint of the thumb is flexed. The nondominant hand must be kept close to the lower lip to ensure an unobstructed path in the midline for the trachlight. The device is then switched on and the ETT–TL is inserted into the oropharynx and positioned in the midline, such that the distal (bent portion) ETT is resting gently against the posterior oropharynx in the midline. The operator's vision is not transitioned to the anterior neck until it is certain that the ETT–TL is in this midline position, resting against the posterior oropharynx. The device is then rocked on the fulcrum created by the bend in the tube, allowing the distal end of the tube to traverse an imaginary arc and enter the glottis. The natural inclination is to push the device as is done with conventional intubation. This approach will only serve to push the ETT–TL into the esophagus.

The jaw lift helps to elevate the epiglottis and enhance the passage of the ETT–TL under the epiglottis into the glottic opening. When the tip of the ETT–TL enters the glottic opening, a well-defined circumscribed glow can be seen at the anterior neck slightly below the laryngeal prominence. Retracting the rigid stylet 5 cm makes the distal portion of the ETT–TL more pliable and facilitates its advance into the trachea (Fig. 11-3). The tip of the ETT is advanced until the glow appears in the sternal notch. At this point, the tip of the ETT is midway between the vocal cords and carina. Now the ETT connector is released from the locking device on the Trachlight and the device is removed from the ETT. In certain lighting conditions, or with particularly dark-skinned or thick-necked patients, it may be desirable to test the transillumination before proceeding through the glottis. After the Trachlight has been placed against the posterior oropharynx as previously described, the ETT–TL is then rocked (not pushed) gently to the right pyriform recess and the intensity of the transilluminated glow through the neck is noted. The intensity of this glow will approximate that found in the midline with successful placement of the device in the trachea. If necessary, room lights may be dimmed after this test shows that the transillumination might be insufficient in ambient lighting.

COMPLICATIONS

Success rates in the hands of experienced users are consistent with or exceed those associated with conventional laryngoscopy. Limited experience with this device has not identified isolated or persistent complications. The complications would be expected to be similar to those for conventional intubation, but less common because the technique is less traumatic and does not require insertion of a laryngoscope.

EVIDENCE

This technique produces a higher success rate than conventional laryngoscopy with a shorter time to intubation when wielded by skilled intubators. It takes about 10 intubations to become familiar with Trachlight intubation and 20 to become facile (1). Most have found that this technique is easier to teach and has a higher level of skill retention than conventional laryngoscopy (2,3), though one study found the opposite (4). The evidence as to whether lighted stylet intubation produces less autonomic stimulation than conventional laryngoscopy is conflicting, though the weight of evidence suggests that this is indeed the case (5–9). The device does appear to produce less trauma to the airway than conventional laryngoscopy. There is evidence that the device is useful in managing difficult airways, particularly anterior airways (10–12). It has been suggested that cricoid pressure may adversely affect the success rate with this device (13), though the weight of evidence suggests that this is not the case (10,11). The device can be coupled with other intubating techniques such as nasal intubation (14–16), intubation through a laryngeal mask (17,18), and with conventional laryngoscopy (19) to facilitate successful tracheal intubation.

REFERENCES

1. Hung OR, Pytka S, Morris I, et al. Clinical trial of a new lightwand (Trachlight™) to intubate the trachea. *Anesthesiology* 1995;83:509–514.
2. Hung OR, Murphy MF. Lightwands, lighted stylets and blind techniques of intubation. In: Sandler AN, Doyle DJ, eds. The difficult airway. *Anaesthesia Clinics NA,* vol 13, Toronto: WB Saunders, 1995.
3. Hung OR, Stewart RD. Lightwand intubation: I. A new intubating device. *Can J Anaesth,* 1995;42:820–825.
4. Soh CR, Kong CF, Kong CS, et al. Tracheal intubation by novice staff: the direct vision laryngoscope or the lighted stylet (Trachlight)? *Emerg Med J* 2002;19:292–294.
5. Hung OR, Pytka S, Murphy MF, et al. Comparative hemodynamic changes following laryngoscopic or lightwand intubation. *Anesthesiology* 1993;79:A497.
6. Kanaide M, Fukusaki M, Tamura S, et al. Hemodynamic and catecholamine responses during tracheal intubation using a lightwand device (Trachlight) in elderly patients with hypertension. *J Anesth* 2003;17:161–165.
7. Kihara S, Brimacombe J, Yaguchi Y, et al. Hemodynamic responses among three tracheal intubation devices in normotensive and hypertensive patients. *Anesth Analg* 2003;96:890–895.
8. Hirabayashi Y, Hiruta M, Kawakami T, et al. Effects of lightwand (Trachlight) compared with direct laryngoscopy on circulatory responses to tracheal intubation. *Br J Anaesth* 1998;81:253–255.
9. Takahashi S, et al: Hemodynamic responses to tracheal intubation with the laryngoscope versus lightwand intubating device (Trachlight®) in adults with normal airway. *Anesth Analg* 2002;95:480–484.
10. Hung OR, Stevens SC, Pytka S, et al. Clinical trial of a new lightwand device for intubation in patients with difficult airways. *Anesthesiology* 1993;79:A498.
11. Hung OR, Pytka S, Morris I, et al. Lightwand intubation: II. Clinical trial of a new lightwand to intubate patients with difficult airways. *Can J Anaesth,* 1995;42:826–830.
12. Latto IP: Management of difficult intubation. In: Latto IP, Rosen M, eds. Difficulties in tracheal intubation. London: Bailliere Tindall, 1987:99–141.
13. Hodgson RE, Goplan PD, Burrows RC, et al: Effect of cricoid pressure on the success of endotracheal intubation with a lightwand. *Anesthesiology* 2001;94:259–262.
14. Yamamura H, Yamamoto T, Kamiyama M: Device for blind nasal intubation. *Anesthesiology* 1959;20:221.
15. Hung OR. Nasal intubation with the Trachlight. *Can J Anaesth* 1999;46:908.
16. Agro F, Brimacombe J, Marchionni L, et al. Nasal intubation with the Trachlight. *Can J Anaesth* 1999;46:907–908.
17. Agro F, Brimacombe J, Carassiti M, et al: Use of a lighted stylet for intubation via the laryngeal mask airway. *Can J Anaesth* 1998:45:556–560.
18. Fan KH, Hung OR, Agro F. A comparative study of tracheal intubation using an intubating laryngeal mask (Fastrach) alone or together with a lightwand (Trachlight). *J Clin Anesth* 2000;12:581–585.
19. Agro F, Benumof JL, Carassiti M, et al. Efficacy of a combined technique using the Trachlight together with direct laryngoscopy under simulated difficult airway conditions in 350 anesthetized patients. *Can J Anaesth* 2002;49:525–526.

12

Flexible Fiberoptic Intubation

Michael F. Murphy

DESCRIPTION

Endotracheal intubation over a fiberoptic bronchoscope has emerged as an invaluable technique in airway management, particularly in patients for whom standard laryngoscopy and orotracheal intubation have failed or are anticipated to be difficult or impossible. No discussion of difficult or emergency airway management is complete without a review of the use of fiberoptic devices to perform diagnostic procedures in the upper airway and endotracheal intubation.

Although fiberoptic bronchoscopes are becoming more widely available in emergency departments, and published studies have described their use in the emergency department, few emergency practitioners have extensive experience with them for diagnostic procedures in the upper airway, and fewer still have done fiberoptic intubations.

INDICATIONS AND CONTRAINDICATIONS

Indications for fiberoptic endoscopy in emergency airway management include the following:

- Intubation of the patient who is predicted to be a difficult intubation. The most frequent candidates are those with supraglottic causes of upper airway obstruction such as angioedema, oropharyngeal abscess or hematoma, Ludwig's angina; or those with slowly progressive laryngeal lesions such as lingual and laryngeal cancers.
- Direct-vision laryngoscopy and intubation is recommended for patients with laryngeal trauma and tracheal disruption. The fiberscope meets this indication.
- Cervical spine immobility required, particularly if the airway is predicted to be difficult.
- Anatomic abnormalities, such as patients with restricted mouth opening or severely hypoplastic mandibles or the morbidly obese.
- Failed intubation in the can't intubate, *can* oxygenate scenario, when continuing deterioration of the airway is not anticipated.

Contraindications to fiberoptic intubation are mostly relative and may include the following:

- Excessive blood and secretions in the upper airway, which have the great potential to obscure the view and reduce the success rate with the fiberoptic technique. Some experienced bronchoscopists use the fiberscope like a Trachlight (see Chapter 11) in situation such as these, using transillumination to indicate entry into the trachea and only then looking through the scope to verify the position of the fiberscope in the trachea.

- High-grade upper-airway obstruction (due to foreign bodies or other lesions) where the procedure may precipitate total airway obstruction. If a patient has a high-grade supraglottic airway obstruction, the delays and risks of precipitating complete airway obstruction or laryngospasm argue strongly against fiberoptic intubation and in favor of cricothyrotomy.
- Inadequate oxygenation by bag and mask does not permit fiberoptic intubation because of the time required (can't intubate, can't ventilate/oxygenate).

TECHNIQUE

Overview

Fiberoptic intubation is a technical challenge that requires initial training, then skill maintenance activities to maintain speed and success. Manual dexterity in manipulating the fiberscope is essential to performing fiberoptic intubation in a timely fashion. This skill is best learned by attending fiberoptic intubation workshops with expert instruction and then practicing on intubation manikins or high-fidelity human patient simulators before one attempts to intubate a patient. This is particularly true of patients with difficult airways. The manufacturers of fiberscopes can usually provide training videos, product support personnel, and manikins to support this endeavor.

The requisite psychomotor skills cannot be developed without practice, and lack of training, practice, and experience constitute the most common cause of failed fiberoptic intubation. A reasonable level of dexterity in bronchoscopic manipulation can be achieved within three to four hours of independent practice using an intubation model. Recent studies have shown that the technique can also be learned in real-life situations by the performance of upper-airway endoscopy when diagnostic opportunities, such as searching for foreign bodies, evaluating the causes of hoarseness, evaluation of severe sore throat, and other upper-airway conditions present themselves. As is the case with many of the specialized airway techniques, semiemergent intubations, such as overdose victims without anticipated difficult airways and who are easily ventilated with a normal oxygen saturation, may be appropriate candidates for fiberoptic intubation. Because success depends on familiarity and skill in using the device, gaining experience in routine cases is invaluable before one is required to perform a difficult fiberoptic intubation in a crisis.

Preparation

Though the emergency difficult or failed airway situation often does not permit lengthy preparation and a methodical approach, maximal success with this technique requires both psychological and pharmacologic patient preparation. When the procedure is to be done "awake" (see Chapter 7), optimizing the chances for success includes the following:

- Educating the patient as to what to expect
- Administering an antisialogogue, such as glycopyrrolate 0.01 mg/kg, at least 20 minutes in advance of the procedure, to minimize obscuring secretions and maximize the effect of topically applied local anesthesia
- Achieving profound local anesthesia of the airway. A fiberoptic intubation requires as much sedation and topical anesthesia as is necessary for awake direct laryngoscopy.
- Administering adequate sedation (Chapter 7)

Scope Selection

Instrument selection for the emergency department (ED) is an important issue. Affordable and durable scopes are easily available from a variety of manufacturers. Selection of a manufacturer may be guided by existing service contracts in your specific institution. These instruments, although expensive, find several uses in the ED to justify such an expenditure:

- Endotracheal intubation, both nasal and oral
- Diagnostic laryngoscopy.
- Oropharyngeal foreign-body location and extraction
- Pulmonary toilette, particularly when ICU patients are "held over" in the ED

The scope should be of sufficient caliber and stiffness to guide the passage of an endotracheal tube (ETT) over itself through the angles of the airway without kinking and resist being flipped out of the trachea, while at the same time maintaining flexibility and ease of manipulation. Most fiberscope manufacturers produce intubation-specific devices that have added stiffness of the fiber bundle to allow ETTs to be guided into the trachea over the scope. This feature allows scopes that are small enough (3 to 4 mm in tip diameter) to be painlessly and atraumatically passed through a topically anesthetized nose for diagnostic work to also be used for fiberoptic intubation. Neonatal and pediatric fiberscopes (2 to 3 mm tip diameter) are also available.

The fiberoptic bundle should be long enough (600 mm) to allow bronchoscopy and airway toilette in the ED. Standard bronchoscopes are 600 mm in length. Some manufacturers produce 400-mm intubating fiberscopes that are not long enough for pulmonary care. A separate channel for the injection of local anesthetic or saline and suctioning is essential, though the smaller neonatal and pediatric fiberscopes may not have them owing to their small size. A formerly recommended practice, the insufflation of oxygen through the suction apparatus to maintain saturations and blow secretions out of the way, is now considered contraindicated following several cases of gastric insufflation, perforation, and death. A new generation of fiberoptic scopes with battery-powered portable self-contained light sources promises to be much more compact and may be preferable for ED applications.

Care of the Instrument

Some general precautions to prevent damage to the scope and its relatively delicate fiberoptic bundles:

- Don't drop the scope.
- Use a bite-block (e.g., oral airway) to protect the scope. Most oral fiberoptic intubation guides incorporate this feature (e.g., the Berman intubating/pharyngeal airway, also called the Berman breakaway airway) and are invaluable aids to successful oral fiberoptic intubation (see Fig. 12-1).
- Avoid acute bending or kinking of the fiber bundle, especially when sliding the ETT over the scope into the trachea.
- If rotation of the ETT during intubation is necessary, rotate both the ETT and the scope to avoid damage to the fibers.
- Lubricate the ETT by spraying local anesthetic agent or other water-soluble material down the tube to allow easy removal of the scope after the ETT is in place. Lubricating the scope makes it slippery and difficult to manipulate.

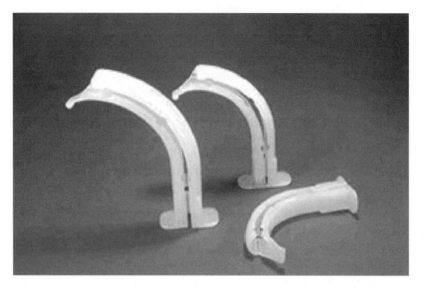

FIG. 12-1. Berman intubating/pharyngeal airways come in three sizes: 8, 9, and 10 cm.

• Clean the device, including the working channel, immediately after use. The best routine is to suction one liter of saline through the device immediately after use. Manufacturers and endoscopy units will provide instructions for acceptable cleaning routines.
• Don't flex the tip against undue resistance to manipulate the direction of an ETT or use it to move tissue out of the way.

The Technique of Fiberoptic Intubation

The fiberscope has two main components: a body (handpiece) housing the controls and accessories and a fiber bundle (Fig. 12-2). Scope tip control is simple: Flexion forward and backward is achieved with the thumb toggle on the body of the fiberscope; rotation clockwise and counterclockwise is done by rotating the wrist of the hand that is holding the body of the fiberscope (not the entire upper body).

The vast majority of EDs will not have a video-capable system, so this description assumes the operator is holding the eyepiece to his of her eye. When looking through the eyepiece of the fiberscope, select visual targets as you advance the scope using the hand holding the fiber bundle to pull the hand holding the body of the scope along. Move toward these targets slowly but steadily using small manipulations forward and back (toggle) and left and right (wrist flexion and extension) to keep successive targets in the center of the visual image. The hand–eye coordination needed for successful fiberoptic intubation has been likened to the kind of hand–eye coordination used to play a video game.

Preparation for the task depends on how much time is available. Generally, most things should be in a state of instantaneous readiness on the difficult and failed airway cart:

1. Gather all your equipment (usually preassembled on a tray):
   a. Topical airway anesthesia supplies and equipment, including three 5-mL syringes loaded with 4% lidocaine to inject into the airway through the scope as needed
   b. Fiberscope, ETTs, airways, bite-blocks
   c. Tonsil suction

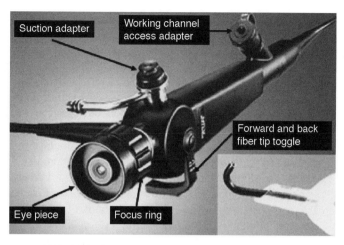

FIG. 12-2. The body of a fiberoptic bronchoscope.

   d. Lubricant and silicone liquid drops (prevents fogging)
   e. Additional airway management equipment as indicated in case of patient deterioration and need for rapid intervention
2. Obtain an able and knowledgeable assistant.
3. Prepare the patient:
   a. Antisialogogue, such as glycopyrrolate 0.01 mg/kg IM or IV
   b. Vasoconstrictor for the nose (if nasal route chosen)
   c. Local airway anesthesia
   d. Sedation as appropriate
   e. Preoxygenate the patient as for rapid sequence intubation (see Chapter 3) as much as is possible
4. Lubricate the tube (as earlier) and slide it over the scope up to the handpiece. Press the ETT connector to the handpiece firmly to hold it in place or tape it there. Lubricating the scope makes it slippery and too hard to manipulate.
5. Put a drop of silicone liquid on the tip of the scope or place the tip of the fiber bundle in a bottle of warmed saline (usually available in the warming cabinets of most EDs) for one minute to prevent fogging.
6. Insert a bite-block if the oral route is chosen, or, preferably, use an intubating guide such as a Berman intubating/pharyngeal airway. If a Berman guide is used, mount the ETT in the guide, ensuring that the tip of the ETT is at the end of the tubular portion of the airway before inserting the guide into the mouth, and then insert the fiberscope through the ETT.
7. Stand up straight, either at the head of, the side of, or facing the patient. Operator positioning is mostly a matter of personal preference and patient tolerance.
8. *Oral technique:* Stay in the midline, stay in the midline, stay in the midline! The best way is to place the long or ring finger in the middle of the upper lip to maintain a reference point and hold the fiber bundle with the index finger and thumb. Gentle traction on the tongue by an assistant using a gauze bandage helps open the airway and prevent the patient from using the tongue to obstruct access to the airway. Custom-made airways such as the Berman intubating/pharyngeal airway are very helpful in keeping the scope in the midline and obviate the need for the tongue traction maneuver. If such an adjunct is used, insert

the ETT into the airway and then insert the scope through the airway/ETT combination, obviating the need to jam or tape the ETT connector onto the scope handpiece.

Nasal technique: Soften the nasotracheal tube by placing the ETT in a bottle of warmed saline or sterile water from the warming closet for 3 to 5 minutes before inserting the ETT through the nostril. It is helpful to dilate the chosen anesthetized nostril by gently and slowly inserting increasingly large nasopharyngeal airways or a lubricated and gloved small finger into the nostril as far as possible immediately before inserting the ETT. Advance the lubricated nasal tube to the nasopharynx and then pass the scope through the tube.

9. Hold the body of the fiberscope in the same hand as your dominant eye. This allows one to turn slightly to the side when using the scope, an important detail in keeping the fiber bundle of the scope straight during the procedure for reasons described later. Some advocate holding the body of the scope in the left hand to facilitate clearance of the light source cable and suction tubing, which exit the body of the scope on its left side (Fig. 12-2). Use your thumb to toggle the tip control lever up and down. The index finger can be used to depress and activate the suction feature. Flexing and extending the wrist moves the tip of the fiber bundle left and right, though the fiber bundle must be held straight with mild tension between the two hands to optimize this maneuver. Slackness in the fiber bundle will not permit wrist motion to rotate its tip. The nondominant hand advances, withdraws, and manipulates the fiber bundle and maintains a midline oral position if the oral route is chosen. The operator should move the hands and arms, not the whole torso, to manipulate the fiber bundle into the airway.

10. The assistant should have a tonsil suction available to aspirate oral secretions and blood. The working channel of the scope may provide insufficient suction to clear the volume of secretions that may be present during the procedure. Should the tip become soiled or fogged obscuring clear vision, bouncing the tip gently against the mucosa may be sufficient to clear it.

11. Get your bearings: At the head of the bed, the base of the tongue is up; beside or in front of the patient it is down. Advance slowly while flexing the tip up to pass over the back of the tongue. The epiglottis comes into view. Keep it above you. You will see the white cords opening and closing with respiration.

12. It may be difficult to coordinate it, but attempt to advance the scope through the vocal cords during inspiration when they are open. You may need to inject 5 mL of 4% lidocaine through the working channel onto the larynx to obtund the cough or closure reflex and permit entry into the trachea.

13. If you get lost, withdraw to the oropharynx and find a landmark.

14. Once the tip of the fiber bundle is through the vocal cords, advance the scope almost to the carina. Now slowly advance the ETT over the scope into the trachea, being careful not to kink the scope. A laryngoscope may be useful to straighten out the angle of approach to the glottis. Gentle rotation of the scope/tube unit through 180 degrees may be necessary if the ETT catches on the cords. Newer ETT tip designs may facilitate passage of the ETT through the cords. (e.g. Parker Tube)

15. If coughing is a persistent problem, inject 5 mL of lidocaine 4% aqueous through the scope.

16. After the ETT has been successfully passed into the trachea, the scope can be used to correctly position the ETT in the midportion of the trachea. Push the tip of the scope through the ETT until it is just distal to the end of the ETT and flex it gently forward. Grasp both the fiberscope and the ETT and move them together until light transilluminates the sternal notch. The light is shining forward immediately beyond the tip of the ETT, so this corresponds to the midtracheal position.

COMPLICATIONS

Patient complications with this technique are uncommon and include mucosal damage to the airway and epistaxis. As with all techniques, damage to the vocal apparatus is possible but rare. The most frequent complication is damage to the scope from biting, twisting, kinking, or dropping. In the past it was taught that oxygen ought to be insufflated down the working channel of the scope to blow secretions out of the way and provide an element of oxygenation for the patient. This practice has been associated with gastric insufflation and rupture leading to death and is no longer recommended.

EVIDENCE

Intubating over a fiberoptic bronchoscope, nasally and orally, is a well-established technique for managing difficult airways (1–4). It has been demonstrated that the technique is easily learned and the skill maintained (5), and that nonhuman models are useful in teaching the manipulative skills that are key to successful intubation (6). It is recognized as a skill important to the training of residents in emergency medicine (7). Levitan et al. surveyed academic emergency departments (EDs) in 1999 attempting to determine what alternative airway management devices were available for difficult airway management (8). Sixty-four percent of them had fiberoptic bronchoscopes. Several studies have demonstrated a success rate for ED fiberoptic intubation by emergency physicians in the 70% to 99% range, depending on training and frequency of use (9–13). Both fiberoptic nasal (adults and children) and oral intubation in the ED have been described in the literature (14,15). Emergency fiberoptic intubation has been used in blunt and penetrating head and neck trauma, laryngeal malignancies, tracheal stenosis, and other difficult airway situations (16–20). As mentioned earlier, the practice of insufflating oxygen down the working channel of the scope has been associated with gastric insufflation and rupture leading to death (21) and is no longer recommended (22).

REFERENCES

1. Morris IR. Fiberoptic intubation. *Can J Anesth* 1994;41:996–1008.
2. Messeter MD, Pettersson KI. Endotracheal intubation with the fiberoptic bronchoscope. *Anaesthesia* 1980;35:294–298.
3. Dellinger RP. Fiberoptic bronchoscopy in adult airway management. *Crit Care Med* 1990;18:882–887.
4. Patel VU. Oral and nasal fiberoptic intubation with a single lumen tube. *Anesthesiol Clin NA* 1991;9:83–95.
5. Ovassapian A, Yelich SJ. Learning fiberoptic intubation. *Anesthesiol Clin NA* 1991;9:175–185.
6. Naik VN, et al: Fiberoptic orotracheal intubation on anesthetized patients. *Anesthesiology* 2001;95:343–348.
7. Gallagher EJ, Coffey J, Lombardi G, et al. Emergency procedures important to the training of emergency medicine residents: who performs them in the emergency department? *Acad Emerg Med* 1995;2:630–633.
8. Levitan RM, Kush S, Hollander JE. Devices for difficult airway management in academic emergency departments: results of a national survey. *Ann Emerg Med* 1999;33:694–698.
9. Afilalo M, Guttman A, Stern E, et al. Fiberoptic intubation in the emergency department: a case series. *J Emerg Med* 1993;11:387–391.
10. Mlinek EJ, Clinton JE, Plummer D, et al. Fiberoptic intubation in the emergency department. *Ann Emerg Med* 1990;19:359–362.
11. Schafermeyer RW. Fiberoptic laryngoscopy in the emergency department. *Am J Emerg Med* 1984;2:160–163.
12. Blanda M, Gallo UE. Emergency airway management. *Emerg Med Clin North Am* 2003;21:1–26.
13. Hamilton PH, Kang JJ. Emergency airway management. *Mt Sinai J Med* 1997;64:292–301.
14. Delaney KA, Hessler R. Emergency flexible fiberoptic nasotracheal intubation. A report of 60 cases. *Ann Emerg Med* 1988;17:919–926.
15. Rucker RW, Silva WJ, Worcester CC. Fiberoptic bronchoscopic nasotracheal intubation in children. *Chest* 1979;76:56–58.
16. Mulder DS, Wallace DH, Woolhouse FM. The use of the fiberoptic bronchoscope to facilitate endotracheal intubation following head and neck trauma. *J Trauma* 1975;15:638–640.

17. Wei WI, Siu KF, Lau WF, et al. Emergency endotracheal intubation under fiberoptic endoscopic guidance for malignant laryngeal obstruction. *Otolaryngol Head Neck Surg* 1988;98:10–13.
18. Wei WI, Siu KF, Lau WF, et al. Emergency endotracheal intubation under fiberoptic endoscopic guidance for stenosis of the trachea. *Surg Gynecol Obstet* 1987;165:547–548.
19. Mandavia DP, Qualls S, Rokos I. Emergency airway management in penetrating neck injury. *Ann Emerg Med* 2000;35:221–225.
20. Edens ET, Sia RL. Flexible fiberoptic endoscopy in difficult intubations. *Ann Otol Rhinol Laryngol* 1981;90:307–309.
21. Hershey MD, Hannenberg AA. Gastric distention and rupture from oxygen insufflation during fiberoptic intubation. *Anesthesiology* 1996;85:1479–1480.
22. Ovassapian A, Mesnick PS, Hannenberg AA, et al. Oxygen insufflation through the fiberscope to assist intubation is not recommended. *Anesthesiology* 1997;87:183–184.

13

Rigid and Semirigid Fiberoptic Intubation

Michael F. Murphy and J. Adam Law

DESCRIPTION

Rigid and semirigid indirect laryngoscopes permit visualization of the glottis indirectly (in contrast to the direct line of sight of direct laryngoscopy) through an image transmitted to an eyepiece via a fiberoptic bundle. Unlike flexible fiberoptic devices, the fiberoptics in rigid devices are usually enclosed in an often J- or L-shaped blade. This preformed blade is easily inserted into the hypopharynx and enables the clinician to look around the tongue, thus "seeing around the corner." Therein lies the chief advantage of these rigid laryngoscopes: Anatomic features such as the anterior larynx, limited head and neck mobility, and limited mouth opening become less of an issue. The semirigid devices have a fiberoptic bundle or camera lens imbedded in a partly malleable stylet that is somewhat amenable to being shaped to conform to the patient's airway.

Examples of rigid indirect laryngoscopes include the **Bullard** Laryngoscope (Circon Corporation, Santa Barbara, CA), the **Upsherscope** (Mercury Medical, Clearwater, FL), and the **WuScope** (Achi Corporation, Fremont, CA). The semirigid devices include the **Shikani Optical Stylet** (SOS; Clarus Medical, Minneapolis, MN) and the **Bonfils** Retromolar Intubation Fiberscope (Karl Stortz Endoscopy, Tuttlingen, Germany). Other malleable intubating stylets are appearing on the market at regular intervals. Two additional laryngoscopes with video capability have recently been introduced:

* **The GlideScope** (Saturn Biomedical, Burnaby, British Columbia, Canada)
* **The Video Macintosh Intubating Laryngoscope System** (VMS; Karl Stortz Endoscopy, Tuttlingen, Germany)

Few of these devices have found their way into the armamentarium of emergency physicians or into emergency airway management. However, there is a growing interest in these devices as rescue devices for the failed and difficult airway, and their clear advantages over direct laryngoscopy suggest that they will come into increasing use, even for "routine" emergency airways.

There is more experience and literature about the Bullard Laryngoscope than the others and therefore the narrative for this device is somewhat longer. However, the other devices all have devotees and are growing in popularity in emergency airway management circles, particularly the Upsherscope, Shikani Optical Stylet, and Bonfils Retromolar Intubation Fiberscope. The video laryngoscope systems will likely gain a foothold as airway teaching devices and in the management of the difficult airway.

BULLARD LARYNGOSCOPE

Invented by American anesthesiologist Roger Bullard, the Bullard Laryngoscope (BL) is a rigid fiberoptic laryngoscope that incorporates a fiberoptic bundle into a long, curved, nonmalleable intubating blade. Once rotated into the hypopharynx, it is designed to sit in the appropriate intubating position, where it affords the clinician a fiberoptically delivered view of the larynx. An endotracheal tube (ETT) mounted on an attached stylet can then be advanced off the stylet into the trachea under visual control.

The BL is available in adult, pediatric, and infant sizes (Fig. 13-1). Incorporated centrally on the posterior aspect of this blade are three channels: one each carrying fiberoptic bundles for light source and image visualization, while the third is a hollow working channel. This Luer-lock fitted working channel can be used for the application of suction, instillation of local anesthetic, or insufflation of oxygen. A viewing arm leading off the blade ends in a viewing lens with variable focus capability. Located between the viewing arm and the proximal end of the working channel is an anchor for a detachable rigid introducing stylet.

The BL uses a standard laryngoscope battery handle similar to that used in an ordinary direct laryngoscope, and a video system can be attached to the viewing objective for teaching purposes. There are two different types of attachable introducing stylets that can be directly mounted on the Bullard Laryngoscope. These are designed to aid with passage of the ETT.

Blade Tip Extender. The distal end of the BL blade is most often used to pick up the epiglottis. In larger patients, the blade may prove too short to do this consistently. A nylon blade tip extender has been made available by the manufacturer to extend the length of the blade to aid in picking up the epiglottis. Many practitioners use it routinely in all male patients, and some use it in all patients. *It is imperative to ensure that the extender when applied (open*

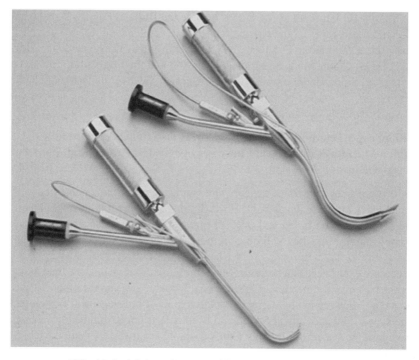

FIG. 13-1. Adult and neonatal Bullard Laryngoscopes.

notch down) clicks firmly on the end of the BL blade. Failure to do this can result in loss of the extender into the patient's hypopharynx. When properly clicked into place, it is very difficult to remove.

Indications and Contraindications

Indications for using a device such as the Bullard include:

- Predicted difficult intubation
- Rigid cervical spine immobilization is required. The operator sees the glottis via the fiberoptic eyepiece, so movement of the head and neck to align the axes of intubation for direct visualization is not required.
- Limited mouth opening. Because the image is conveyed fiberoptically, the intubator does not have to see in through the mouth, which need only be opened 2 cm to permit passage of the blade and tube.
- Failed intubation in the can't intubate, *can* oxygenate scenario in which the problem was inability to visualize the glottis

Contraindications include the following:

- Excessive blood and secretions in the upper airway can obscure the view and reduce the success rate with any fiberoptic technique; the Bullard Laryngoscope is no exception.
- The design of the device is dependent on normal upper-airway anatomy to maximize success. Upper-airway obstruction due to foreign bodies or other lesions is a relative contraindication.
- Can't intubate, can't ventilate/oxygenate scenario, unless the device is immediately available and does not delay the performance of a surgical airway

Technique

1. Preoxygenate the patient to the extent possible.
2. Attach the blade extender to the device.
3. Fogging can be prevented by warming the blade before insertion into the patient or putting a drop of antifog on the fiberoptic lens.
4. Oxygen can be insufflated down the working channel of the BL. Alternatively or additionally, nasal prongs can be used to deliver oxygen nasally or orally in the spontaneously breathing patient during the intubation attempt.
5. Load the ETT onto the stylet with the stylet protruding through the Murphy eye. (Some operators do not use the Murphy eye and simply load the ETT as with a standard stylet. It is worth noting that this is the only technique where a stylet is permitted to protrude beyond the end of the ETT because of the direct-vision nature of the technique.
6. Lubricate the blade and tube.
7. Hold the device in the left hand.
8. The patient's head and neck should be in the neutral position. The blade/stylet/ETT device is inserted into the mouth in the horizontal plane (Fig. 13-2**A**) over the top of the tongue, and then rotated caudad in the saggital plane into the posterior pharynx (Fig. 13-2**B**). The device follows the natural curve of the oro- and hypopharynx, and force is unnecessary to place the device.
9. Visualize the epiglottis through the fiberoptic viewer as the device is advanced, pick it up, and lift it anteriorly. This is done by lifting the handle away from the chin (Fig. 13-2**C**) and not by fulcruming. Visualize the glottic opening and advance the ETT off the stylet

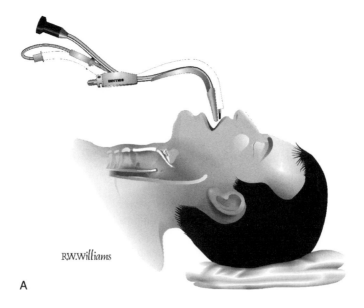

A

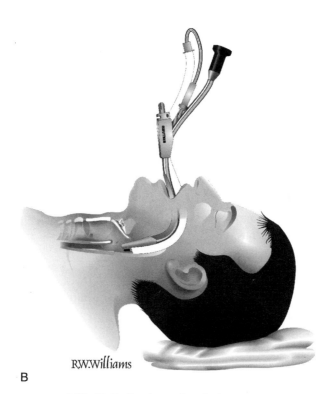

B

FIG. 13-2. See legend on facing page.

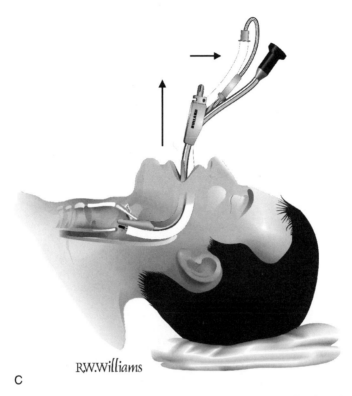

R.W.Williams

C

FIG. 13-2. Technique of insertion of the Bullard Laryngoscope. The body of the device is initially horizontal to insert the blade into the mouth (**A**) and then rotated over the back of the tongue to seat the device (**B**). The tip of the blade usually picks up the epiglottis. The entire device may need to be lifted (**C**) to enable passage of the ETT into the trachea.

into the airway (Fig. 13-3**A**). It may be necessary to lift up on the handle of the device and rock slightly forward until only the posterior aspect of the glottis is visible to get the ETT to enter the glottis. Alternatively, it may be easier to freehand an ETT loaded onto a stylet and "hockey sticked" with a sharp 90-degree bend distally, corresponding to the shape of the blade. Once the cords have been visualized, the ETT is inserted into the hypopharynx. Once its tip is visualized at the glottic opening, the ETT is advanced through the cords by advancing it off the stylet (as distinct from simply withdrawing the stylet).

10. Rock the BL to remove it from the mouth (Fig. 13-3**B**).

Success Rates and Complications

This device requires some practice, though those with experience with fiberoptic intubation catch onto the view presented and become oriented to the device relatively quickly.

Damage to teeth and airway structures is possible:

- If the device is forcefully inserted or manipulated
- If the tip of the stylet is not kept in view and prevented from skewering soft tissues

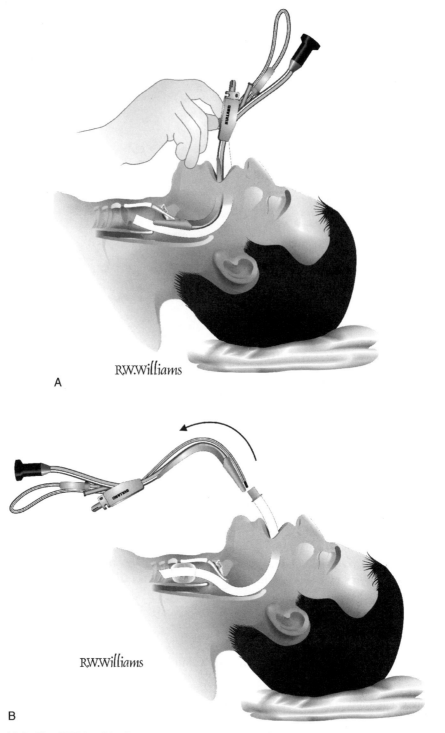

FIG. 13-3. The ETT is slid off the loaded stylet into the trachea (**A**) and the device is rotated out of the airway (**B**).

WU SCOPE

The WuScope is a rigid fiberoptic system available in two adult sizes. Though it can be used to facilitate either oral or nasal intubation, it is usually used orally. Also featuring a J-shaped rigid main blade, in this system a second bivalve blade is positioned with the main blade to form two round passageways (Fig. 13-4). An ETT is passed through one of the passageways and a flexible fiberoptic nasopharyngoscope, serving as the optical system, through the other. The exoskeleton provides an element of protection for the lens of the optical system from blood, secretions, or redundant soft tissues. There is a separate channel for insufflation of oxygen, and suction can be accomplished by passing a suction catheter through the ETT. This catheter can also be used as an intubation guide.

This device has yet to gain widespread use in the airway management community for a number of reasons:

- It can be awkward and time consuming to assemble the various parts.
- It is physically a large device and generates some degree of trepidation when inserted in the airway.
- The system requires purchasing both a nasopharyngoscope and the WuScope, so is significantly more expensive than other rigid devices.

Indications and Contraindications

Indications for using the WuScope include:

- Anticipated difficult airway, or a failed airway if time permits.
- Rigid cervical spine immobilization is required.

Contraindications to the use of the device include:

- Less than 25 mm of mouth opening

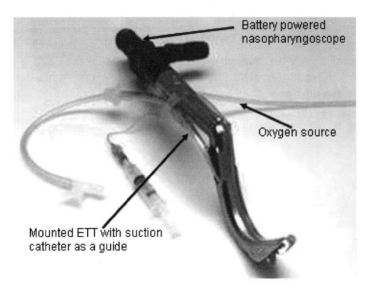

Battery powered nasopharyngoscope

Oxygen source

Mounted ETT with suction catheter as a guide

FIG. 13-4. The WuScope.

- Can't intubate, can't ventilate/oxygenate scenario, unless the device is immediately available and does not delay the performance of a surgical airway

Technique

The WuScope is designed to facilitate tracheal intubation with the patient's head in the ***neutral*** position without necessitating tongue displacement, head extension, or neck movement:

1. Introduce the properly assembled WuScope into the patient's mouth in the midline (Fig. 13-5**C**, view *A*). A minimum mouth opening of 20 to 25 mm is required.
2. Look through the eyepiece as the blade passes the uvula, the posterior pharyngeal wall, (Fig. 13-5**C**, view *B*), and the epiglottis toward the larynx (Fig. 13-**5C,** view *C*).
3. With the suction catheter as a guide, align the ETT with the glottis by gently moving the blade sideways, or withdrawing, advancing, or lifting up the device slightly.
4. When the ETT and the glottis are properly aligned, advance the ETT over the suction catheter and into the glottis.
5. Remove the bivalve element from the patient's mouth first, and then remove the handle, main blade, and fiberscope as one unit, leaving the ETT in place.

Complications

There is insufficient information about the instrument to identify complications at this time. Cricoid pressure may reduce the intubation success rate with the WuScope.

UPSHER SCOPE

Bearing similarities to the BL, the Upsherscope incorporates a tube-guiding delivery channel posteriorly where an ETT can be placed (Fig. 13-6). The blade differs from the BL blade in being more C-shaped: It is angled to only about 60 degrees and does not contain a working channel for oxygen or local anesthetic insufflation. Compatible with sizes 6.5 to 8.5 ETTs, the scope is available only in an adult version, and use has been limited to the oral route. As with other fiberoptic techniques, attention must be paid to antifogging measures. Insertion technique is similar to that described for the BL. Once the glottis is visualized, the (well-lubricated) ETT is advanced down the delivery channel and through the cords. As the ETT advances, it tends to move posteriorly and to the right: use of a gum elastic bougie within the lumen of the ETT may help with tube passage through the cords. A recent modification of the design has added a flange to the inferior portion of the channel to help guide the ETT anteriorly into the airway. Following intubation, the tube can be disengaged from the tube channel and the scope withdrawn.

SHIKANI OPTICAL STYLET

The Shikani Optical Stylet (SOS) is a semirigid stylet containing fiberoptic bundles for light and vision transmission (Fig. 13-7). The stylet, bent distally at about 45 degrees, ends proximally in an eyepiece. A bright halogen light is supplied from a battery-powered handle, but the stylet is also compatible with Green-specification fiberoptic laryngoscope handles or remote light sources via fiberoptic cable. A video camera can be applied proximally to the eyepiece. An adjustable tube stop holds the endotracheal tube on the SOS. The tube

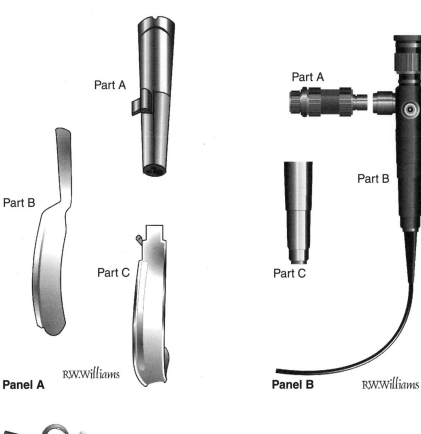

Part A

Part B

Part C

R.W.Williams

Panel A

Part A

Part B

Part C

R.W.Williams

Panel B

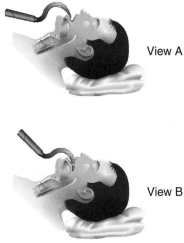

View A

View B

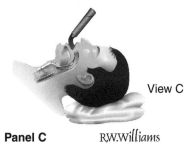

View C

Panel C R.W.Williams

FIG. 13-5. Panel A: The parts of the WuScope. Part *C* inserts into part *A* and locks into place. The clamshell type flange *B* then fits into part *C*, forming two channels: a small one for the fiberoptic nasopharyngoscope (**Panel B,** part *B*) and the other for the ETT. **Panel B:** Part *A* is a battery light source for the fiberscope and part *C* is a mounting device that fits onto the top of part *A* in panel **A. Panel C:** The WuScope being rotated into position.

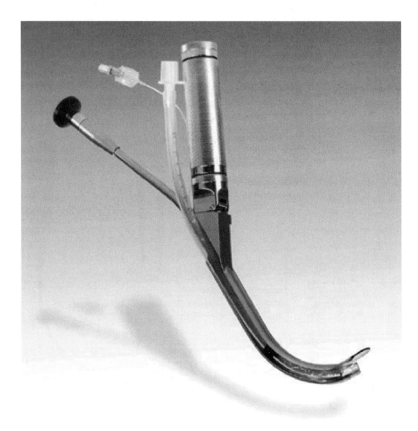

FIG. 13-6. The Upsherscope. Note the channel through which the ETT slides.

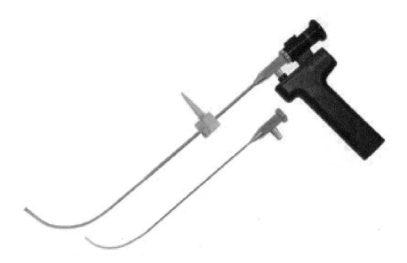

FIG. 13-7. Adult and pediatric Shikani Optical Stylet.

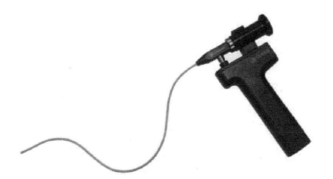

FIG. 13-8. The FAST (Flexible Airway Scope Tool).

stop incorporates an O_2 port, permitting insufflation of oxygen if indicated. The malleable distal section of the SOS stylet can be adjusted by hand to conform to the patient's anatomy.

To use the SOS, an ETT is loaded on the stylet, with the distal end of the stylet positioned just proximal to the ETT tip. The ETT can be stabilized in this position by using the tube stop proximally. The ETT–stylet combination can then be inserted into the mouth and hypopharynx under direct vision. An aggressive jaw lift/tongue pull during insertion will help maintain visual orientation through the scope. Alternatively, the instrument can be used in conjunction with direct laryngoscopy. For example, given an unanticipated Grade III laryngoscopy (epiglottis only), the ETT–SOS stylet combination can be inserted under the epiglottis under direct vision, whereupon the glottic opening can be sought through the eyepiece. With either technique, the ETT–stylet is advanced through the cords, and then the ETT is slid off the stylet into the trachea. The SOS stylet is advertised as being useful for the management of difficult and routine airways, with the video capability facilitating airway management teaching. The distal light source and mounted ETT suggest that it might be useful in light-guided intubation (similar to the Trachlight) though there is no literature to support this contention.

FAST (Flexible Airway Scope Tool; Fig. 13-8) is a fully flexible fiberoptic stylet attachment that is interchangeable with the semirigid SOS intubating stylet. It can be used to visually confirm the placement of ETTs, Combitubes, and LMA-Fastrach.

BONFILS RETROMOLAR INTUBATION FIBERSCOPE

Like the Shikani Optical Stylet, the Bonfils system is also a stylet containing fiberoptic bundles for light and vision transmission (Fig. 13-9). Intubation is performed in an identical manner to the SOS technique. The stylet, bent distally at about 45 degrees, ends proximally in an eyepiece, which unlike the SOS is moveable, permitting ease of use. This confers a substantial technical advantage for the Bonfils over the Shikani Optical Stylet. A small device on the shaft of the stylet enables the loaded ETT to be fixed at a position of the clinician's choice on the stylet. The continuous insufflation of oxygen prevents fogging during use. It can be used in conjunction with direct laryngoscopy or on its own.

Light sources may take the form of a laryngoscope handle or an external fiberoptic power source. A video adapter is also available. The video adapter seems particularly helpful for learning how to use the Bonfils.

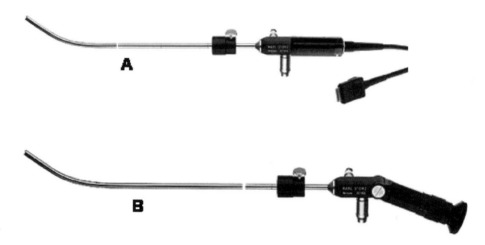

FIG. 13-9. The Bonfils Retromolar Intubation Fiberscope. **A:** The video equipped configuration. **B:** The direct-vision eyepiece. Note that the eyepiece has a swivel attachment.

The Bonfils is touted by the manufacturer as a device to be used in managing the difficult airway and has been used extensively in Europe and in a few North American sites. There is insufficient literature to draw conclusions about its performance in large series or to permit comparisons with other devices.

FIBEROPTIC AND VIDEO EQUIPPED CONVENTIONAL LARYNGOSCOPES

Two devices that incorporate a video capability in a conventional appearing Macintosh style laryngoscope blade are currently entering the marketplace:

- the Video Macintosh Intubating Laryngoscope System (VMS) (Karl Stortz Endoscopy, Tuttlingen, Germany)
- the GlideScope (Saturn Medical, Burnaby, British Columbia, Canada)

The VMS device adds a fiberoptic bundle to an exterior channel running along the back of a Macintosh laryngoscope blade. The fiber bundle emerges where the bulb is normally situated and connects proximally to a high-resolution color video monitor. The image provided is a wide-angle view of what the end of the laryngoscope blade encounters. The view of the larynx is remarkably clear.

The GlideScope has a high-resolution video camera embedded within the laryngoscope style blade (Fig. 13-10). A clear image is captured by the camera and displayed on a 7-in. LCD black and white monitor screen. A light-emitting diode (LED) light source mounted beside the camera provides continuous illumination during the intubation. Once the larynx is visualized, an ETT loaded onto a stylet and "hockey sticked" to a similar right angle as for the Trachlight can then be inserted freehand into the airway. Interestingly, although the GlideScope yields a consistently excellent view of the glottic aperture, it can be difficult to get the tube tip correctly positioned in the field of view. The manufacturer recommends a smooth, C-shaped curve for this purpose, but often, the right-angle "hockey stick" as for the Trachlight makes for easier insertion and better distal control.

Both the GlideScope and the VMS are reusable and are easily cleaned and sterilized. In addition, the devices:

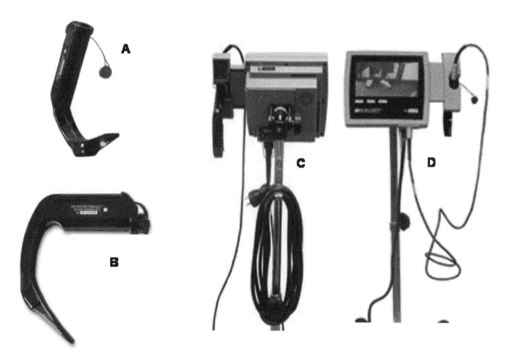

FIG. 13-10. The GlideScope. **A** and **B** depict the laryngoscope with the imbedded fiberoptic camera. A cable attaches the camera to a black and white video screen (**C** and **D**) that is mounted on wheels for positioning at the time of intubation and ease of transfer among intubating locations.

- Usually provide an unobstructed view of the glottis
- Are easy to learn how to use, particularly by someone accustomed to using a laryngoscope
- Are wonderful teaching tools

SUMMARY

It would appear that the appeal of rigid fiberoptic devices has retreated, or at the very least stalled, over the last few years. This may be due to many factors including cost (all of them), difficulty in maintaining skill and facility with the devices, complexity with the technique or the equipment, failure rates higher than expected (particularly in difficult airways), and finally, competition from the semirigid devices such as the Shikani and the Bonfils.

One of the assets of the rigid devices through the 1990s was the ability to display an intubation on a video monitor. This was an unparalleled teaching capability. Now all of the fiberoptic devices enjoy that capability, and the video laryngoscopes have the added advantage of doing so in a design format that looks, feels, and is used in a time-tested and familiar way.

Most airway management experts are of the opinion that the solution to failed intubation is entwined in the development of a fiberoptic visual assist device that, when combined with some other technology, will seek out and find the trachea in a fail-safe manner. The Bonfils, the Shikani, and other prototype devices are a step along that road.

In summary, the literature somewhat supports the use of the rigid fiberoptic devices in the management of the difficult airway, particularly when cervical spine immobilization is present. There is no evidence to support the use of any of these devices in the can't intubate, can't ventilate failed airway.

EVIDENCE

1. Bullard Laryngoscope: The Bullard was the first of the rigid fiberoptic laryngoscopes to be introduced into clinical use. This unique device gained early notoriety as perhaps being useful in the difficult airway (1–4), and was demonstrated to have some usefulness in airways such as these (3,4). National bodies recommended the device as an alternative that might be used in a difficult airway (5), and a few emergency departments acquired the device (6). However, it was not long before it was recognized that, although the device gave a stellar view of the glottis, it was a challenge to get the tube to go through the cords, and tricks and tips populated the literature (7–9). The initial enthusiasm for the device waned though it remained useful in managing the patient with an immobilized cervical spine (10–14), a common method of simulating a difficult airway (11). The device has performed well in a head-to-head comparison with flexible fiberoptic intubation for patients with immobilized cervical spines (14). Dislodgement of the blade extender has emerged as a real risk (15). On balance, the technical difficulties experienced by Bullard users, the acceptance of rapid sequence intubation with in-line stabilization for patients with potential cervical spine injuries and the introduction of newer devices has pushed the Bullard from the forefront of rigid fiberoptic devices.

2. WuScope: The WuScope was initially designed for the difficult airway (16), and early case studies suggested it might be useful for some causes of difficult airway such as expanding neck hematomas and other causes of upper-airway compression and in trauma (17–19). Like the Bullard, it was also touted to be of use in the cervical spine-immobilized patient (20–22). Success rates suffer when cricoid pressure is in place (23), suggesting that its role in emergency airway management might be limited.

3. Upsherscope: Few studies have been published on the use of the Upsherscope. Fridrich compared use of the Upsherscope with direct laryngoscopy in a randomized controlled trial and found that the Upsherscope resulted in a longer time to intubation, needed more attempts, and had a higher incidence of failure (24). A second study assessing the Upsherscope in 200 patients resulted in successful intubation of 95% of the patients, with the intubation being judged as straightforward in just under half the patients (25). Both studies noted difficulty in picking up the epiglottis, perhaps because of inadequate angulation of the blade. Some authorities have included the Upsherscope on a list of devices that are potentially useful in the difficult airway (26). The intubating stylet has been coupled with the Upsherscope to enhance success (27). At present, there is insufficient literature to support its use in emergency airway management.

4. Shikani Optical Stylet, Bonfils Retromolar Intubation Fiberscope, Video Macintosh Intubating Laryngoscope System, and the GlideScope: References are provided for the reader's review (28–33), though presently there is no literature regarding the use of any of these devices for managing airways in the emergency department.

REFERENCES

Bullard Laryngoscope

1. Borland LM, Casselbrandt M. The Bullard laryngoscope. A New indirect oral laryngoscope (pediatric version). *Anesth Analg* 1990;70:105–108.

2. Cohn AI, McGraw SR, King WH. Awake intubation of the adult trachea using the Bullard laryngoscope. *Can J Anaesth* 1995;42:246–248.
3. Gorback MS. Management of the challenging airway with the Bullard laryngoscope. *J Clin Anesth* 1991;3:473–477.
4. Cohn AI, Hart RT, McGraw SR, et al. The Bullard laryngoscope for emergency airway management in a morbidly obese parturient. *Anesth Analg* 1995;81:872–873.
5. Crosby ET, Cooper RM, Douglas MJ, et al. The unanticipated difficult airway with recommendations for management. *Can J Anaesth* 1998;45:757–776.
6. Levitan RM, Kush S, Hollander JE. Devices for difficult airway management in academic emergency departments: results of a national survey. *Ann Emerg Med* 1999;33:694–698.
7. Crosby ET. Techniques using the Bullard laryngoscope. *Anesth Analg* 1995;81:1314–1315.
8. Habibi A, Bushell E, Jaffe RA, et al. Two tips for users of Bullard intubating laryngoscope. *Anesth Analg* 1998;87:1206–1208.
9. Dunn SM, Shulman GB, Cohn AI. More tips for users of the Bullard laryngoscope. *Anesth Analg* 1999;89:267.
10. Cohn AI, Zornow MH. Awake endotracheal intubation in patients with cervical spine disease: a comparison of the Bullard laryngoscope and the fiberoptic bronchoscope. *Anesth Analg* 1995;81:1283–1286.
11. MacQuarrie K, Hung OR, Law JA. Tracheal intubation using a Bullard laryngoscope for patients with a simulated difficult airway. *Can J Anaesth* 1999;46:760–765.
12. Hastings RH, Vigil AC, Hanna R, et al. Cervical spine movement during laryngoscopy with the Bullard, MacIntosh, and Miller laryngoscopes. *Anesthesiology* 1995;82:859–869.
13. Watts ADJ, Gelb AW, Bach DB, et al. Comparison of the Bullard and MacIntosh laryngoscopes for endotracheal intubation of patients with a potential cervical spine injury. *Anesthesiology* 1997;87:1335–1342.
14. Shulman GB, Connelly NR. A comparison of the Bullard laryngoscope versus the flexible fiberoptic bronchoscope during intubation in patients afforded inline stabilization. *J Clin Anesth* 2001;13:182–185.
15. Marshall KA, James CF. Complication of Bullard laryngoscope: dislodgment of blade-extender resulting in an upper airway foreign body. *Anesthesiology* 1998;89:1604–1605.

WuScope

16. Wu TL, Chou HC. A new laryngoscope—the combination intubating device. *Anesthesiology* 1994;81:1085–1087.
17. Wu TL. Use of the WuScope tubular fiberoptic laryngoscope in post-carotid endarterectomy airway obstruction. In: Problems in Airway Management. *Anesthesiology News* 2000 (Oct);128–131.
18. Chou HC, Wu TL. Long and narrow pharyngolaryngeal passage in difficult airway. *Anesth Analg* 2002;94:478.
19. Wu TL, Chou HC. Use of the WuScope in the trauma patient. In: Trauma Anesthesia Quarterly. *Anesthesiology News* 1995(Oct);40–42.
20. Sandhu NS, Schaffer S, Capan LM, et al. Comparison of the WuScope and Macintosh #3 blade in normal and cervical spine stabilized patients. *Anesthesiology* 1999;91:A480.
21. Smith CE, Pinchak AB, Sidhu TS, et al. Evaluation of tracheal intubation difficulty in patients with cervical spine immobilization: fiberoptic (WuScope) versus conventional laryngoscopy. *Anesthesiology* 1999;91:1253–1259.
22. Wu TL, Chou HC. WuScope versus conventional laryngoscope in cervical spine immobilization. *Anesthesiology* 2000;93:588.
23. Smith CE, Boyer D. Cricoid pressure decreases ease of tracheal intubation using fiberoptic laryngoscopy (WuScope System). *Can J Anaesth* 2002;49:614–619.

UpsherScope

24. Fridrich P, Frass M, Krenn CG, et al. The UpsherScope in routine and difficult airway management: a randomized, controlled clinical trial. *Anesth Analg* 1997;85:1377–1381.
25. Pearce AC, Shaw S, Macklin S. Evaluation of the Upsherscope. *Anaesthesia* 1996;51:561–564.
26. Foley LJ, Ochroch EA. Bridges to establish an emergency airway and alternate intubating techniques. *Crit Care Clin* 2000;16:429–444.
27. Yeo V, Chung DC, Hin LY. A bougie improves the clinical utility of the Upsherscope. *J Clin Anesth* 1999;11:471–476.

Shikani Optical Stylet

28. Shikani AH. New "seeing" stylet-scope and method for the management of the difficult airway. *Otolaryngol Head Neck Surg* 1999;120:113–116.
29. Agro F, Cataldo R, Carassiti M, et al. The seeing stylet: a new device for tracheal intubation. *Resuscitation* 2000;44:177–180.

30. Pfitzner L, Cooper MG, Ho D. The Shikani seeing stylet for difficult intubation in children: initial experience. *Anaesth Intensive Care* 2002;30:462–466.

Bonfils Retromolar Intubation Fiberscope

31. Kleeman PP, Jantzen JP, Bonfils P. The ultra-thin bronchoscope in management of the difficult paediatric airway. *Can J Anaesth* 1987;34:606–608.

Video Macintosh Intubating Laryngoscope System

32. Kaplan MB, Ward DS, Berci G. A new video laryngoscope—an aid to intubation and teaching. *J Clin Anesth* 2002;14:620–626.
33. Schwarz U, Weiss M. Endotracheal intubation of patients with Pierre-Robin sequence. Successful use of video intubation laryngoscope. *Anaesthesist* 2001;50:118–121.

14

Video Laryngoscopy

John C. Sakles

DESCRIPTION

Video laryngoscopy is a new technology and concept that has recently been applied to airway management. Several airway devices incorporating a micro video camera have recently been introduced. These include the GlideScope (Saturn Biomedical, Burnaby, British Columbia, Canada), the X-Lite Video by Rusch (Duluth, GA), and the Video Macintosh Laryngoscope by Karl Storz Endoscopy (Tuttlingen, Germany). Only the GlideScope is a true video laryngoscope in the strictest sense. The other video laryngoscopes use fiberoptics to transmit the image to the video camera and thus are more of a hybrid of a fiberoptic and video scope. This discussion focuses on the GlideScope as the protypical video laryngoscope. The GlideScope system, by Saturn Biomedical, consists of several elements. There is a unified plastic handle and curved laryngoscope blade that has a micro video camera embedded on the undersurface of the blade (Fig. 14-1). The video camera is placed about midway down the blade, *not* at the tip as is the case with most optical airway devices. This design allows one to have a greater field of view, which facilitates navigation to the glottis, and additionally, protects the lens from contamination, thus helping to overcome two of the greatest limitations of conventional fiberoptic devices. The laryngoscope attaches to a 7-inch liquid crystal display (LCD) monitor via a video cable that also carries power to two light-emitting diodes (LEDs) mounted alongside the video camera to provide illumination. The monitor displays a black and white image with a resolution of 320×240. The black and white nature of the image actually provides a sharper picture than a comparable color video device. The monitor has a video out port (RCA type) so that the image can be sent to another monitor or to a VCR for recording. The monitor has several on-screen controls that allow the operator to adjust features such as brightness, contrast, orientation, and so on. The monitor is attached to a cradle that allows it to be rotated to the optimal viewing angle, and the cradle rests on a mobile telescoping pole that allows easy adjustment of the height of the monitor (Fig. 14-2). The unit is powered by AC current and must be plugged into a wall socket to function. However, there are currently plans underway to develop a battery-powered unit. The laryngoscope blade has a 60-degree angulation that allows the operator to see quite far anteriorly with a minimum of lifting force. The two small LEDs (one blue and one red) on the laryngoscope blade provide adequate illumination. Because the video camera is black and white, the required illumination, and thus power, is kept to a minimum. The video camera incorporates an antifog device that is of great utility in emergency intubations where excessive secretions are the norm. Currently, only an adult laryngoscope blade is available with the GlideScope unit. A pediatric blade and a neonatal blade have recently been developed and likely will be available in the near future.

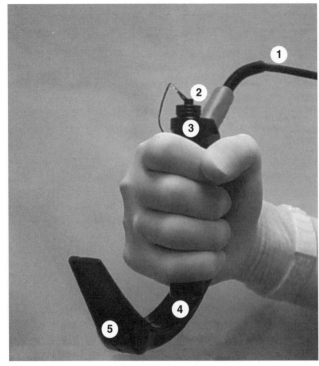

KEY
1 Video cable
2 Terminal protective cap
3 Laryngoscope handle
4 Laryngoscope blade
5 Videocamera

FIG. 14-1. GlideScope laryngoscope.

INDICATIONS AND CONTRAINDICATIONS

The GlideScope can be used for routine intubations and can also be considered an alternative airway device for difficult or failed airways. It is ideally suited to visualize and intubate an anterior larynx where direct laryngoscopy has proven unsuccessful. Because it does not require direct visualization of the larynx through the mouth, it is useful when cervical mobility or mouth opening is limited. Patients in whom it is desirable to minimize movement of the neck are excellent candidates as very little force is needed to expose the glottis with the laryngoscope blade. The GlideScope performs very well in the presence of secretions, blood, and vomit and thus is a good choice in these circumstances.

The only absolute contraindication to use of the GlideScope is restricted mouth opening of less than 18 mm, as this is the width of the widest portion of the blade. Relative contraindications to use of the GlideScope are situations in which the tube must be placed rapidly, for example, in a patient who desaturates very quickly or a patient with massive pulmonary edema requiring aggressive suctioning during intubation. Although glottic visualization is achieved very rapidly in almost all cases, insertion of the endotracheal tube (ETT) takes longer than is the case with direct laryngoscopy because of difficulty negotiating the angle to the anteriorly positioned glottis.

TECHNIQUE

The GlideScope is used in the following manner to perform tracheal intubation. The handle is grasped with the left hand, in the same fashion as a conventional laryngoscope, and the

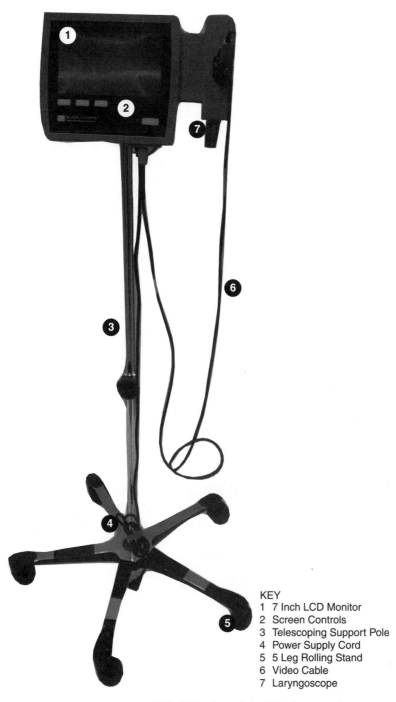

KEY
1 7 Inch LCD Monitor
2 Screen Controls
3 Telescoping Support Pole
4 Power Supply Cord
5 5 Leg Rolling Stand
6 Video Cable
7 Laryngoscope

FIG. 14-2. Complete GlideScope unit.

tip of the laryngoscope blade is gently inserted between the teeth under direct vision. Occasionally it is necessary to use a scissor technique to open the mouth or perform a jaw thrust to lift the tongue anteriorly so that the blade can pass underneath it. The critical point here is to start out in the *midline* of the tongue. There is **no** sweeping of the tongue to the left as is done with conventional laryngoscopy. It is very difficult to identify landmarks if the blade is off midline. As soon as the tip of the laryngoscope blade passes the teeth, the operator should direct his or her attention to the video monitor and use the landmarks on the video screen to navigate to the glottic aperture. Typically the uvula will be seen if the blade is correctly situated in the midline. The operator should then continue to walk the blade down the tongue, past the uvula, with a slight elevating motion until the epiglottis is seen. At the point, it is best to continue advancing the blade in the vallecula, with some gentle upward force, to lift the epiglottis out of the way (Fig. 14-3**A**). The blade should ultimately be seated in the vallecula much in the same way that a Macintosh blade would be. If the glottic view is insufficient, often a gentle tilt of the handle will expose it fully, in contradistinction to the lifting motion with a conventional laryngoscope. If the glottic aperture still cannot be exposed, the blade can be withdrawn a bit, placed under the epiglottis, and used like a Miller blade to physically displace the epiglottis up and out of the way (Fig. 14-3**B**). The problem with doing this is that this tends to tilt the larynx more sharply, making advancement of the tube into the trachea technically more challenging. Identifying and exposing the glottis is the easy part of using the GlideScope. The challenging

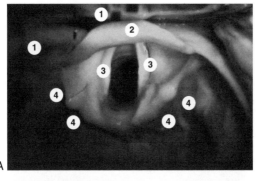

KEY
1 GlideScope blade
2 Epiglottis
3 Vocal cords
4 Arytenoids

A

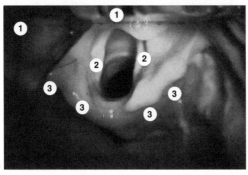

KEY
1 GlideScope blade
2 Vocal cords
3 Arytenoids

B

FIG. 14-3. A: View of the glottis with the GlideScope seated in the vallecula, similar to use of a curved Macintosh laryngoscope blade. **B:** View of the glottis using the GlideScope as a straight blade (Miller) and directly displacing the epiglottis upwards.

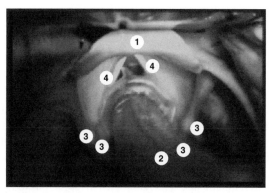

KEY
1 Epiglottis
2 Endotracheal tube
3 Arytenoids
4 Vocal cords

FIG. 14-4. View of endotracheal tube entering the trachea aperture as seen through the GlideScope.

part is actually directing the ETT toward the image of the glottis the operator is seeing on the video screen. This is technically difficult for two reasons. The first is that the GlideScope video camera is directed at an angle of 60 degrees and thus the angle of attack of the tube is quite steep, compounded by the fact that the GlideScope tends to tilt the glottis inferiorly, further increasing the acuity of the angle of entry. The second issue is that using the screen to navigate to the glottis requires some stereoscopic skill and hand–eye coordination that may not come naturally to all operators. The key to getting the tube to enter the trachea has to do with forming the ETT in the right shape before inserting it into the patient's mouth. There are two options. The manufacturer recommends bending the ETT to conform to the shape of the GlideScope blade: a gentle curve of 60 degrees. An alternative approach is to bend the tube at a right angle just proximal to the cuff, similar to the configuration of the tube when using the Trachlight (see Chapter 11). The tube is then inserted into the right corner of the mouth and rotated upward, at which point the tip of the tube should be pointing at the glottis. Gentle forward rotation of the tube on the apex of the bend, which is sitting on the posterior pharyngeal wall, will then allow the operator to align the tip of the tube perfectly with the glottic entrance. Advancement of the tube then allows the tip to pass through the cords under direct video visualization (Fig. 14-4). At this point, because of the extreme angulation, it is very difficult to continue advancing the tube into the trachea, and thus it is wise to **withdraw the stylet** several centimeters, or even completely, while maintaining gentle steady forward pressure on the tube in a manner analogous to that for the Trachlight. Additionally, if the **GlideScope is withdrawn** about 2 cm, the larynx drops down, lessening the sharp angle and greatly facilitating further advancement of the tube. Standard methods of tube confirmation can then be performed, including mandatory end-tidal carbon dioxide (CO_2) determination.

The GlideScope laryngoscope blade must be cleaned and disinfected after each use. Gross contaminants and large debris can be scrubbed off with a surgical scrub brush or enzymatically removed with a proteolytic compound such as Enzyme or Medzyme. For sterilization of the blade, Steris, Sterrad, ethylene oxide, pasteurization, or glutaraldehyde are all acceptable and safe. The electrical connector cap should be placed over the electrical contact port on the laryngoscope handle to prevent corrosion of the contacts. The only method of sterilization that is absolutely contraindicated is autoclaving, which involves exposure of the device to very high temperatures that will damage the video camera element. In fact, the laryngoscope blade has a silver temperature indicator that turns black if the device is exposed to temperatures exceeding 80° Celsius.

COMPLICATIONS

The complications of GlideScope intubation have not been well documented, as the device is fairly new. It is anticipated that the complications will likely mirror those of conventional laryngoscopy, but may be somewhat reduced because the GlideScope does not require the lifting force of conventional laryngoscopy to permit direct visualization of the glottis from outside the patient's mouth. The incidence of failed intubation is not yet known, but in almost every instance, the glottis will be visualized and failure will occur because of inability to pass the tube through the vocal cords into the trachea. The direct visualization during insertion and intubation suggests that there is very little likelihood of laryngeal trauma from the GlideScope. There can be some minor laryngeal trauma from the tip of the ETT as one attempts to navigate the tube between vocal cords. It is not unusual for novice GlideScope users to hit the arytenoids while trying to direct the tube between the cords, underscoring the need for gentle technique as for all intubations.

EVIDENCE

The GlideScope has only recently been introduced into clinical practice, so there is little research on the device. In a letter to the editor, Agro et al. compared the glottic exposure achieved with the GlideScope to the view obtained with a Macintosh blade in 15 patients with cervical immobilization (1). They found that the GlideScope improved the Cormack-Lehane view of the glottis by one grade in 14 out of 15 patients. In one patient, who was a grade III airway, the GlideScope did not improve the view of the glottis and the patient was intubated with the aid of a bougie. The glottic views in this series of patients were poor during conventional laryngoscopy, when compared to a routine operating room (OR) population or to previous intubation studies, suggesting a difficulty airway cohort, although the author did not report this. For example, using a standard Macintosh blade, one patient was a grade 4, 9 patients were grade 3, 5 patients were grade 2, and no patients were grade 1. Thus in this small series the vocal cords could be identified in only 5 out of 15 patients (33%), compared with 95% in routine OR series. In an abstract by Sakles et al. the GlideScope (GS) was compared to two fiberoptic airway devices, the UpsherScope (US) and the Seeing Optical Stylet (SOS; Chapter 13) (2). Emergency medicine residents with no prior experience with these devices were asked to intubate manikins, and the success rate for each device and the time needed to perform the intubation was evaluated. The GlideScope was successful 100% of the time and on average required one attempt and 65 seconds to perform the intubation. The US had a success rate of 71% and on average required 1.4 attempts and 65 seconds. The SOS was successful in only 43% of the cases and on average required 2.2 attempts and 128 seconds. If the results of this small pilot study are validated by a larger investigation, one would have to conclude that the GlideScope has a shorter learning curve than the other devices when applied to manikin training. The authors hypothesized that the greater success rate and faster time to intubation with the GlideScope may have been due to the similarity of the device and technique to conventional laryngoscopy. In summary, there has been very little formal evaluation of the GlideScope to date, and no controlled studies have yet been published. Preliminary evidence supports clinical experience that this device may prove to be a highly effective emergency airway device, particularly in patients with poor laryngoscopic view by conventional laryngoscopy.

REFERENCES

1. Agro F, Barzoi G, Montecchia F. Tracheal intubation using a Macintosh laryngoscope or GlideScope in 15 patients with cervical spine immobilization [Letter]. *Brit J of Anaesthesia* 2003;90:705–706.
2. Sakles JC, Tolby N, VanderHeyden TC, et al. Ability of emergency medicine residents to use alternative optical airway devices. Paper presented at: the Western Meeting of the Society for Academic Emergency Medicine; April 2003; Phoenix, AZ.

ADDITIONAL READING

Cooper RM. Use of a new videolaryngoscope (GlideScope) in the management of the difficult airway. *Can J Anesth* 2003;50:611–613.

15

Surgical Airway Techniques

Robert J. Vissers and Aaron E. Bair

I. Surgical airway management

Surgical airway management is defined as the creation of an airway by an invasive technique. All other methods of airway management use existing anatomic portals of access to the trachea (i.e., nasopharynx, oropharynx). Surgical airway management involves the creation of an opening to the trachea by surgical means. This opening is then used to provide ventilation and oxygenation. There is some confusion engendered by use of the term *surgical airway management*. In some discussions, surgical airway management includes both cricothyrotomy and needle cricothyrotomy with percutaneous transtracheal ventilation. Other discussions limit *surgical airway management* to cricothyrotomy and consider percutaneous transtracheal ventilation to be simply another airway management technique. For the purposes of discussion in this chapter, *surgical airway management* is deemed to include cricothyrotomy, percutaneous transtracheal ventilation, and placement of a surgical airway using a cricothyrotome, which is a device intended to place a surgical airway percutaneously without performance of formal cricothyrotomy. The cricothyrotomes may be considered as an alternative to cricothyrotomy; however, most of the available cricothyrotomes use an uncuffed tube and therefore do not afford airway protection and are limited in the amount of positive airway pressure that they can generate.

Some newer kits have added a cuffed tube and represent a better choice of cricothyrotome in the emergency setting. Similarly, percutaneous transtracheal ventilation does not protect the airway and should be considered a temporizing measure only. A kit has recently been developed that offers all the instruments and equipment to perform either the Seldinger percutaneous cricothyrotome or an open cricothyrotomy, using a cuffed tube for both methods (Melker Universal Cricothyrotomy Catheter Kit, Cook Critical Care, Bloomington, IN). In children 12 years of age or under, however, percutaneous transtracheal ventilation is the method of choice for surgical airway management because of the technical difficulties of cricothyrotomy and cricothyrotome placement (see later). Each of the surgical airway techniques is described in detail in the sections that follow.

A. Description

Cricothyrotomy is the establishment of a surgical opening in the airway through the cricothyroid membrane and placement of a cuffed tracheostomy tube or endotracheal tube (ETT).

A cricothyrotome is a kit or device that is intended to establish a surgical airway without resorting to formal cricothyrotomy. These kits use two basic approaches. One approach relies on the Seldinger technique, in which the airway is accessed via a small needle through which a flexible guide wire is passed. The airway device, with a dilator, is then passed over this guide wire and into the airway in a manner analogous with that of central line placement by the Seldinger technique. The other type of technique relies on the direct percutaneous placement of an airway device without the use of a Seldinger technique. There have been no clinical studies to date demonstrating the superiority of one approach over another or of any of these devices over formal surgical cricothyrotomy. However, certain attributes of the devices make them intuitively more, or less, hazardous for insertion (see the *Evidence* section later).

B. Indications and contraindications

The primary indication for cricothyrotomy is when a failed airway has occurred (see Chapter 2) and the patient cannot be adequately ventilated or oxygenated with a bag and mask, or the patient is adequately oxygenated but there is not another available device (e.g., fiberoptic scope, lighted stylet, intubating laryngeal mask airway (LMA), etc.) that is felt to be appropriate for that patient. A second indication is a method of primary airway management in patients for whom nasotracheal or orotracheal intubation is contraindicated or felt to be impossible. Thus, cricothyrotomy should be thought of as a rescue technique in most circumstances, and only infrequently will it be used as the primary method of airway management. An example of a circumstance in which cricothyrotomy is the primary method of airway management is the patient with severe lower facial trauma in whom access through the mouth or nose would be too time-consuming or impossible. This patient requires immediate airway management because of the risk of aspiration of blood and secretions, and cricothyrotomy is indicated.

Providers must recognize that often the main hurdle to performing cricothyrotomy is simply recognizing when it is necessary to proceed with surgical airway management, abandoning further attempts at laryngoscopy or the use of an alternative device. Rapid sequence intubation, augmented by a variety of noninvasive airway management methods, is so successful that cricothyrotomy is often viewed as a method of last resort, to be undertaken only after multiple noninvasive attempts or techniques have failed. However, the relentless (unsuccessful) pursuit of a noninvasive airway along with the resultant delay in the initiation of a surgical airway can readily result in hypoxic disaster. This fact is particularly true in the can't intubate, can't oxygenate circumstance, when surgical airway management is immediately indicated and must not be delayed while attempts are made with other devices.

Once the decision to initiate surgical airway management has been made, there are a few fundamental considerations:

a) Will accessing the cricothyroid membrane be *effective*? In other words, will an incision at the level of the cricothyroid membrane bypass the obstruction and solve the problem? If the obstructing lesion is significantly distal to the cricothyroid membrane, performing a cricothyrotomy is a critical waste of time (see Chapter 32).

b) Will the patient's anatomy or pathological process make cricothyrotomy *difficult* to perform? Placement of the initial skin incision is based on palpating the pertinent anatomy. If adiposity, burns, trauma, or infection make this procedure difficult, then the strategy should be adjusted accordingly. A mnemonic for difficult cricothyrotomy (SHORT) is shown in Box 15-1.

c) Which *type* of invasive technique will most readily be used (i.e., open surgical or percutaneous)? This consideration takes into account provider preference based on previous experience and equipment availability.

> **Box 15-1.** Mnemonic for Difficult Cricothyrotomy
>
> **S**urgery (history of neck surgery, presence of surgical scar)
> **H**ematoma
> **O**besity
> **R**adiation (history or evidence of radiation therapy)
> **T**rauma (direct laryngeal trauma with disrupted landmarks)

Contraindications for surgical airway management are few and, with one exception, are relative. That one exception is young age. Children have a small, pliable, mobile larynx and cricoid cartilage, making cricothyrotomy extremely difficult. For children under 12 years of age, unless they are teenage or adult sized, percutaneous transtracheal ventilation should be used as the surgical airway management technique of choice (see Chapters 19 and 20). Relative contraindications include preexisting laryngeal or tracheal pathology such as tumor, infections, or abscess in the area in which the procedure will be performed; hematoma or other anatomic destruction of the landmarks that would render the procedure difficult or impossible; coagulopathy; and lack of operator expertise. Cricothyrotomy has been performed successfully after systemic thrombolytic therapy. Cricothyrotomy has a very high success rate when performed in the emergency department (ED) setting. The presence of an anatomic barrier in particular should prompt consideration of alternative techniques that might result in a successful airway. However, in cases in which no alternative method of airway management is likely to be successful or timely enough, cricothyrotomy should be performed without hesitation. The same principles apply for both the cricothyrotome and for percutaneous transtracheal ventilation.

Percutaneous transtracheal ventilation is not contraindicated in small children and, in fact, is the surgical airway method of choice for children under 12 years of age. The cricothyrotomes have not been demonstrated to improve success rates or time or to decrease complication rates when compared with surgical cricothyrotomy. As with formal cricothyrotomy, experience, skill, knowledge of anatomy, and adherence to proper technique are essential for success when a cricothyrotome is used.

C. TECHNIQUE

1. Anatomy and landmarks

The cricothyroid membrane is the anatomical site of access in the emergent surgical airway, regardless of the technique used. It has several advantages over the trachea in the emergent setting. The cricothyroid membrane is more anterior than the lower trachea, and there is less thyroid and soft tissue between the membrane and the skin. There is less vascularity and less chance of significant bleeding.

The cricothyroid membrane is identified by first locating the laryngeal prominence (notch) of the thyroid cartilage. Approximately one fingerbreadth below the laryngeal prominence, the membrane may be palpated in the midline of the anterior neck, as a soft depression between the inferior aspect of the thyroid cartilage above and the hard cricoid ring below. The relevant anatomy may be easier to appreciate in males, because of the more prominent thyroid notch. The thyrohyoid space, which lies above the laryngeal prominence, and the hyoid bone, which resides high in the neck, should also be identified. This will prevent the misidentification of the thyrohyoid membrane as the cricothyroid membrane, which would lead to misplacement of the tracheostomy tube above the vocal cords. In children, the cricothyroid membrane is disproportionately smaller because of a greater overlap of the thyroid cartilage over the cricoid cartilage. For this reason, cricothyrotomy is not recommended in children age 12 or less.

Unfortunately, the same anatomic or physiologic abnormalities (i.e., trauma, morbid obesity, congenital anomalies) that necessitated the surgical airway also may hinder easy palpation of landmarks. One way to estimate the location of the cricothyroid membrane is by placing four fingers on the neck, oriented longitudinally, with the small finger in the sternal notch. The membrane is approximately located under the index finger and can serve as a point at which the initial incision is made. Except as described later in the technique for the rapid four-step cricothyrotomy, a vertical skin incision is preferred, and particularly so if anatomic landmarks are not readily apparent. Palpation through this vertical incision can then confirm the location of the cricothyroid membrane. Alternatively, identification may be assisted by using a locator needle attached to a syringe containing saline or lidocaine. Aspiration of air bubbles suggests entry into the airway, but will not distinguish between the cricothyroid membrane and a lower tracheal placement.

2. **Cricothyrotomy technique**
   a. **The no-drop technique**
      The cricothyrotomy instrument set should be simple, consisting of only that equipment necessary to complete the procedure. A sample listing of recommended contents of a cricothyrotomy tray is shown in Box 15-2.
      (1) Identify the landmarks
          The cricothyroid membrane is identified using the landmarks described previously (Fig. 15-1).
      (2) Prepare the neck
          If time permits, apply appropriate antiseptic solution. Local anesthesia is desirable if the patient is conscious. Infiltration of the skin and subcutaneous tissue of the anterior neck with 1% lidocaine solution will provide adequate anesthesia. If time permits and the patient is conscious and responsive, anesthetize the airway by injecting lidocaine by transcricothyroid membrane puncture (see Chapter 7). The patient will cough briefly, but the airway will be reasonably adequately anesthetized.
      (3) Immobilize the larynx
          Throughout the procedure, the larynx must be immobilized (Fig. 15-2). This is best done by placing the thumb and long finger on opposite sides of

---

Box 15-2. Recommended Contents of Cricothyrotomy Tray

a. Trousseau dilator
b. Tracheal hook
c. Scalpel with no. 11 blade
d. Cuffed, nonfenestrated, no. 4 tracheostomy tube
e. Optional equipment may include several 4 × 4 gauze sponges, two small hemostats, and surgical drapes.

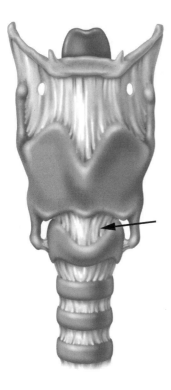

FIG. 15-1. Anatomy of the larynx. The cricothyroid membrane (*arrow*) is bordered above by the thyroid cartilage and below by the cricoid cartilage.

the superior laryngeal horns, the posterior superior aspect of the laryngeal cartilage. With the thumb and long finger thus placed, the index finger is ideally positioned anteriorly to relocate and reidentify the cricothyroid membrane at any time during the procedure.

(4) Incise the skin

A 2-cm vertical midline skin incision should be used (Fig. 15-3). Care should be taken to avoid cutting the deeper structures of the neck. The cricothyroid membrane is separated from the outside world only by skin, subcutaneous tissue, and anterior cervical fascia. An overly vigorous incision risks damage to the larynx, cricoid cartilage, and the trachea.

(5) Reidentify the membrane

With the thumb and long finger maintaining immobilization of the larynx, the index finger can now palpate the anterior larynx, the cricothyroid membrane, and the cricoid cartilage without any interposed skin or subcutaneous tissue (Fig. 15-4). The landmarks thus confirmed, the index finger can be left in the wound by placing it on the inferior aspect of the anterior larynx, thus providing a clear indicator of the superior extent of the cricothyroid membrane.

(6) Incise the membrane

The cricothyroid membrane should be incised in a horizontal direction, with an incision at least 1 cm long (Fig. 15-5A). It is recommended to try to incise the lower half of the membrane rather than the upper half because of the relatively superior location of the superior cricothyroid artery and vein (Fig. 15-5B).

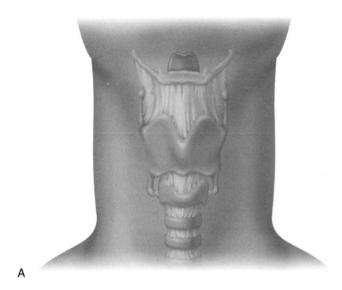

A

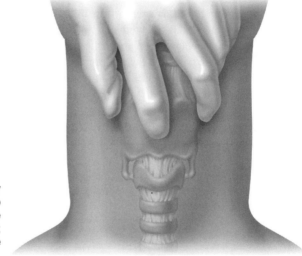

B

FIG. 15-2. A: Surface anatomy of the airway. **B:** The thumb and long finger immobilize the superior cornua of the larynx; the index finger palpates the cricothyroid membrane.

(7) Insert the tracheal hook

The tracheal hook is rotated so that it is oriented in the transverse plane, passed through the incision, and then rotated again so that the hook is oriented in a cephalad direction. The hook is then applied to the inferior aspect of the thyroid cartilage, and gentle upward and cephalad traction is applied to bring the airway immediately out to the skin incision (Fig. 15-6). If an assistant is available, this hook may be passed to the assistant to maintain immobilization of the larynx.

(8) Insert the Trousseau dilator

The Trousseau dilator may be inserted in one of two ways. One method is to insert the dilator well in through the incision, directing the blades of the dilator longitudinally down the airway. The second method, which is

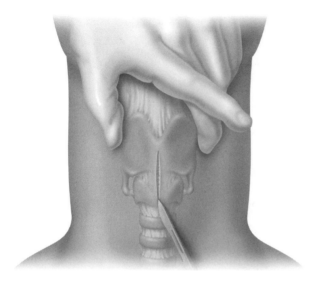

FIG. 15-3. With the index finger moved to the side but continued firm immobilization of the larynx, a vertical midline skin incision is made, down to the depth of the laryngeal structures.

preferred, is to insert the dilator minimally into the anterior wound with the blades oriented superiorly and inferiorly, allowing the dilator to open and enlarge the vertical extent of the cricothyroid membrane incision, which is often the anatomically limiting dimension (Fig. 15-7). When this technique is used, care must be taken not to insert the dilator too deeply

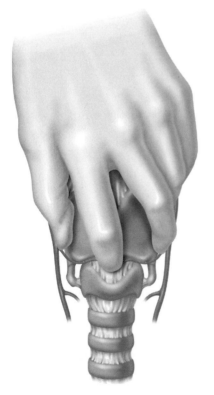

FIG. 15-4. With skin incised, the index finger can now directly palpate the cricothyroid membrane.

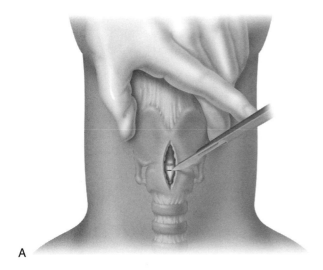

A

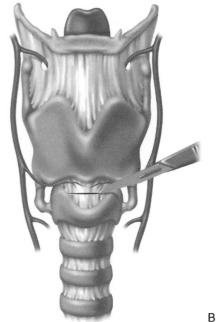

FIG. 15-5. A: A horizontal membrane incision is made near the inferior edge of the cricothyroid membrane. The index finger may be swung aside or may remain in the wound, palpating the inferior edge of the thyroid cartilage, to guide the scalpel to the membrane. **B:** A low cricothyroid incision avoids the superior cricothyroid vessels, which run transversely near the top of the membrane.

B

into the airway, as it will impede subsequent passage of the tracheostomy tube. Some techniques have also described removing the dilator before insertion of the tube.

(9) Insert the tracheostomy tube

The tracheostomy tube, with its inner cannula *in situ,* is gently inserted through the incision between the blades of the Trousseau dilator. As the tube is advanced gently following its natural curve, the Trousseau dilator is rotated to allow the blades to orient longitudinally in the airway (Fig. 15-8). The tracheostomy tube is advanced until it is firmly seated against the anterior neck. The Trousseau dilator is then carefully removed.

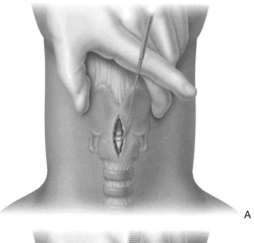

A

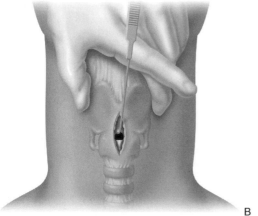

B

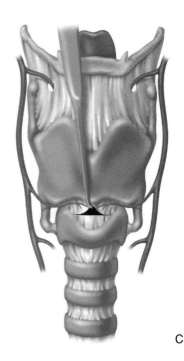

C

FIG. 15-6. A: The tracheal hook is oriented transversely during insertion. **B, C:** After insertion, cephalad traction is applied to the inferior margin of the thyroid cartilage.

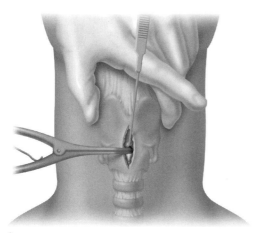

A

FIG. 15-7. A: The Trousseau dilator is inserted a short distance into the incision. **B:** In this orientation, the dilator enlarges the opening vertically, the crucial dimension.

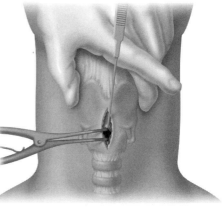

B

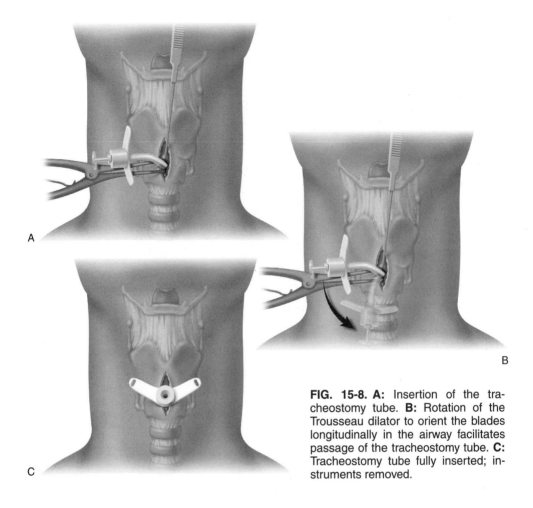

FIG. 15-8. A: Insertion of the tracheostomy tube. **B:** Rotation of the Trousseau dilator to orient the blades longitudinally in the airway facilitates passage of the tracheostomy tube. **C:** Tracheostomy tube fully inserted; instruments removed.

(10) Inflate the cuff and confirm tube position

With the cuff inflated, the tracheostomy tube position can be confirmed by the same methods as the ETT position. Carbon dioxide detection will reliably indicate correct placement of the tube and is mandatory, as for endotracheal intubation. Immediate subcutaneous emphysema with bagging suggests probable paratracheal placement. If doubt remains, rapid passage of a nasogastric tube through the tracheostomy tube will result in easy passage if the tube is in the trachea and obstruction if the tube has been placed through a false passage into the tissues of the neck. Auscultation of both lungs and the epigastric area is also recommended, although esophageal placement of the tracheostomy tube is exceedingly unlikely. Chest radiography should be performed to assist in the assessment of tube placement and to evaluate for the presence of barotrauma.

b. The rapid four-step technique

This abbreviated cricothyrotomy method has been developed and adopted for training purposes at some centers. As with all techniques, the patient should be maximally oxygenated and, if given sufficient time, the anterior neck may be prepared and locally anesthetized as for the no-drop method. From a *position at*

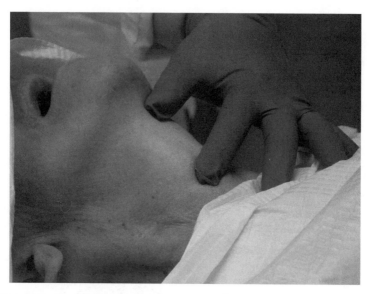

FIG. 15-9. Palpation: the operators thumb is on the hyoid bone, while the cricothyroid membrane is identified using the index finger.

the head of the bed, the rapid four-step technique for cricothyrotomy proceeds sequentially:

(1) *Palpate and identify landmarks*

The cricothyroid membrane should be identified as described previously (Fig. 15-9). If the key landmarks are unable to be identified by palpation through the soft tissue, then a vertical skin incision is required to permit accurate identification.

(2) *Skin incision*

Once the pertinent palpable anatomy is identified, the cricothyroid membrane is incised. If the anatomy is fully appreciated through the intact skin, and there is no uncertainty about landmarks or location, then incise the skin and cricothyroid membrane simultaneously with a single horizontal incision of approximately 1.5 cm in length (Fig. 15-10A). For this type of incision, a no. 20 scalpel yields an incision that requires little widening, once used to puncture the skin and cricothyroid membrane. If the anatomy is not readily and unambiguously identified through the skin, then an initial vertical incision should be created to allow more precise palpation of the anatomy and identification of the cricothyroid membrane. In either situation, the cricothyroid membrane is incised with the no. 20 blade that is maintained in the airway while a tracheal hook (preferably a blunt hook) is placed parallel to the scalpel on the caudad side of the blade (Fig. 15-10B). The hook is then rotated to orient it in a caudad direction to put gentle traction on the cricoid ring. The scalpel is then removed from the airway. At no time during this procedure is the incision left without instrument control of the airway. This detail is particularly important in a scenario where the patient still has the ability to respond or swallow. The newly created stoma could be irretrievably lost if the airway is uncontrolled and moves

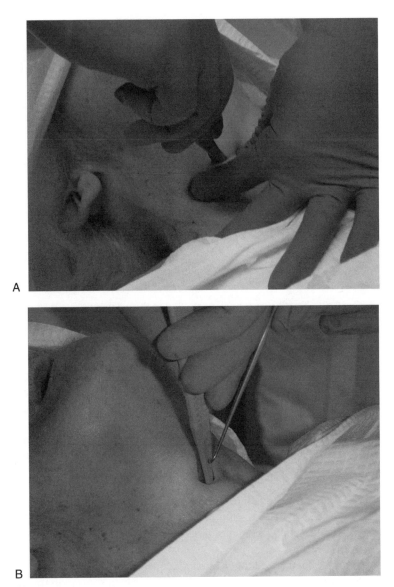

FIG. 15-10. Incision: **A:** a horizontal incision is initiated while stabilizing the larynx. **B:** before removing the scalpel from the airway, a hook is placed on the caudal side of the scalpel, parallel to the blade.

relative to the skin incision. Additionally, as is the case for the no-drop method, this is a technique that relies exclusively on palpation of key structures. Bleeding will inevitably obscure visualization of the anatomy. No time should be wasted using suction or gauze or manipulating the overhead lighting.

(3) *Traction*

The tracheal hook that has been rotated caudally and is controlling the cricoid ring is now used to lift the airway toward the skin incision. This action provides modest stoma dilation. The direction of hook pull is reminiscent of

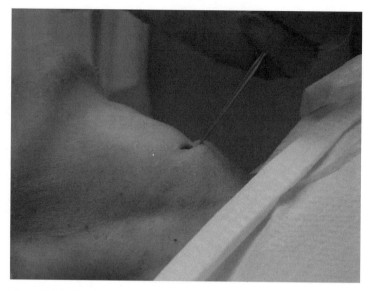

FIG. 15-11. Traction: the hook is applied to the cricoid ring and lifted.

the up and away direction used with laryngoscopy (Fig. 15-11). The amount of traction force required for easy intubation (18 newtons or 4.05 pounds force) is significantly lower than the force that is associated with breakage of the cricoid ring (54 newtons or 12.14 pounds force). Use of the hook in this direction generally provides sufficient widening of the incision, and a Trousseau dilator is usually not required. The technique of pulling the airway upward in this way also minimizes the possibility of intubating the pretracheal potential space.

(4) *Intubation*

With adequate control of the airway using the hook placed on the cricoid ring, an ETT is readily placed into the airway and secured (Fig. 15-12). Confirmation techniques proceed as described in the no-drop technique.

c. Complications

Since the common adoption of rapid sequence intubation (RSI), cricothyrotomy is infrequently performed in emergency departments, so reports of complications are difficult to evaluate. In the National Emergency Airway Registry (NEAR II) study, less than 1% of more than 7,700 ED intubations involved cricothyrotomy.

The most important complication for the patient in the context of surgical airway management is when delayed decision making after initial intubation failure leads to prolonged, ineffective intubation attempts that result in hypoxic injury. Failure to rapidly place the tracheotomy tube into the trachea or to misplace the tube into the soft tissues of the neck is more a failure of technique than a complication and must be recognized immediately, as is the case with any misplaced ETT. Complications such as pneumothorax, significant hemorrhage requiring operative intervention, laryngeal or tracheal injury, and long-term complications, such as subglottic stenosis or permanent voice change, are relatively infrequent and usually minor. The potential for these complications to occur in no way outweighs the need to establish the airway. In general, the

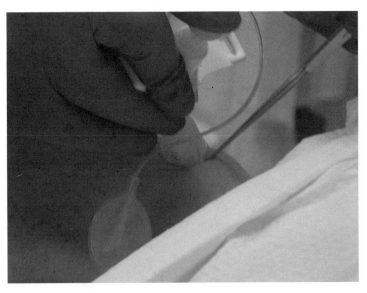

FIG. 15-12. Intubation: the endotracheal tube is passed into the incision as the hook stabilizes the cricoid ring.

incidence of all complications, both immediate and delayed, major or minor, is approximately 20%. Most of these complications are minor, particularly when compared to the consequences of a persistently failed airway. Box 15-3 lists complications of surgical airway management.

3. Cricothyrotome technique

a. Seldinger technique

Numerous commercial cricothyrotome devices are available. Several of them use a modified Seldinger technique to assist in the placement of a tracheal airway (Fig. 15-13). This method is similar to the one commonly used in the placement of central venous catheters and offers some familiarity to the operator uncomfortable with or inexperienced in the surgical cricothyrotomy technique described earlier. Devices that incorporate an inflatable cuff are recommended.

Box 15-3. Complications of Surgical Airway Management

1. Hemorrhage
2. Pneumomediastinum
3. Laryngeal/tracheal injury
4. Cricoid ring laceration
5. Barotrauma (TTJV)
6. Infection
7. Voice change
8. Subglottic stenosis

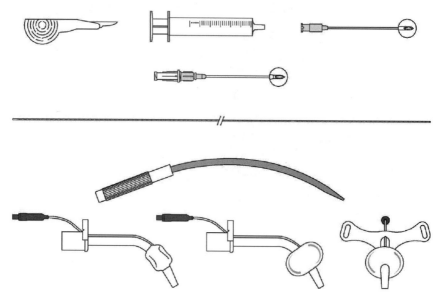

FIG. 15-13. Commercial devices used to perform cricothyrotomy with a modified Seldinger technique. Access is achieved percutaneously through the cricothyroid membrane. The tract is dilated and the airway is established with a cuffed tracheostomy tube inserted over the wire guide. (Melker emergency cricothyrotomy catheter sets, Cook Critical Care, Bloomington, IN.)

(1) *Identification of landmarks*

The cricothyroid membrane is identified by the method described previously. The nondominant hand is used to control the larynx and maintain identification of the landmarks.

(2) *Neck preparation*

Antiseptic solution is applied to the anterior neck, and, if time permits, infiltration of the site with 1% lidocaine with epinephrine is recommended.

(3) *Locator needle insertion*

The introducer needle (18 gauge) is then inserted into the cricothyroid membrane in a slightly caudal direction. The needle is attached to a syringe and advanced with the dominant hand, while negative pressure is maintained on the syringe. The sudden aspiration of air indicates placement of the needle into the tracheal lumen.

(4) *Guide wire insertion*

The syringe is then removed from the needle. A soft-tipped guide wire is inserted through the needle into the trachea in a caudal direction. The needle is then removed, leaving the wire in place. Control of the wire must be maintained at all times.

(5) *Skin incision*

A small skin incision is then made adjacent to the wire. This facilitates passage of the airway device through the skin. Alternatively, the skin incision may be made vertically over the membrane before insertion of the needle and guide wire.

(6) *Insertion of the airway and dilator*

The airway catheter [3 to 6 mm internal diameter (ID)] with an internal dilator in place is inserted over the wire into the trachea. If resistance is met, the skin incision should be deepened and a gentle twisting motion applied to the airway device. When the airway device is firmly seated in the trachea, the wire and dilator are removed together.

(7) *Tube location confirmation*

If the device has a cuff, inflate it at this time. Tube location can then be confirmed as for surgical cricothyrotomy, including mandatory end-tidal carbon dioxide (CO_2) detection. The devices are radiopaque on radiographs. The airway must then be secured properly.

b. Direct airway placement devices

Several direct airway devices (e.g., Nu-Trake, Pertrach) are commercially available. These generally involve multiple steps in the insertion, using a large device that functions as both introducer and airway. The details of the operation of these devices may be obtained from the manufacturer and are provided as inserts with the kits. These devices offer no clear advantage in technique, are rarely (if ever) as easily placed as is claimed, and are considered more likely to cause traumatic complications during their insertion than those that use a Seldinger technique, primarily because of the cutting characteristics of the airway device. In particular, cricothyrotomes recommended for children should be approached with extreme caution and are not recommended.

4. Percutaneous transtracheal jet ventilation technique

Needle cricothyrotomy with percutaneous transtracheal jet ventilation (TTJV) is a surgical airway that may be used to temporize in the can't intubate, can't ventilate situation, particularly in children. Although TTJV is rarely performed in the emergency setting, it is a simple, relatively effective means of supporting oxygenation. Advantages of this technique over cricothyrotomy may include speed, a simpler technique, and less bleeding. It can also provide an alternative for operators unable to perform a cricothyrotomy. Age is not a contraindication to TTJV, which is the surgical airway of choice for children under 12 years old.

Several other aspects of this technique that differ from cricothyrotomy are important to consider. To provide ventilation, supraglottic patency must be maintained to allow for exhalation. In the case of complete upper-airway obstruction, air stacking from TTJV will cause barotrauma, therefore cricothyrotomy is preferable. Another significant difference is that the catheter in TTJV does not provide airway protection. Also, suctioning cannot be adequately performed through the percutaneous catheter. TTJV has been associated with a significant incidence of barotrauma and is less commonly used as a rescue device, particularly with the widespread use of other devices such as the LMA. TTJV is therefore best considered a temporizing means of rescue oxygenation until a more definitive airway can be obtained.

a. Procedure

(1) *Identification of the landmarks*

The anatomy and landmarks used in needle cricothyrotomy are identical to those described earlier for a surgical cricothyrotomy. If there are no contraindications, the head of the patient should be extended. Placing a towel under the shoulders may facilitate cervical hyperextension. The area overlying the cricothyroid membrane should be prepared with an antiseptic solution and, if time permits, anesthetized with 1% lidocaine and epinephrine.

(2) *Immobilize the larynx*

Use the thumb and the middle fingers of the nondominant hand to stabilize the larynx and cricoid cartilage while the index finger palpates the cricothyroid membrane (Fig. 15-14A). It is essential to maintain control of the larynx throughout the procedure.

(3) *Transtracheal needle insertion*

A large-bore intravenous catheter (12 to 16 gauge) is attached to a 20-mL syringe, which may be empty or partially filled with a clear liquid. A 15-degree angle can be created by bending the needle/catheter combination 2.5 cm from the distal end of the intravenous catheter, or a commercially available catheter can be employed (see Equipment later). The commercial catheter is preferred, because it is reinforced with wire coils to prevent kinking. The dominant hand holds the syringe with the needle directed caudally in the long axis of the trachea at a 30-degree angle to the skin (Fig. 15-14B). While maintaining negative pressure on the syringe, the needle is inserted through the cricothyroid membrane into the trachea. As soon as the needle enters the trachea, the syringe will easily fill with air. If a liquid is used, bubbles will appear. Any resistance implies that the catheter remains in the tissue. In the awake patient, lidocaine may be used in the syringe and then injected into the tracheal lumen to suppress the cough reflex.

(4) *Catheter advancement*

Once entry into the trachea is confirmed, the catheter can be advanced. The needle may be partially or completely withdrawn before advancement; however, the needle should not be advanced with the catheter (Fig. 15-14C). A small incision can assist with catheter advancement if there is resistance at the skin.

(5) *Confirmation of location*

The catheter should be advanced to the hub and controlled by hand at all times. Air should be reaspirated to confirm once again the location of the catheter within the trachea (Fig. 15-14D,E).

(6) *Connection to jet ventilation*

The catheter is then connected to the female end of the tubing of the jet ventilation system by a Luer lock. The hub should not be secured in place by anything other than a human hand until a definitive airway is established. Firm, constant pressure must be applied by hand to ensure that proper positioning is maintained and to create a seal at the skin to minimize air leak.

(7) *Technique of jet ventilation*

In the adult, the jet ventilation system should be connected to an oxygen source of 50 pounds per square inch (psi) with a continuously adjustable regulator to allow the pressure to be titrated, so that the lowest effective pressure (often about 30 psi) required to safely deliver a tidal volume is used. In general, inspiration is less than 1 second followed by 2 to 3 seconds of expiration. Because the gas flow through a 14-gauge needle at 50 psi is 1,600 mL/sec, less than 1 second of inspiratory time is required for an adequate tidal volume in a normally compliant lung. Exhalation depends on the elastic recoil of the lung, which is a relatively low driving pressure. Therefore the recommended inspiratory-to-expiratory ratio (I:E) is 1:3. It is very important to maintain upper-airway patency to allow for exhalation and avoid air trapping and barotrauma. All patients should have an oral and nasal airway placed. For small adults and children, oxygen pressure should

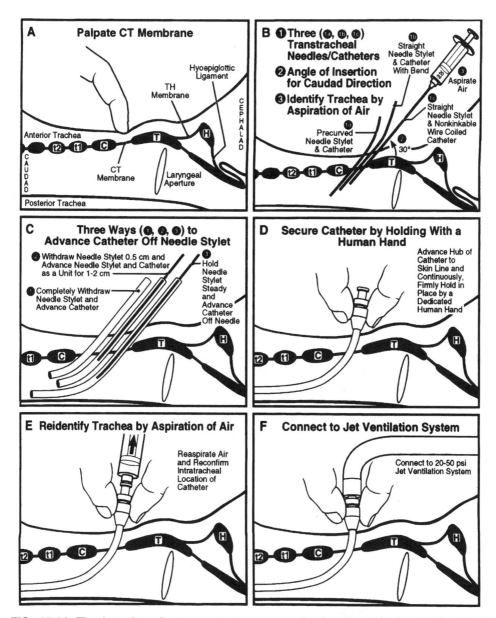

FIG. 15-14. The insertion of a percutaneous transtracheal catheter for jet ventilation. **A:** Cricothyroid membrane is identified and the larynx is controlled. **B:** Needle catheter is inserted percutaneously. **C:** Catheter is advanced. **D:** Catheter must be secured at all times by hand. **E:** Intratracheal location is reconfirmed. **F:** Connection to a jet ventilation system. (Abbreviations: T, thyroid cartilage; H, hyoid bone; C, cricoid cartilage; t1, first tracheal cartilage.) (Adapted from Benumof JL. Trans-tracheal jet ventilation via percutaneous catheter and high-pressure source. In: Benumof JL, ed. *Airway management: principles and practice.* St Louis: Mosby, 1996, with permission.)

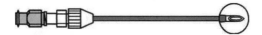

FIG. 15-15. Nonkinkable wire-coiled transtracheal jet ventilation catheter. (Cook Critical Care, Bloomington, IN.)

be down-regulated to less than 20 to 30 psi if possible. For children under 5 years old, a bag should be used for ventilation, connected to the catheter using the ETT adapter from a 3.0-mm-ID ETT.

b. Equipment

(1) Transtracheal catheters

A large-bore intravenous catheter is acceptable. The proper placement is made easier by placing a small angle 2.5 cm from the tip. Commercially available devices include precurved (Acutronic, Germany) and nonkinkable wire-coiled (Cook Critical Care, Bloomington, IN) catheters (Fig. 15-15). The wire-coiled catheter will not kink when bent, therefore providing a more secure airway.

(2) Transtracheal jet ventilation systems

The TTJV system consists of a high-pressure oxygen source (usually central wall oxygen pressure of 50 psi); high-pressure oxygen tubing; a regulator to control the driving pressure; an on/off valve to control inspiratory time; high-pressure tubing; and a Luer lock to connect to the catheter (Fig. 15-16).

A regulator to control the driving pressure is optional but highly recommended. This device is particularly useful where barotrauma is a concern and in pediatrics, where the inspiratory pressures should be reduced to less than 20 to 30 psi if possible. Although a system can be assembled inexpensively from readily available materials, a commercially made, preassembled system is recommended. The reliability and control inherent in the commercial devices are well worth the marginal increase in cost.

A TTJV system can also be connected to a low-flow portable oxygen tank when circumstances require mobility. When the flow is set at the maximal 15 L/min and no flow is allowed, the pressure temporarily increases to 120 psi. Once flow is released, high flow occurs momentarily and then rapidly decreases to the steady state of 5 to 10 psi. Adequate tidal volumes may be achieved through a 14-gauge catheter in the first 0.5 second. A shorter I:E ratio of 1:1 is recommended.

Another setup using manual ventilation with a self-inflating reservoir bag has been described, using standard equipment found in any emergency department. Bag ventilation may be connected directly to the percutaneous transtracheal catheter in two ways. The male end of a 15-mm ETT adapter from a 3-mm-ID ETT will fit directly into the catheter. Alternatively the male end of a plungerless 3-mL syringe will fit into the catheter, and the male end of an 8-mm-ID ETT adapter will then insert into the female end of the empty syringe. Ventilation is temporary at best, and partial arterial pressure (P_{ACO_2}) will increase at a rate of 4 mm Hg/min. Even the simple assembly of this system is too time-consuming to be done during the event, so it must be preassembled. This arrangement may have particular utility in the pediatric patient less than 5 years old when excessive pressures may be delivered via a TTJV device, even when a regulator to control inspiratory

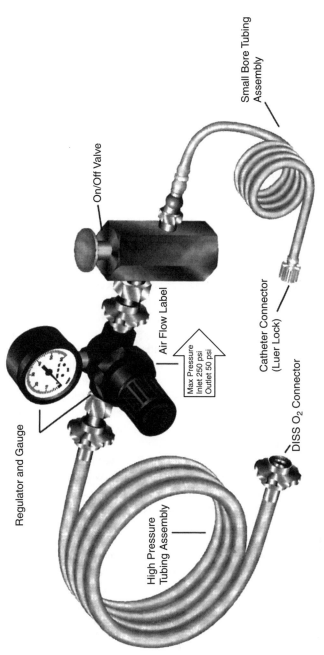

FIG. 15-16. Jet ventilator system with high-pressure oxygen tubing, on/off valve, PVC tubing with Luer lock, and pressure regulator with gauge. (Manufactured by Instrumentation Industries, Inc., Bethel Park, PA.)

pressures is available. In general, children under 5 years old should receive TTJV via a ventilation bag; age 5 to 12 years old at less than 30 mm Hg and greater than 12 years to adult at 30 to 50 mm Hg. A catheter of less than 3 mm ID will be insufficient to adequately ventilate/oxygenate the adult patient using a bag, and 50 psi pressurized oxygen is required.

  c. Complications specific to TTJV
  - Subcutaneous emphysema
  - Barotrauma
  - Reflex cough with each ventilation (may be aborted with lidocaine)
  - Catheter kinking
  - Obstruction from blood or mucus
  - Esophageal puncture
  - Mucosal damage if nonhumidified gas is used

II. Tips and pearls

Surgical airway management is rarely the method of first choice for patients in the emergency department. However, there is a population of patients for whom surgical airway management will literally make the difference between life and death. Therefore, emergency physicians and others who provide care for patients requiring emergency airway management must be proficient with surgical airway management.

There may be little advantage to using a cricothyrotome rather than a formal, surgical cricothyrotomy set. Time of performance of the procedure, complication rates, degree of difficulty, and success rates are all comparable between the two methods. Of the available cricothyrotomes, those that use the Seldinger technique and use a cuffed tube are preferable. Personal preference should also guide selection. A new kit offers all instruments and equipment to perform both the Seldinger-based cricothyrotome insertion and a formal, open, cricothyrotomy by either the no-drop or rapid four-step technique (Melker Universal Cricothyrotomy Catheter Kit, Cook Critical Care, Bloomington, IN). There is no evidence that any cricothyrotome can be placed in a child under 10 to 12 years of age with acceptable success and safety, regardless of the design of the device or the claims of the manufacturer.

Percutaneous transtracheal ventilation is virtually never indicated in the adult patient. In adults, establishment of a more functional surgical airway using a cricothyrotome or by formal cricothyroidotomy is vastly preferable. However, percutaneous transtracheal ventilation remains a useful temporizing measure. In children under 12, the opposite is true. In this age group, percutaneous transtracheal ventilation is the primary surgical airway management method of choice, and cricothyrotomy and cricothyrotomes should be avoided. Despite the extreme infrequency of use of percutaneous transtracheal ventilation in the emergency department, it is important to have a percutaneous transtracheal ventilation set readily available and to be familiar with how to connect and use it. The wire-coiled catheter designed for TTJV is preferable to standard IV catheters because of the tendency for the latter to kink.

Of the methods described in this chapter, only a formal surgical cricothyrotomy and variations of the recently modified Melker kit (Cook Critical Care) results in the placement of a cuffed tube within the trachea. All the other techniques described here must be considered temporary at best. Placement of a tracheostomy tube or ETT through a formal surgical cricothyrotomy incision results in an airway that can be used as a definitive airway for the patient.

The no. 4 cuffed tracheostomy tube, which has an inside diameter of 5 mm, should be used for virtually all cases of adult cricothyrotomy in the emergency department. The tube is of adequate size to provide ventilation in virtually all circumstances, and its outside dimensions are such that it will almost always be easily inserted. For very large adult men, a no. 6 can be used.

EVIDENCE

1. Which technique is best? There is almost no literature that effectively compares different techniques of invasive surgical airway management. The relatively rare performance of an emergency surgical airway, compounded with the urgency of the circumstance, may explain the absence of any controlled clinical trials comparing techniques in the emergency setting. Comorbid injuries or illness often precludes long-term assessment of sequelae, and the few studies performed do not compare or identify specific invasive techniques (1). As such, the current level of evidence for or against a particular technique exists as expert consensus based on collective experience, limited descriptive series, or studies in cadaveric and animal models (2–10).

Several studies have directly compared the percutaneous, wire-guided technique to the traditional open, or no-drop technique in cadavers (11–13). Eisenberger *et al.* studying the performance of intensive care trainees, and Chan *et al.* in a similar study of emeregency residents and attendings, compared the two techniques in randomized, crossover studies and found no difference in times to completion between groups (11,12). Immediate complications were also similar. Interestingly, the majority of participants in Chan's study stated a preference for the percutaneous, wire-guided technique (12).

2. Rapid four-step or no-drop technique for open cricothyrotomy? Each approach has its proponents. The no-drop technique has been in use for decades and has withstood the test of time. The rapid four-step technique is proposed to be an improvement over the no-drop technique based on the following:

1. The rapid four-step technique requires only one person to perform the procedure. Ideally, the no-drop technique requires *two* people (i.e., one operator and one assistant). The assistant is responsible for not dropping the tracheal hook as it stabilizes the trachea. Without an assistant, the operator must maintain the no-drop approach with the Trousseau dilator while inserting the tube; not a desirable circumstance.
2. The rapid four-step technique can be readily performed from the head of the bed without having to move to the patient's side, where the operator is best positioned for the no-drop technique.
3. The rapid four-step technique requires only a simple hook and a scalpel, which may be available even in the absence of a formal cricothyrotomy kit. This is a minimal advantage because the standard cricothyrotomy kit is also simple containing only three basic instruments (scalpel, hook, and dilator.)

There are no controlled human trials comparing these approaches; however, case series suggest RFST is an acceptable approach in the emergency setting (10,14,15). In a randomized, crossover, cadaveric study comparing the two techniques, Holmes *et al.* found the RFST to be significantly faster (43s versus 134s, $p < 0.001$) without a significant difference in immediate complications (16). Davis *et al.* in a similar study also found the RFST to be faster (17).

Potential disadvantages of the rapid four-step technique.

The RFST relies on a single, relatively small incision to hasten the placement of the endotracheal tube. Although literature exists that supports the routine use of this technique, it is important to point out the location of the initial incision is of critical importance (10,14,15). Most of the reported complications related to the RFST in patients have been related to the initial incision being made too small and then requiring time consuming revision of the incision (10). If the initial incision is misplaced or initially made too small and subsequently requires revision, then any proposed time saving advantage is lost. Concerns over a possible higher incidence of cricoid ring damage and esophageal perforation have been raised but, larger studies are needed to see if this possibility is real (16,17). The use of a double hook may significantly reduce the potential for cricoid ring injury (17,18).

Overall, choice of the RFST versus the no-drop method will be made by the operator on the basis of training, experience, and judgement, and either approach is acceptable, each having some advantages and disadvantages and neither being clearly superior.

3. Can a procedure done so rarely be taught, retained and used successfully? Ultimately, any discussion of the technical merits of a procedure will be irrelevant if hesitancy on the part of the provider results in significant delay in establishing a definitive airway. Fortunately, this potential hesitancy is readily overcome with technical proficiency. However, as an infrequently used technique, proficiency will require a concerted effort to acquire and maintain it. Anyone responsible for emergency airway management should choose an invasive method, learn it, and practice it at regular intervals to maintain proficiency.

Recent articles regarding the popularity and success of RSI have prompted editorials concerned with the current problem of gaining and maintaining competency in invasive airway management (19–21). Retrospective studies suggest a current cricothyrotomy rate of approximately 1% of all emergency airways. The reasons for this low incidence have been attributed to emergency resident training, the success of RSI, and reduced transport rate for blunt traumatic arrests (19,21). Regardless of the cause, this incidence is felt to be too low to ensure adequate training, yet highlights the probability that all emergency physicians will be called on to perform an invasive airway at some point in their career.

To address this issue, some authors have advocated the performance of invasive airway techniques on the newly dead (22). Many physicians have received cricothyrotomy and endotracheal intubation training on the recently deceased without consent from the family. This practice, however, has raised ethical concerns and is no longer considered an acceptable practice at many institutions (23). Olsen *et al.* studied the feasibility of obtaining family consent for teaching cricothyrotomy on the newly dead in the emergency department. Consent was obtained for postmortem cricothyrotomy in 20 of 51 deaths (39%) in a large teaching hospital over a seven month period (23). It is unclear how feasible this approach would be in other settings, but does represent a potential opportunity to practice in a way that most closely approximates the true anatomy.

To ensure familiarity with the equipment and technique, it is likely that practice must take place outside the clinical setting. Koppel reported that although 80% of anesthesiology programs instruct their residents on cricothyrotomies, 60% use lectures only, a poor teaching technique for developing proficiency in manual skills (24). One study attempted to determine the minimum training required to perform cricothyrotomy in 40 seconds or less in a mannequin. One hundred and two physicians performed 10 procedures, and by the fifth attempt 96% plateaued in their success (25).

There are no studies that have identified the optimal interval between training episodes for retention, although one small report suggested increased retention when repeated monthly versus every three months (26). Studies in cadavers performed primarily to compare different techniques have also identified a similarly rapid learning curve, however, the time to procedure completion was greater (73 to 102 seconds) (11,13).

There are no studies examining the clinical correlation of these training techniques; however, the high success rates of emergency cricothyrotomies suggests retention and application has occurred. Based on the limited available literature, we make the following recommendations regarding the learning and retention of invasive airway techniques:

1. Identify a preferred method of invasive airway management to learn; select one that is immediately available to you.
2. Practice the technique one to two times per year on live animal models, animal tracheas, patient simulators, or manikins, depending on the availability.
3. Practice the procedure five times at each training session.
4. When appropriate, consider requesting consent for cricothyrotomy on the newly dead.

Tracheas may be ordered from a slaughter house at relatively low cost, and the technique may be attempted multiple times on each specimen. Simulators represent a significant purchase cost but are useful for training multiple critical skills and are increasingly commonly available at teaching institutions as prices have become much lower. Models specifically for cricothyrotomy training are also available. Live animal models and cadavers are generally used only in formal residency training sessions and specialized procedural courses because of significant expense and limited access.

REFERENCES

1. McGill J, Clinton JE, Ruiz E. Cricothyrotomy in the emergency department. *Ann Emerg Med* 1982;11:361–364.
2. Esses BA, Jafek BW. Cricothyrotomy: a decade of experience in Denver. *Ann Otol Rhinol Laryngol,* 1987;96:519–524.
3. Walls RM. Cricothyroidotomy In: Campbell WH, ed. *Emergency Medicine Clinics of North America.* Philadelphia: WB Saunders, 1988.
4. Elandson MJ, Clinton JE, Ruiz E, et al. Cricothyrotomy in the emergency department revisited. *J Emerg Med* 1989;7:115–118.
5. DeLaurier GA, Hawkins ML, Treat RC, et al. Acute airway management: role of cricothyroidotomy. *Am Surg* 1990;56:12–15.
6. Salvino CK, Dries D, Gamelli R, et al. Emergency cricothyroidotomy in trauma victims. *J Trauma* 1993;34:503–505.
7. Hawkins ML, Shapiro MB, Cue JI, et al. Emergency cricothyroidotomy: a reassessment. *Am Surg* 1995;61:52–55.
8. Bair AE, Filbin MR, Kulkarni RG, et al. Failed intubation in the emergency department: analysis of prevalence, rescue techniques and personnel. *J Emerg Med* 2002;23:131–140.
9. Bair AE, Panacek EA, Wisner DH, et al. Cricothyrotomy: a 5-year experience at one institution. *J Emerg Med* 2003;24:151–156.
10. Isaacs JH. Emergency cricothyrotomy: long-term results. *Am Surg* 2001;67:346–349.
11. Eisenberger P, Laczika K, List M, et al. Comparison of conventional surgical versus Seldinger technique emergency cricothyrotomy performed by inexperienced clinicians. *Anesthesiology* 2000;92:687–690.
12. Chan TC, Vilke GM, Bramwell KJ, et al. Comparison of wire-guided cricothyrotomy versus standard surgical cricothyrotomy technique. *J Emerg Med* 1999;17:957–962.
13. Johnson DR, Dunlap A, McFeely P, et al. Cricothyrotomy performed by prehospital personnel: a comparison of two techniques in a human cadaver model. *Am J Emerg Med* 1993;11:207–209.
14. Brofeldt BT, Panacek EA, Richards JR. An easy cricothyrotomy approach: the rapid four-step technique. *Acad Emerg Med* 1996;3:1060–1063.
15. Brofeldt BT, Osborn ML, Sakles JC, et al. Evaluation of the rapid four-step cricothyrotomy technique: an interim report. *Air Med J* 1998;17:127–130.
16. Holmes JF, Panacek EA, Sakles JC, et al. Comparison of 2 cricothyrotomy techniques: standard method versus rapid 4-step technique. *Ann Emerg Med* 1998;32:442–447.
17. Davis DP, Bramwell KJ, Hamilton RS, et al. Safety and efficacy of the rapid four-step technique for cricothyrotomy using a Bair Claw. *J Emerg Med* 2000;19:125–129.
18. Bair AE, Laurin EG, Karchin A, et al. Cricoid ring integrity: implications for emergent cricothyrotomy. *Ann Emerg Med* 2003;41:333–337.
19. Chang RS, Hamilton RJ, Carter WA. Influence of an emergency medicine residency on the role of cricothyrotomy. *Acad Emerg Med* 1996;3:534.
20. Knopp RK, Waeckerle JF, Callaham ML. Rapid sequence intubation revisited. *Ann Emerg Med* 1998;31:398–400.

21. Chang RS, Hamilton RJ, Carter WA. Declining rate of cricothyrotomy in trauma patients with an emergency medicine residency: implications for skills training. *Acad Emerg Med* 1998;5:247–251.
22. Knopp RK. Practicing cricothyrotomy on the newly dead. *Ann Emerg Med* 1995;25:694–695.
23. Olsen J, Spilger S, Windisch T. Feasibility of obtaining family consent for teaching cricothyrotomy on the newly dead in the emergency department. *Ann Emerg Med* 1995;25:660–665.
24. Koppel J, Reed A. Formal instruction in difficult airway management. *Anesthesiology* 1995;83:1343–1346.
25. Wong DT, Prabhu AJ, Coloma M, et al. What is the minimum training required for successful cricothyrotomy? *Anesthesiology* 2003;98:349–353.
26. Prabhu AJ, Correa R, Wong DT, et al. What is the optimal training interval for a cricothyrotomy? *Can J Anesth* 2001;48:A59.

16

Pretreatment Agents

Robert E. Schneider and David A. Caro

I. Drugs used in the pretreatment phase of RSI
A. General approach

During the preparation phase of rapid sequence intubation (RSI), a decision must be made about administration of specific pretreatment drugs that will attenuate the normal physiologic and pathophysiologic reflex responses caused by airway manipulation (laryngoscopy) and the insertion of an endotracheal tube (intubation). These reflex responses are initiated by stimulation of afferent receptors in the posterior pharynx, hypopharynx, and larynx, which results in increased afferent traffic and central stimulation of the brain leading, in turn, to increases in intracranial pressure (ICP), stimulation of the autonomic nervous system with increases in heart rate and blood pressure, and stimulation of the upper and lower respiratory tract resulting in increases in airway resistance. It has been shown that the duration and aggressiveness of laryngoscopy and intubation, particularly stimulation of the carina, correlates strongly with the magnitude of these reflex responses. The central nervous system, cardiovascular system, and respiratory system all respond predictably to these stimuli, and in selected patients, the resultant physiologic manifestations may adversely affect the patient's outcome. Even though well-controlled outcome studies have not been done, it seems reasonable, given the available data, that all attempts should be made to attenuate these responses and to use pharmacologic agents that mitigate the patient's underlying or presenting problems.

The central nervous system responds to airway manipulation by increasing cerebral metabolic oxygen demand, increasing cerebral blood flow, and, if intracranial elastance is compromised, increasing ICP. This response is important in situations in which there is loss of autoregulation such that blood flow to the brain or regions of the brain is pressure passive (i.e., increases in blood pressure result in increases in ICP).

The cardiovascular system responds to the sympathetic nervous system actuation triggered by airway stimulation. In children this process is seen primarily as a monosynaptic reflex promoting vagal stimulation of the sinoatrial (SA) node that results in bradycardia. In adults, a polysynaptic event predominates, whereby impulses travel afferently via the 9th and 10th cranial nerves to the brain stem and spinal cord, and then return efferently through the cardioaccelerator nerves and sympathetic ganglia. This results in norepinephrine release from the adrenergic nerve terminals, epinephrine release from the adrenal glands, and activation of the renin-angiotensin system, which further leads to increases in blood pressure. This overall increase in heart rate and blood

183

pressure to levels as high as twice normal may be detrimental in those patients with myocardial ischemia, with known aortic or intracerebral aneurysm or dissection, or in penetrating trauma where any increase in shear pressure may reactivate previous hemorrhage. In similar fashion, increases in blood pressure may result in significant increases in ICP if autoregulation has been lost (e.g., in head injury or intracerebral hemorrhage (see Chapter 24).

The respiratory system responds in two important ways to airway stimulation. There is activation of the upper-airway reflexes that can lead to laryngospasm and coughing, both of which compromise the patient. Of these, the former may be more significant in that it may produce difficulty with intubation. However, if laryngospasm occurs, it can be abolished by neuromuscular blockade. Coughing may be significant in cases of increased ICP, unstable cervical spine injury, or penetrating globe injuries. In all patients, there is actuation of the lower-airway reflexes that leads to increases in airway resistance. This reaction is most often manifested by bronchospasm, which can be reflex, irritant, or antigenic in nature and can result in significant morbidity.

Whether control of these adverse reflexes improves patient outcome is not known, but the body of knowledge that is currently available argues for the use of specific pretreatment drugs capable of mitigating potentially harmful physiologic effects. To optimize their effect, all these pretreatment agents should be administered 3 minutes before induction, if possible. The goal is to achieve peak drug concentration at the precise time the patient is undergoing laryngoscopy and intubation. The uses of the individual drugs in specific clinical circumstances are described in Chapters 23 to 33. The useful agents are most easily remembered by the mnemonic *LOAD,* which stands for *L*idocaine, *O*pioid, *A*tropine, and *D*efasciculating agent. This chapter provides a general discussion of the appropriate pharmacologic agents and their relevant properties.

B. The LOAD approach

1. Lidocaine (Xylocaine)

The literature is replete with articles that debate the efficacy of lidocaine in the pretreatment phase of tracheal intubation. It has been shown unequivocally that 1.5 mg/kg of lidocaine IV 3 minutes before intubation suppresses the cough reflex and attenuates the increase in airway resistance that is irritant in origin (endotracheal tube). Its effect on antigenic bronchospasm is more controversial. The literature is likewise supportive of lidocaine's mitigating effect on potential increases in ICP at 1.5 mg/kg IV 3 minutes before tracheal intubation. This result is ascribed to lidocaine's ability to increase the depth of anesthesia, decrease cerebral metabolic oxygen demand globally, decrease cerebral blood flow, and increase cerebrovascular resistance. The literature is indecisive and indeed contradictory regarding lidocaine's effect on attenuating the sympathetic response to laryngoscopy, and therefore lidocaine cannot be recommended for this purpose.

a. Recommendation

Lidocaine, 1.5 mg/kg IV, 3 minutes before induction is advocated for all patients with reactive airways disease ('tight lungs', Chapter 25) or elevated ICP ('tight brain', Chapter 24). Lidocaine is thus being used to mitigate:

• The reflex rise in ICP that occurs in response to the stimulation of the laryngoscopy and intubation in patients with elevated ICP, and

• The reflex bronchospasm that occurs in response to the stimulation of laryngoscopy and intubation in patients with reactive airways disease

Lidocaine has a wide safety profile at 1.5 mg/kg IV. The primary toxic effect is the development of seizures, which should occur only at much greater doses.

The effect of topical lidocaine on ICP or airway reactivity is incompletely studied, and this agent should be reserved for use during awake intubation techniques (Chapter 7).

2. Opioid—fentanyl (Sublimaze)

Given in sufficiently high doses, most anesthetic agents, with the exception of ketamine, will attenuate the reflex sympathetic (catecholamine) response to laryngoscopy. However, the doses and depth of anesthesia that are required to achieve substantial attenuation will produce significant hypotension. The opioids, specifically fentanyl, significantly attenuate this sympathetic response with minimal side effects, except for respiratory depression. Although fentanyl has no direct effect on ICP, increasing doses of any of the opioids will suppress ventilation, resulting in hypercarbia, cerebrovasodilation, and subsequent increases in ICP. Fentanyl does not release histamine and has no direct effect on the pulmonary response to laryngoscopy. Fentanyl has been shown to have a partial attenuating effect on the reflex sympathetic response to laryngoscopy at doses as low as 2 mcg/kg (.002 mg/kg) IV. A greater response with moderate attenuation is seen at 6 mcg/kg (0.006 mg/kg) IV, and almost complete attenuation at 11 to 15 mcg/kg (0.011 to 0.015 mg/kg) IV, a rather large dose and one usually reserved for patients undergoing cardiac surgery.

In the emergency department (ED), a dose of 3 mcg/kg (0.003 mg/kg) of fentanyl IV 3 minutes before intubation is indicated for patients who might be adversely affected by a systemic discharge of catecholamines with the resulting transient, but significant, increase in heart rate and blood pressure (Chapters 24 and 27). Patients with elevated ICP, intracranial hemorrhage ischemic heart disease, known or suspected cerebral or aortic aneurysm, aortic dissection, and perhaps hemodynamically stable penetrating trauma are all candidates for pretreatment with fentanyl. The approach is to consider whether the patient may have an adverse effect from a surge in blood pressure (shear pressure).

Fentanyl should be given as the last of the pretreatment drugs, over an interval of 30 to 60 seconds. Caution must be used when fentanyl is given as a pretreatment agent because significant respiratory depression and hypotension (central sympathectomy) may occur. In particular, since fentanyl is being given precisely to reduce sympathetic tone, great caution must be used if the patient is dependent on sympathetic tone to maintain hemodynamic stability (e.g., hypovolemia). Muscle wall rigidity is a unique and idiosyncratic response to opioids and is probably related to the dose and speed of opioid administration, the concomitant use of nitrous oxide, and the presence or absence of muscle relaxants. It is not reversible with naloxone (Narcan). It is usually seen with fentanyl doses well in excess of 500 mcg (0.5 mg) and primarily affects the chest and abdominal wall musculature. The rigidity has rarely been reported in conscious patients. It tends to occur very quickly after the patient begins to lose consciousness. Rigidity has not been reported with the ED use of fentanyl. Rigidity can be attenuated or prevented with defasciculating doses of a nondepolarizing neuromuscular blocking agent or by the administration of paralyzing doses of succinylcholine (SCh) once the abnormality is recognized. Avoiding the rapid administration of large doses of opioids is the most reliable way of preventing this very uncommon, but important, complication.

a. Recommendation

In the operating room, fentanyl is used as an induction agent at doses of 15 to 30 mcg/kg (0.015 to 0.03 mg/kg) IV. In the ED, fentanyl is a pretreatment agent, not an induction agent. Fentanyl has its greatest use in those patients at risk from increasing blood pressure [i.e., increases in ICP, myocardial pressure (ischemia), or vascular shear pressure (aneurysmal disease, dissection, penetrating vascular trauma)]. In these patients any further increase in sympathetic stimulation from laryngoscopy and intubation might be detrimental to the patient's outcome. In such patients, fentanyl 3 mcg/kg (0.003 mg/kg) is administered intravenously over 30 to 60 seconds as the final pretreatment drug. If the patient is overtly hypotensive, or minimally stable and dependent on sympathetic drive, fentanyl should not be used. One must be prepared for dose-related hypotension and respiratory depression that may occur with fentanyl administration.

3. Atropine

Atropine is indicated in only one clinical situation in the ED. All children less than 10 years of age should be pretreated with atropine 0.02 mg/kg IV 3 minutes before the administration of SCh to prevent bradycardia induced by SCh and laryngoscopic manipulation.

4. Defasciculating Agents

Succinylcholine causes a significant rise in ICP when given to patients with elevated ICP (see Chapter 24). This rise in ICP can be abolished completely by prior administration of a full dose of a competitive neuromuscular blocking agent and mitigated significantly by administration of a defasciculating dose of the same competitive agent. Vecuronium, pancuronium, and rocuronium are the defasciculating agents that are potentially useful in the pretreatment phase of RSI. Their greatest usefulness is mitigating potential increases in ICP caused by SCh; therefore they should be considered for use in all medical and trauma situations in which increases in ICP are a concern and SCh is selected as the muscle relaxant (Chapter 24). These drugs do not attenuate the reflex sympathetic response to laryngoscopy, nor do they attenuate increases in airway resistance. The appropriate defasciculating dose for any of these agents is 10% of the normal paralyzing dose. Note that the paralyzing dose and the intubating dose are different. The paralyzing dose is usually roughly 50% of the intubating dose (e.g., 1.0 mg/kg is the intubating dose, 0.6 mg/kg is the paralyzing dose for rocuronium.) Defasciculating doses of SCh (0.15 mg/kg) given as a pretreatment drug will also inhibit fasciculations, but whether this specific pretreatment mitigates any potential rise in intracranial or intraocular pressure is not known.

  With any of the nondepolarizing neuromuscular blocking agents, the defasciculating dose may uncommonly cause muscular weakness or even apnea. Active support of the patient's oxygenation and ventilation with a bag and mask may be needed throughout the completion of induction, paralysis, and intubation. Pancuronium can produce tachycardia through cardiac muscarinic blockade, which may preclude its use in certain clinical situations. Vecuronium or rocuronium may be the preferred drug for those patients in whom tachycardia may worsen their underlying clinical condition. Both drugs are much more expensive than pancuronium and vecuronium requires reconstitution at the time of use.

a. Recommendation

Administer a defasciculating dose of a competitive neuromuscular blocking agent (e.g., 0.06 mg/kg of rocuronium, or 0.01 mg/kg of vecuronium or pancuronium) as a pretreatment agent 3 minutes before administration of succinylcholine in patients with elevated ICP who are undergoing RSI with succinylcholine.

II. Summary

Pretreatment agents are used to attenuate the adverse physiologic responses to laryngoscopy and intubation.

LOAD is the mnemonic used to stimulate recall of lidocaine, opioids, atropine, and defasciculating agents for pretreatment.

Ideally, any pretreatment agent should be administered 3 minutes before induction to match peak drug effect with airway manipulation. It is recommended that pretreatment agents be given even if the time to airway manipulation is compressed or prolonged.

The following drugs should be considered as pretreatment for the specific clinical situations listed.

- **LIDOCAINE:** Lidocaine (Xylocaine) 1.5 mg/kg IV 3 minutes before airway manipulation for patients at risk for increased ICP—medical or trauma (tight brain) or those with bronchospastic disease (tight lungs—i.e., asthma, chronic obstructive pulmonary disease, possibly cardiac asthma)
- **OPIOID:** Fentanyl (Sublimaze) 3 mcg/kg (0.003 mg/kg) IV 3 minutes before induction for patients at risk for increased ICP—medical or trauma (tight brain), ischemic heart disease (tight heart), aneurysm or dissection, or those at risk for recurrent hemorrhage in penetrating vascular trauma but who are hemodynamically stable (shear pressure)
- **ATROPINE:** Atropine 0.02 mg/kg IV 3 minutes before induction for any child less than 10 years of age undergoing RSI with SCh.
- **DEFASCICULATION:** Vecuronium (Norcuron), pancuronium (Pavulon), or rocuronium (Zemuron) at 10% of the normal paralyzing dose 3 minutes before induction for patients at risk for increased ICP—medical or trauma, who will be receiving SCh.

Adult patients with increased ICP are candidates to receive three of the four pretreatment drugs (lidocaine, fentanyl, defasciculation) and often are the most pharmacologically sophisticated intubations in the ED.

Beta-blockers [e.g., esmolol (Brevibloc)] have been shown to be beneficial in attenuating the sympathetic response to laryngoscopy. They are not effective in attenuating any rise in ICP. They may increase airway resistance, especially in patients with reactive airways disease. The main concern with beta-blockers is that they are negative inotropes; in clinical situations in which maximum cardiac output is mandatory, these agents are contraindicated. With the availability of other, more appropriate drugs (especially fentanyl), the beta-blockers have little use in RSI in the ED.

EVIDENCE

1. Lidocaine use for elevated ICP. Lidocaine's role in RSI for the head-injured patient is hotly contested (1). Unfortunately, there are no studies to date that directly address this question. It is unlikely that such a prospective study can be carried out with current technology, as the measurement of ICP without an invasive manometer in the acutely ill patient is not possible. However, the role of lidocaine in blunting reflex ICP response to other airway maneuvers (e.g., endotracheal suctioning, bronchoscopy) has been studied, with a number of studies showing some protective effect from lidocaine use (2,3), and others showing no effect at all (4). Importantly, no direct harm has been noted with lidocaine use in these circumstances. The rationale for lidocaine use in the RSI algorithm rests on the possible upside benefit with minimal to no downside in the doses recommended. See also Chapter 24.

2. Lidocaine use for bronchoconstriction. The use of lidocaine in the bronchospastic patient has also been disputed. Intravenous lidocaine has been shown to be beneficial in blunting reflex bronchospasm caused by airway manipulation (5,6,7), although this concept has been challenged (8). Nebulized lidocaine can be used to anesthetize the airway for awake evaluations, and causes minimal change in bronchoconstriction (9–13). Again, it would appear that the potential benefits of lidocaine in reactive airways disease significantly outweigh its minimal potential for adverse effects (see Chapter 25).

3. Atropine use in children undergoing RSI. Atropine is a standard pretreatment drug for any child less than 10 years old undergoing intubation, as it blunts the reflex cholinergic stimulation caused by airway manipulation and also counteracts the intense cholinergic stimulation caused by succinylcholine (see Chapter 19). This recommendation has been based on accumulated clinical experience, but has not been subjected to randomized study.

4. Muscle rigidity and stiff-man syndrome with fentanyl. When administered rapidly and in relatively high doses (greater than 500 mcg, 0.5 mg), fentanyl can result in laryngospasm and muscular rigidity that can make a patient difficult to ventilate. Both are resistant to naloxone reversal and usually require rapid neuromuscular blockade (14).

5. Defasciculation. Most of the non-depolarizing neuromuscular blocking agents have proven effective in reducing SCh-induced fasciculations (15) with some suggestion that rocuronium might be the best (16). The relationship between defasciculation and ICP response is discussed in Chapter 24. Although small doses of SCh will also reduce fasciculation from later paralyzing doses, the effect of this approach on ICP is unknown (17).

REFERENCES

1. Robinson N, Clancy M. In patients with head injury undergoing rapid sequence intubation, does pretreatment with intravenous lignocaine/lidocaine lead to an improved neurological outcome? A review of the literature. *Emerg Med J* 2001;18:453–457.
2. Grover VK, Reddy GM, Kak VK, et al. Intracranial pressure changes with different doses of lignocaine under general anaesthesia. *Neurol India* 1999;47:118–121.
3. Bedford RF, Persing JA, Pobereskin L, et al. Lidocaine or thiopental for rapid control of intracranial hypertension? *Anesth Analg* 1980;59:435–437.
4. Samaha T, Ravussin P, Claquin C, et al. Prevention of increase of blood pressure and intracranial pressure during endotracheal intubation in neurosurgery: esmolol versus lidocaine. *Ann Fr Anesth Reanim* 1996;15(1):36–40.
5. Nishino T, Hiraga K, Sugimori K. Effects of i.v. lignocaine on airway reflexes elicited by irritation of the tracheal mucosa in humans anaesthetized with enflurane. *Br J Anaesth* 1990;64:682–687.
6. Groeben H, Silvanus MT, Beste M, et al. Combined intravenous lidocaine and inhaled salbutamol protect against bronchial hyperreactivity more effectively than lidocaine or salbutamol alone. *Anesthesiology* 1998;89:862–868.
7. Groeben H, Foster WM, Brown RH. Intravenous lidocaine and oral mexiletine block reflex bronchoconstriction in asthmatic subjects. *Am J Respir Crit Care Med* 1996;154(Pt 1):885–888.
8. Maslow AD, Regan MM, Israel E, et al. Inhaled albuterol, but not intravenous lidocaine, protects against intubation-induced bronchoconstriction in asthma. *Anesthesiology* 2000;93:1198–2204.
9. Groeben H, Schlicht M, Stieglitz S, et al. Both local anesthetics and salbutamol pretreatment affect reflex bronchoconstriction in volunteers with asthma undergoing awake fiberoptic intubation. *Anesthesiology* 2002;97:1445–1450.
10. Udezue E. Lidocaine inhalation for cough suppression. *Am J Emerg Med* 2001;19:206–207.
11. Groeben H, Silvanus MT, Beste M, et al. Combined lidocaine and salbutamol inhalation for airway anesthesia markedly protects against reflex bronchoconstriction. *Chest* 2000;118:509–515.
12. Groeben H, Silvanus MT, Beste M, et al. Both intravenous and inhaled lidocaine attenuate reflex bronchoconstriction but at different plasma concentrations. *Am J Respir Crit Care Med* 1999;159:530–535.
13. Groeben H, Grosswendt T, Silvanus M, et al. Lidocaine inhalation for local anaesthesia and attenuation of bronchial hyper-reactivity with least airway irritation. Effect of three different dose regimens. *Eur J Anaesthesiol* 2000;17:672–679.
14. Miller RD [Ed.]: Anesthesiology, 5th edition. Churchill-Livingstone, 2000;291–292.
15. Harvey SC, Roland P, Bailey MK, Tomlin MK, Williams A. A randomized, double-blind comparison of rocuronium, d-tubocurarine, and "mini-dose" succinylcholine for preventing succinylcholine-induced muscle fasciculations. *Anesth Analg* 1998;87:719–722.
16. Martin R, Carrier J, Pirlet M, Claprood Y, Tetrault JP. Rocuronium is the best non-depolarizing relaxant to prevent succinylcholine fasciculations and myalgia. *Can J Anaesth* 1998;45:521–525.
17. Koenig KL. Rapid-sequence intubation of head trauma patients: prevention of fasciculations with pancuronium versus minidose succinylcholine. *Ann Emerg Med* 1992;21:929–932.

17

Sedative and Induction Agents

Robert E. Schneider and David A. Caro

Induction agents are among the most potent agents used in medicine today. The ideal induction agent would smoothly and quickly render the patient unconscious, unresponsive, and amnestic in one arm/heart/brain circulation time. Such an agent would also provide analgesia, maintain stable cerebral perfusion pressure and cardiovascular hemodynamics, be immediately reversible, and have few, if any, adverse side effects. Unfortunately, such an induction agent does not exist. Most induction agents meet the first criterion because they are highly lipophilic and therefore have a rapid onset within 15 to 30 seconds of intravenous administration. Their clinical effect is likewise terminated quickly as the drug rapidly redistributes to less-well-perfused tissues. All the induction agents have the potential to cause myocardial depression and subsequent hypotension. These effects depend on the particular drug, the patient's underlying physiologic condition, and the dose and speed of injection of the drug. The faster the drug is administered [intravenous (IV) push], the larger the concentration of drug that saturates those organs with the greatest blood flow (i.e., brain and heart) and the more pronounced the effect. Because rapid sequence intubation (RSI) requires rapid administration of the sedative/induction agent, the choice of drug and the dose must be individualized to capitalize on desired effects, while minimizing those that might adversely affect the patient. Some patients are so unstable that the goal is to produce amnesia rather than anesthesia because to produce the latter might lead to hypotension and organ hypoperfusion.

Anesthetic induction is intended to rapidly render the patient unable to appreciate, respond to, or recall noxious stimuli, and is therefore toward the extreme of a continuum that ranges from anxiolysis and mild sedation on one end to deep-plane general anesthesia on the other. The induction agents are therefore appropriately classified as sedative/hypnotic agents and include ultra-short-acting barbiturates: thiopental (Pentothal) and methohexital (Brevital); benzodiazepines: principally midazolam (Versed); and miscellaneous agents: etomidate (Amidate), ketamine (Ketalar), and propofol (Diprivan). Other agents, such as the opioid analgesic fentanyl (Sublimaze), can function as anesthetic induction agents when used in very large doses (e.g., for fentanyl 30 mcg/kg, 0.03 mg/kg) but are rarely, if ever, used for that purpose during emergency intubation, so are not discussed here.

All of the induction agents discussed in this chapter share important pharmacokinetic characteristics: As mentioned previously, they are highly lipophilic and therefore a standard induction dose of each in a euvolemic, normotensive patient will onset within 30 seconds. The observed clinical duration of each drug is measured in minutes and is due to the drugs' redistribution half-life ($t_{1/2}\alpha$) characterized by redistribution of the drug from the central circulation (brain) to larger, well-perfused tissues, for example, fat and muscle. The elimination half-life ($t_{1/2}\beta$, usually measured in hours) is characterized by each drug's reentry from fat and lean muscle into plasma down a concentration gradient followed by hepatic metabolism that precedes renal excretion. Generally it requires four to five elimination half-lives to clear the drug completely from the body.

Because the target organ is the brain, and the desired effect is produced rapidly following bolus injection of the drug, dosing of induction agents in normal-sized and obese adults should be based on ideal body weight in kilograms. This amount can be estimated based on the patient's actual body weight, or a rough approximation can be obtained by subtracting 100 from the patient's height in centimeters; that is, 6 feet 4 inches = 76 inches $\times$ 2.54 centimeters/inch = 193 centimeters $-$ 100 = 93 kilograms. This approach provides a very acceptable estimate of ideal body weight, and the administered induction dose can then be adjusted based on the clinical status of the patient. Further dosing guidelines are provided in Chapters 19 and 20 for pediatric patients and in Chapter 31 for morbidly obese patients.

Aging affects the pharmacokinetics of induction agents. In the elderly, lean body mass and total body water decrease while total body fat increases, resulting in an increased volume of distribution, an increase in $t_{1/2}\beta$, and an increased duration of drug effect. The elderly are also much more sensitive to the hemodynamic and respiratory depressant effects of these agents, and consequently, most induction doses should be reduced.

I. Ultra-short-acting barbiturates
A. Thiopental Sodium (Pentothal)

Induction dose (mg/kg)	onset (sec)	$t_{1/2}\alpha$ (min)	duration (min)	$t_{1/2}\beta$ (hr)
3–6	<30	2–4	5–10	10–12

1. Clinical Pharmacology

Thiopental is the prototypical barbiturate used for anesthetic induction. These agents act at the barbiturate receptor, which forms part of the GABA-receptor complex to enhance and mimic the action of GABA (γ-aminobutyric acid). Thiopental decreases GABA dissociation from its receptor, which enhances GABA's neuroinhibitory activity, directly opens the chloride channel, and at higher drug concentrations, causes hyperpolarization of this chloride channel resulting in global depression of neuronal excitation and subsequent patient obtundation.

Thiopental is cerebroprotective causing a dose-dependent decrease in cerebral metabolic oxygen consumption and a parallel decrease in cerebral blood flow and intracranial pressure, provided cerebral perfusion pressure is maintained.

2. Indications and Contraindications

Thiopental's primary use as an induction agent is for patients suspected of having increased intracranial pressure or status epilepticus, as it has significant anticonvulsant activities in addition to the cerebroprotective properties outlined earlier. Thiopental and all of the other barbiturates are absolutely contraindicated in patients with acute intermittent porphyria, or variegate porphyria, as they can activate the enzyme responsible for precipitating an acute attack, which can be life-threatening. The barbiturates are not contraindicated in other types of porphyria.

Thiopental releases histamine (see later), and so is relatively contraindicated in patients with reactive airways disease.

3. Dosage and Clinical Use

The dosing of thiopental depends on the hemodynamic status of the patient and the concomitant use of other agents in the RSI algorithm. Thiopental is a potent venodilator and myocardial depressant. Consequently, the dose must be decreased in patients with decreased intravascular volume, those with compromised myocardial function, the elderly, and whenever thiopental is used with other drugs that affect sympathetic tone or cardiovascular function. In euvolemic, normotensive adults, the recommended induction dose is 3 to 5 mg/kg IV. For most emergency intubations, the lower dose of this range, that is, 3 mg/kg, achieves excellent sedation and intubating conditions with less tendency to cause hypotension that often occurs with the 5 mg/kg dose.

In the adult patient who is suspected of hypovolemia, myocardial dysfunction, or compromised hemodynamic status, the dose of thiopental should be reduced to 1 to 2 mg/kg IV. Thiopental should be avoided entirely in frankly hypotensive patients for whom other drugs, especially etomidate or ketamine, may preserve greater hemodynamic stability. With the widespread adoption of etomidate, which has significant cardiovascular stability, thiopental has seen limited use as an induction agent for emergent RSI.

4. Adverse Effects

As with any induction agent, inadequate dosing leaves the patient more lightly sedated and makes laryngoscopy more difficult, even in the context of use of a muscle relaxant. The chief side effects of thiopental include central respiratory depression, venodilation, and myocardial depression. These latter two may be manifested by hypotension that tends to be greater in both treated and untreated hypertensive patients compared with normotensive patients. Both can be detrimental in many patients in whom optimal preload is required to maintain cardiac output and prevent organ ischemia. Thiopental causes a dose-related release of histamine that in most situations is not clinically significant, but may cause or exacerbate bronchospasm in patients with reactive airways disease. Ketamine is the preferred induction agent for patients with reactive airways disease. There is a 10% to 20% incidence of nausea and vomiting that occurs during recovery from thiopental. Thiopental crosses the placenta, but there is reported fetal safety to a maternal dose of 6 mg/kg IV. Larger doses may produce fetal cardiovascular depression. One to two percent of patients will experience pain on injection of thiopental, especially if small veins on the dorsum of the hand are used. Inadvertent intraarterial injection or subcutaneous extravasation of thiopental can result in chemical endarteritis and distal thrombosis, ischemia, and tissue necrosis due to its highly alkaline pH (>10). Should extravasation occur, 40 to 80 mg of papaverine (Cerespan) in 20 mL normal saline or 10 mL of 1% lidocaine (Xylocaine) should be injected intraarterially proximal to the site.

B. Methohexital (Brevital)

Induction dose (mg/kg)	Onset (sec)	$t_{1/2\alpha}$ (min)	Duration (min)	$t_{1/2\beta}$ (hr)
1–3	<30	5–6	5–10	2–5

1. Clinical Pharmacology

Methohexital shares similar clinical pharmacologic properties with thiopental. It is two to three times more potent than thiopental, 1.5 mg of methohexital being equal to 4 mg of thiopental. The mechanism of action on the GABA-receptor complex and the cerebroprotective effects are identical to thiopental. The $t_{1/2}\ \beta$ for methohexital is two to three times shorter than that for thiopental.

2. Indications and Contraindications

The indications for use of methohexital are the same as thiopental. Methohexital is often used in those patients undergoing cardioversion or electroconvulsive therapy where its rapid onset of amnesia and a short duration of action are desirable. Similar to thiopental, methohexital is absolutely contraindicated in patients with acute intermittent porphyria, or variegate porphyria.

3. Dosage and Clinical Use

The onset of methohexital is more rapid and the duration of action shorter than with thiopental. The recommended induction dose in the euvolemic, normotensive patient is 1.5 mg/kg IV. If the patient is hypovolemic or hypotensive, the dose is reduced to 0.5 to 1.0 mg/kg IV. As with thiopental, the availability of etomidate has diminished the use of methohexital as an induction agent for emergency department RSI.

4. Adverse Effects

Methohexital causes more excitatory phenomena (twitching, hiccups) than thiopental. In about 5% of patients there is pain on drug injection, and as with thiopental, methohexital crosses the placenta. Ten to twenty percent of patients receiving methohexital will experience nausea and vomiting during recovery.

II. Benzodiazepines

	Induction dose (mg/kg)	Onset (sec)	$t_{1/2}\alpha$ (min)	Duration (min)	$t_{1/2}\beta$ (hr)
midazolam	0.2–0.3	30–60	7–15	15–30	2–4
lorazepam	0.03–0.06[a]	60–120	3–10	60–120	10–20
diazepam	0.3–0.6[a]	45–60	10–15	15–30	20–40

[a]Not recommended for use as an induction agent for emergency RSI.

1. Clinical Pharmacology

Although chemically distinct from the barbiturates, the benzodiazepines also exert their effects via the GABA-receptor complex. Benzodiazepines specifically stimulate the benzodiazepine receptor, which in turn modulates GABA, the primary neuroinhibitory transmitter. The benzodiazepines provide amnesia, anxiolysis, central muscle relaxation, sedation, anticonvulsant effects, and hypnosis. Although the benzodiazepines generally have similar pharmacologic profiles, they differ in selectivity, which makes their clinical usefulness variable. The benzodiazepines have potent, dose-related amnestic properties, perhaps their greatest asset in the emergency department. The lipophilicity of the benzodiazepines varies widely. Greater lipid solubility confers a more rapid onset of action because of the brain's high lipid content. The three benzodiazepines of interest to emergency physicians are midazolam (Versed), diazepam (Valium), and lorazepam (Ativan). Of the three, midazolam (Versed) is the most lipid soluble and is the only benzodiazepine suitable for use as an induction agent for emergent RSI. Midazolam has a slightly more rapid onset (30 to 60 seconds) than diazepam (Valium; 45 to 60 seconds), which in turn has a more rapid onset than lorazepam (Ativan; 60 to 120 seconds). Regardless, the time to clinical effectiveness of benzodiazepines is longer than any of the other induction agents, which mitigates their role in emergent RSI. The termination of action of these drugs is due to initial redistribution and subsequent hepatic metabolism via microsomal oxidation for midazolam and diazepam and glucuronide conjugation for lorazepam. The innate structure of each parent compound will determine the precise mechanism of hepatic degradation and the production of active or inactive metabolites, both of which will dictate the eventual elimination half-life of each drug. Midazolam has one insignificant active metabolite and a $t_{1/2}\beta$ of 2 to 4 hours. Diazepam has two active metabolites, both of which can prolong its sedative effect but more importantly are metabolized and excreted more slowly than diazepam and account for its prolonged $t_{1/2}\beta$ of 20 to 40 hours. Lorazepam has five inactive metabolites and a $t_{1/2}\beta$ of 10 to 20 hours. The benzodiazepines do not release histamine, and allergic reactions are very rare.

2. Indications and Contraindications

The primary indications for benzodiazepines are to promote amnesia and sedation. In this regard, the benzodiazepines are unparalleled. Midazolam's primary use in the emergency department is for procedural sedation, lorazepam is used primarily for treatment of seizures and alcohol withdrawal, and all three of these agents are used for sedation and anxiolysis in a variety of settings, including postintubation.

Because of their dose-related reduction in systemic vascular resistance and direct myocardial depression, dosage must be adjusted in volume-depleted or hemodynamically compromised patients. Studies have shown that normal induction doses of midazolam, 0.3 mg/kg, are rarely administered during emergent RSI. Unlike the other induction agents, including those that cause hypotension, midazolam is generally significantly underdosed during emergency RSI. It is postulated that this is due to the clinicians' familiarity with sedating doses of midazolam from experience with procedural use and lack of familiarity with the dosing and pharmacokinetics of midazolam as an induction agent.

3. Dosage and Clinical Use

The correct induction dose of midazolam for hemodynamically stable patients is 0.2 to 0.3 mg/kg IV push; the dose should be reduced to 0.1 mg/kg in hemodynamically compromised patients. Midazolam should be limited to amnestic dosing (i.e., 0.02 mg/kg) or avoided altogether in patients in frank shock (Chapter 28). Diazepam and lorazepam are not recommended for emergency department RSI because of their slower onset and are rarely used for this purpose.

4. Adverse Effects

Except for midazolam, the benzodiazepines are insoluble in water and are usually in solution in propylene glycol. Unless injected into a large vein, pain and venous irritation on injection can be significant.

III. Miscellaneous agents

A. Etomidate (Amidate)

Induction dose (mg/kg)	Onset (sec)	$t_{1/2}\alpha$ (min)	Duration (min)	$t_{1/2}\beta$ (hr)
0.3	15–45	2–4	3–12	2–5

1. Clinical Pharmacology

Etomidate is an imidazole derivative that is primarily a hypnotic and has no analgesic activity. With the exception of ketamine, etomidate is the most hemodynamically stable of the currently available induction agents. It exerts its effect by enhancing GABA activity at the GABA-receptor complex, inhibiting excitatory stimuli. Etomidate attenuates underlying elevated intracranial pressure by

decreasing cerebral blood flow and cerebral metabolic oxygen demand. Its hemodynamic stability preserves cerebral perfusion pressure. Etomidate is metabolized
in the liver, yielding an inactive metabolite that is excreted primarily by the kidneys.

Etomidate does not release histamine and is safe for use in patients with reactive airways disease. However, it lacks the direct bronchodilatory properties of
ketamine, which may be a preferable agent in these patients.

2. Indications and Contraindications

Etomidate has become the induction agent of choice for most emergent RSIs because of its rapid onset, its profound hemodynamic stability, its positive CNS
profile, and its rapid recovery. There are no contraindications to its use, but as with
any induction agent, dosage must be adjusted in hemodynamically compromised
patients. Etomidate is not FDA approved for use in children, but many series report
safe and effective use in pediatric patients (Chapters 19 and 20).

3. Dosage and Clinical Use

In euvolemic and hemodynamically stable patients, the normal induction dose of
etomidate is 0.3 mg/kg IV push. In compromised patients, the induction dose should
be reduced commensurate with the patient's clinical status.

4. Adverse Effects

Etomidate is associated with nausea and vomiting during recovery in 30% to 40%
of patients undergoing general anesthesia procedures. Its comparable incidence
after emergency RSI is unknown. This has not been an issue in the ED, where
patients are usually kept sedated and paralyzed after tracheal intubation. Pain on
injection is common because of the diluent (propylene glycol) and can be somewhat
mitigated by having a fast-flowing IV solution running in a large vein. Myoclonic
movement during induction is common and has been confused for seizures. It is of
no clinical consequence and generally terminates promptly as the neuromuscular
blocking agent takes effect. The occurrence of hiccups, usually during awakening,
is highly variable, 0% to 70%.

The most significant and controversial side effect of etomidate is its reversible
blockade of 11-beta-hydroxylase, which decreases both serum cortisol and aldos-
terone levels. This side effect has been more common with continuous infusions of
etomidate in the intensive care unit setting rather than with a single-dose injection
used for emergency RSI. Adverse effects due to cortisol suppression have not been
reported in ED patients undergoing RSI, even when specifically sought.

B. Ketamine (Ketalar)

Induction dose (mg/kg)	Onset (sec)	$t_{1/2}\alpha$ (min)	Duration (min)	$t_{1/2}\beta$ (hr)
1–2	45–60	11–17	10–20	2–3

1. Clinical Pharmacology

Ketamine is a phencyclidine (PCP) derivative that provides significant analgesia,
anesthesia, and amnesia with minimal effect on respiratory drive. The amnestic
effect is not as pronounced as that seen with the benzodiazepines. Ketamine is
thought to interact with the N-methyl-D-aspartate (NMDA) receptors at the GABA-
receptor complex, promoting neuroinhibition and subsequent anesthesia. Action on
opioid receptors accounts for its profound analgesic effect. Ketamine releases catecholamines, stimulates the sympathetic nervous system, and therefore augments
heart rate and blood pressure in those patients who are not catecholamine depleted

secondary to the demands of their underlying disease. Ketamine directly stimulates the central nervous system (CNS), increasing cerebral metabolism, cerebral metabolic oxygen demand ($CMRO_2$), and cerebral blood flow (CBF), thus potentially increasing intracranial pressure (ICP) in patients with CNS injury. However, the corresponding increases in mean arterial pressure may offset the rise in ICP, resulting in relatively stable cerebral perfusion pressure, and any risk of increased CNS injury must be considered to be hypothetical. In addition to its catecholamine-releasing effect, ketamine directly relaxes bronchial smooth muscle, producing bronchodilatation. Ketamine is primarily metabolized in the liver, producing one active metabolite, norketamine, which is metabolized and excreted in the urine.

2. Indications and Contraindications

Ketamine is the induction agent of choice for patients with reactive airways disease who require tracheal intubation. Because of its pharmacologic profile, ketamine also should be considered the induction agent of choice for patients who are hypovolemic or hypotensive without evidence of serious brain injury and for patients with hemodynamic instability due to cardiac tamponade or redistributive shock. In normotensive or hypertensive patients with ischemic heart disease, catecholamine release may adversely increase myocardial oxygen demand, but it is not known whether this effect might be important in patients with significant hypotension, who are probably maximally catecholamine stimulated before the ketamine is given. Ketamine's preservation of central respiratory drive makes it appealing for awake upper airway evaluation in the difficult airway patient. The use of ketamine in patients with elevated ICP remains controversial based on the previous discussion (see Chapter 24).

3. Dosage and Clinical Use

The induction dose of ketamine is 1 to 2 mg/kg IV. In patients who are catecholamine depleted, doses greater than 1.5 mg/kg IV may cause myocardial depression. Because of its generalized stimulating effects, ketamine enhances laryngeal reflexes and increases pharyngeal and bronchial secretions. These secretions may precipitate laryngospasm and be bothersome during upper airway examination in the difficult airway patient or during procedural sedation, but are not an issue during RSI. Atropine 0.02 mg/kg IV or glycopyrrolate (Robinul) 0.005 mg/kg IV may be administered in conjunction with ketamine to promote a drying effect.

4. Adverse Effects

The hallucinations that are well known to occur occasionally on emergence from ketamine are more common in the adult than in the child and can be eliminated by the concomitant or subsequent administration of a benzodiazepine, if desired. This is rarely an issue in ED airway management, in which the patient is usually sedated for prolonged periods, often with benzodiazepines.

C. Propofol (Diprivan)

Induction dose (mg/kg)	Onset (sec)	$t_{1/2}\alpha$ (min)	Duration (min)	$t_{1/2}\beta$ (hr)
1.5–3	15–45	2–4	5–10	1–3

1. Clinical Pharmacology

Propofol is an alkylphenol derivative with hypnotic properties. It is highly lipid soluble. Propofol enhances GABA activity at the GABA-receptor complex. It decreases $CMRO_2$ and ICP. Propofol causes a direct reduction in blood pressure through vasodilatation and direct myocardial depression, resulting in a decrease in cerebral perfusion pressure, which may be detrimental to a compromised patient. For these reasons it is rarely, if ever, the induction agent of choice in emergent RSI, where patient instability is the norm. Propofol has pharmacologic properties similar to both thiopental and etomidate. It causes greater myocardial depression and venodilation than thiopental, when used in equivalent doses.

2. Indications and Contraindications

Propofol is an excellent induction agent in a very stable patient. Its adverse potential for hypotension and reduction in cerebral perfusion pressure reduces its role as an induction agent in emergent RSI. There have been reports in the literature of propofol's use as an induction agent during tracheal intubation for reactive airways disease. The pharmacotherapeutics in this specific clinical situation seem to parallel those of ketamine. There are no absolute contraindications to the use of propofol.

3. Dosage and Clinical Use

The induction dose of propofol is 1.0 to 2.0 mg/kg IV in a euvolemic, normotensive patient. Because of its predictable tendency to reduce mean arterial blood pressure, smaller doses are generally used when propofol is given as an induction agent for emergency RSI.

4. Adverse Effects

Propofol causes pain on injection comparable to that of methohexital, less than etomidate, and more than thiopental. This effect can be attenuated by injecting the medication through a rapidly running IV in a large vein (e.g., antecubital). Propofol can cause mild clonus to a greater degree than thiopental, but less than etomidate or methohexital. Venous thrombophlebitis at the injection site is another potential adverse effect of propofol.

EVIDENCE

1. Dosing of midazolam for RSI. The dose of midazolam for induction of anesthesia is 0.1 to 0.3 mg/kg IV. The data to support this dose are from dosing studies conducted in the 1980s after the introduction of midazolam into clinical practice (1–9). Berggren and Eriksson prospectively demonstrated that midazolam 0.36 $\pm$ 0.01 mg/kg provided anesthetic depth similar to that of thiopentone 6.43 $\pm$ 0.21 mg/kg, in 60 female patients undergoing induction for elective abortion (1). Driessen et al. found that 0.2 mg/kg midazolam and 5.0 mg/kg thiopental provided similar depth of anesthesia in 40 women undergoing outpatient anesthesia (2). Jensen et al. found similar results using 0.2 mg/kg midazolam versus 3.0 mg/kg of thiopental for 40 orthopedic surgeries, and Izuora et al. found 0.15 to 0.2 mg/kg midazolam comparable to thiopental 4 to 6 mg/kg in 145 patients undergoing surgical procedures (3,4). Lebowitz et al. found midazolam 0.15 mg/kg and thiopental 3 mg/kg to display similar characteristics in 20 critically ill patients requiring intubation, and Pakkanen and Kanto found comparable results with 0.15 mg/kg of midazolam versus 4.7 mg/kg of pentothal (5,6). Lebowitz et al. compared 20 patients undergoing elective surgery, using 0.25 mg/kg midazolam and 4.0 mg/kg thiopental, again showing similar levels of anesthesia (7). Crawford prospectively evaluated 40 patients undergoing elective cesarean section, using 0.3 mg/kg midazolam and 4.0 mg/kg thiopental, demonstrating similar planes of anesthesia (8). Salonen et al. studied 27 children undergoing elective surgery and found that a dose of 0.6 mg/kg midazolam did not provide anesthesia equivalent to pentothal 5.0 mg/kg (9). Interestingly, Sagarin et al. recently demonstrated that most emergency intubations performed with midazolam generally use doses in the 0.03 to 0.04 mg/kg range (10). The lower dosing appears to be due to inexperience with the larger doses of midazolam used for induction or the concern that hypotension may ensue. Other induction agents, including thiopental and etomidate, were used in recommended doses (10).

2. Hemodynamic stability of induction agents. Use of etomidate results in the least variation in blood pressure and heart rate when compared to the other agents used for rapid induction of anesthesia (11–15). Etomidate also appears to have less effect on cardiac function as determined by echocardiographic findings (15). This effect is seen in children and adults, including the elderly (11–13).

3. Adrenal cortisol suppression after a single dose of etomidate. Etomidate causes reversible adrenocortical suppression by interfering with 11-beta-hydroxylation of 11-deoxy-cortisol, which prevents its conversion to cortisol. Etomidate cannot be used as a long-term infusion because of this side effect (16). Multiple outpatient surgery studies show a similar drop in serum cortisol after a single dose of etomidate. Schenarts et al. demonstrated a similar drop in serum cortisol at 4 hours when ED patients received etomidate; all patients spontaneously recovered adrenal cortical function within 12 hours without intervention (17). Absalom et al. demonstrated similar results in critically ill patients (18). When etomidate is used as an induction agent, the reversible drop in serum cortisol does not require supplemental glucocorticoids.

4. Ketamine use in patients with elevated intracranial pressure. Ketamine has been observed to further increase ICP in patients with elevated ICP (19), even in patients who show an initial transitory decrease (20). Multiple studies are confounded by the use of other induction or premedication agents. Similar effects in ICP rise have been observed in animal studies (21–26). However, a corresponding increase in mean arterial pressure may offset the ICP rise (27–30). The use of ketamine in ED patients with elevated ICP remains controversial and is therefore not recommended. See also Chapter 24.

5. Etomidate use in patients with seizures. Etomidate has been shown to increase activity in certain EEG leads in comparison to other sedatives when given to patients induced for general anesthesia. Thiopental, propofol, and midazolam all suppress EEG activity more quickly and completely than etomidate (31). The use of propofol, midazolam, or pentothal for RSI in the status seizure patient, followed by an infusion in the postintubation phase and ongoing EEG monitoring, is a logical choice. Use of etomidate in the patient with status seizure is not contraindicated, as it does depress the level of consciousness, and long-term sedation with benzodiazepines or propofol will generally follow the intubation.

6. Sedative choice for a severe bronchospasm. Ketamine and propofol both cause bronchodilation when used for induction (32–36). Eames et al. prospectively demonstrated that 2.5 mg/kg of propofol was superior to either 0.4 mg/kg etomidate or 5 mg/kg pentothal in decreasing mean airway pressure during bronchoscopy in 75 patients (32). Simon et al. demonstrated immediate improvement after propofol in 6 of 18 intubated patients with severe asthma on ventilators, compared to 8 of 13 who were placed on halothane anesthesia (33). Hemmingson et al. demonstrated a clinically and statistically significant improvement in respiratory dynamics after prospectively infusing ketamine or placebo to 14 asthmatics on ventilators (3,4). Etomidate causes a mild increase in airway resistance, but thiopental causes a significant rise in bronchospasm and resistance (32,36). Midazolam data is lacking. Ketamine is the recommended drug for patients without coronary artery disease because it is readily available, can be given IV push, and results in an increase in hemodynamic parameters such as heart rate and blood pressure, in contrast to propofol.

7. Importance of sedative choice in improving the laryngoscopic view of the vocal cords. The choice of sedative used for intubation may influence intubation success rates, especially if lower doses of a paralytic agent are used. Thiopental, methohexital, and propofol have each been shown to independently improve first-intubation success rates when using rocuronium 0.6 mg/kg, compared to etomidate, benzodiazepines, ketamine, or no agent (37,38). Propofol was found to be better than etomidate in the research of Skinner et al. as well (39). However, Fuchs-Buder et al. found no difference between thiopental and etomidate with alfentanyl pretreatment and rocuronium 0.6 mg/kg, and Hans et al. found ketamine superior to pentothal with midazolam 2 mg pretreatment and rocuronium 0.6 mg/kg. El-Orbany et al. found no difference between thiopental, propofol, and etomidate when rapacuronium was used as the paralytic agent (40–42) . This is currently a controversial topic; the correct dose of paralytic agent used for RSI may be as important an issue (Chapter 18).

  8. Sedative induction dosing should be made on ideal body weight. The total volume of distribution is increased in an obese patient, but the volume of the central intravenous compartment is not significantly different than in patients near their ideal body weight (43–45). This affects the benzodiazepines and barbiturates, specifically. Initial doses of thiopental and midazolam based on ideal body weight are appropriate (46,47).

  9. Ideal body weight estimation. Ideal body weight can be estimated by the Broca index: height in cm minus 100 for men; height in cm minus 105 for women (43,48,49).

REFERENCES

 1. Berggren L, Eriksson I. Midazolam for induction of anaesthesia in outpatients: a comparison with thiopentone. *Acta Anaesthesiol Scand* 1981;25:492–496.
 2. Driessen JJ, Booij LH, Crul JF, et al. Comparative study of thiopental and midazolam for induction of anesthesia. *Anaesthetist* 1983;32:478–482.
 3. Jensen S, Schou-Olesen A, Huttel MS. Use of midazolam as an induction agent: comparison with thiopentone. *Br J Anaesth* 1982;54:605–607.
 4. Izuora KL, Foulkes-Crabbe DJ, Kushimo OT, et al. Open comparative study of the efficacy, safety and tolerability of midazolam versus thiopental in induction and maintenance of anaesthesia. *West Afr J Med* 1994;13:73–80.
 5. Lebowitz PW, Cote ME, Daniels AL, et al. Cardiovascular effects of midazolam and thiopentone for induction of anaesthesia in ill surgical patients. *Can Anaesth Soc J* 1983;30(Jan):19–23.
 6. Pakkanen A, Kanto J. Midazolam compared with thiopentone as an induction agent. *Acta Anaesthesiol Scand* 1982;26:143–146.
 7. Lebowitz PW, Cote ME, Daniels AL, et al. Comparative cardiovascular effects of midazolam and thiopental in healthy patients. *Anesth Analg* 1982;61:771–775.
 8. Crawford ME, Carl P, Bach V, et al. A randomized comparison between midazolam and thiopental for elective cesarean section anesthesia. I. Mothers. *Anesth Analg* 1989;68:229–233.
 9. Salonen M, Kanto J, Iisalo E. Induction of general anesthesia in children with midazolam—is there an induction dose? *Int J Clin Pharmacol Ther Toxicol* 1987;25:613–615.
10. Sagarin MJ, Barton ED, Sakles JC, et al. National Emergency Airway Registry Investigators. Underdosing of midazolam in emergency endotracheal intubation. *Acad Emerg Med* 2003;10:329–338.
11. Benson M, Junger A, Fuchs C, et al. Use of an anesthesia information management system (AIMS) to evaluate the physiologic effects of hypnotic agents used to induce anesthesia. *J Clin Monit Comput* 2000;16:183–190.
12. Guldner G, Schultz J, Sexton P, et al. Etomidate for rapid-sequence intubation in young children: hemodynamic effects and adverse events. *Acad Emerg Med* 2003;10:134–139.
13. Sokolove PE, Price DD, Okada P. The safety of etomidate for emergency rapid sequence intubation of pediatric patients. *Pediatr Emerg Care* 2000;16(Feb):18–21.
14. Jellish WS, Riche H, Salord F, et al. Etomidate and thiopental-based anesthetic induction: comparisons between different titrated levels of electrophysiologic cortical depression and response to laryngoscopy. *J Clin Anesth* 1997;9(Feb):36–41.
15. Gauss A, Heinrich H, Wilder-Smith OH. Echocardiographic assessment of the haemodynamic effects of propofol: a comparison with etomidate and thiopentone. *Anaesthesia* 1991;46(Feb):99–105.
16. Allolio B, Stuttmann R, Fischer H, Leonhard W, Winkelmann W. Long-term etomidate and adrenocortical suppression. *Lancet* 1983;2:626.
17. Schenarts CL, Burton JH, Riker RR. Adrenocortical dysfunction following etomidate induction in emergency department patients. *Acad Emerg Med* 2001;8(Jan):1–7.
18. Absalom A, Pledger D, Kong A. Adrenocortical function in critically ill patients 24 h after a single dose of etomidate. *Anaesthesia* 1999;54:861–867.
19. Schulte am Esch J, Pfeifer G, Thiemig I, et al. *Acta Neurochir (Wien)* 1978;45:15–25.

20. Albanese J, et al.: Ketamine decreases intracranial pressure and electroencephalographic activity in traumatic brain injury patients during propofol sedation. *Anesthesiology* 1997;87:1328–1334.
21. Schwedler M, Miletich DJ, Albrecht RF. Cerebral blood flow and metabolism following ketamine administration. *Can Anaesth Soc J* 1982;29(May):222–226.
22. Pfenninger E, Dick W, Ahnefeld FW. The influence of ketamine on both normal and raised intracranial pressure of artificially ventilated animals. *Eur J Anaesthesiol* 1985;2:297–307.
23. Pfenninger E, Ahnefeld FW, Grunert A. Intracranial pressure during ketamine administration with spontaneous respiration. *Anaesthesist* 1985;2(Sept):297–307.
24. Pfenninger E, Grunert A, Bowdler I, et al. The effect of ketamine on intracranial pressure during haemorrhagic shock under the conditions of both spontaneous breathing and controlled ventilation. *Acta Neurochir (Wien)* 1985;78:113–118.
25. Langsjo JW, Kaisti KK, Aalto S, et al. Effects of subanesthetic doses of ketamine on regional cerebral blood flow, oxygen consumption, and blood volume in humans. *Anesthesiology* 2003;99:614–623.
26. Klose R, Hartung HJ, Kotsch R, et al. Experimental studies on the intracranial pressure increase by ketamine in haemorrhagic shock. *Anaesthesist* 1982;31(Jan):33–38.
27. Bourgoin A, Albanese J, Wereszczynski N, et al. Safety of sedation with ketamine in severe head injury patients: comparison with sufentanil. *Crit Care Med* 2003;31:711–717.
28. Kolenda H, Gremmelt A, Rading S, et al. Ketamine for analgosedative therapy in intensive care treatment of head-injured patients. *Acta Neurochir (Wien)* 1996;138:1193–1199.
29. Mayberg TS, Lam AM, Matta BF, et al. Ketamine does not increase cerebral blood flow velocity or intracranial pressure during isoflurane/nitrous oxide anesthesia in patients undergoing craniotomy. *Anesth Analg* 1995;81(Jul):84–89.
30. Friesen RH, Thieme RE, Honda AT, et al. Changes in anterior fontanel pressure in preterm neonates receiving isoflurane, halothane, fentanyl, or ketamine. *Anesth Analg* 1987;66:431–434.
31. Reddy RV, Moorthy SS, Dierdorf SF, et al. Excitatory effects and electroencephalographic correlation of etomidate, thiopental, methohexital, and propofol. *Anesth Analg* 1993;77:1008–1011.
32. Eames WO, Rooke GA, Wu RS, et al. Comparison of the effects of etomidate, propofol, and thiopental on respiratory resistance after tracheal intubation. *Anesthesiology* 1996;84:1307–1311.
33. Simon A, Nebel B, Metz G. Emergency intubation and ventilation therapy in severe bronchial asthma. *Pneumologie* 1990;44[Suppl 1]:657–658.
34. Hemmingsen C, Nielsen PK, Odorico J. Ketamine in the treatment of bronchospasm during mechanical ventilation. *Am J Emerg Med* 1994;12:417–420.
35. Conti G, Dell'Utri D, Vilardi V, et al. Propofol induces bronchodilation in mechanically ventilated chronic obstructive pulmonary disease (COPD) patients. *Acta Anaesthesiol Scand* 1993;37(Jan):105–109.
36. Conti G, Ferretti A, Tellan G, et al. Propofol induces bronchodilation in a patient mechanically ventilated for status asthmaticus. *Intensive Care Med* 1993;19:305.
37. Wu RS, Wu KC, Sum DC, et al. Comparative effects of thiopentone and propofol on respiratory resistance after tracheal intubation. *Br J Anaesth* 1996;77:735–738.
38. Sivilotti ML, Filbin MR, Murray HE, et al. Does the sedative agent facilitate emergency rapid sequence intubation? *Acad Emerg Med* 2003;10:612–620.
39. Skinner HJ, et al.: Evaluation of intubating conditions with rocuronium and either propofol or etomidate for rapid sequence induction. *Anaesthesia* 1998;53:702–706.
40. Fuchs-Buder T, Sparr HJ, Ziegenfuss T. Thiopental or etomidate for rapid sequence induction with rocuronium. *Br J Anaesth* 1998;80:504–506.
41. Hans P, et al.: Influence of induction of anaesthesia on intubating conditions one minute after rocuronium administration: comparison of ketamine and thiopentone. *Anaesthesia* 1999;54:266–296.
42. El-Orbany MI, Wafai Y, Joseph NJ, et al. Does the choice of intravenous induction drug affect intubation conditions after a fast-onset neuromuscular blocker? *J Clin Anesth* 2003;15(Feb):9–14.
43. Ogunnaike BO, Whitten CW. Anesthetic management of morbidly obese patients. *Semin Anesth Periop Med Pain* 2002;21:46–58.
44. Blouin RA, Kolpek JH, Mann HJ. Influence of obesity on drug disposition. *Clin Pharm* 1987;6:108–124.
45. Abernethy DR, Greenblatt DJ. Drug disposition in obese humans: an update. *Clin Pharmacokin* 1986;11:199–213.
46. Shenkman Z, Shir Y, Brodsky JB. Perioperative management of the obese patient. *Br J Anaesth* 1993;70:349–359.
47. Jung D, Mayersohn M, Perrier D. Thiopental disposition in lean and obese patients undergoing surgery. *Anesthesiology* 1982;56:269–274.
48. Adams JP, Murphy PG. Obesity in anaesthesia and intensive care. *Br J Anaesth* 2000;85:91–108.
49. McCarroll SM, Saunders PR, Bras PJ. Anesthetic considerations in obese patients. *Prog Anesthesiol* 2000;3:1–12.

18

Neuromuscular Blocking Agents

Robert E. Schneider and David A. Caro

I. Neuromuscular blocking agents

Neuromuscular blocking agents (NMBAs) are the cornerstone of emergency airway management and are used to obtain total control of the patient and to facilitate rapid endotracheal intubation while minimizing the risks of aspiration or other adverse physiologic events. NMBAs do not provide analgesia, sedation, or amnesia, however, and an induction or sedative agent must be used during rapid sequence intubation (RSI) for patients who are not completely unresponsive. Similarly, appropriate sedation is essential when neuromuscular blockade is maintained postintubation.

In order to understand the pharmacology of neuromuscular blocking agents, it is important to understand their effects at the postjunctional cholinergic nicotinic receptors in the neuromuscular junction. Under normal circumstances, the nerve synthesizes acetylcholine (ACH) and stores it in small packages (vesicles). Nerve stimulation results in these vesicles migrating to the nerve surface, rupturing and discharging ACH into the junctional clefts between the nerve and the muscle as well as those clefts that invaginate into the muscle fiber. The ACH attaches to ACH receptors, promoting muscle fiber depolarization that propagates into a muscle contraction. ACH then detaches from the receptor and is hydrolyzed by acetylcholinesterase (ACHE) which also resides in the clefts. NMBAs are either agonists (depolarizers of the motor end plate) or antagonists (nondepolarizers of the motor end plate). The antagonists attach to the receptors and competitively block ACH from accessing ACH receptors. Because they are in competition with ACH for the motor end plate, they can be displaced from the end plate by increasing concentrations of ACH, the end result of reversal agents (e.g. neostigmine) that inhibit ACHE and allow acetylcholine accumulation and neuromuscular retransmission.

In clinical practice there are two classes of neuromuscular blocking agents: the noncompetitive or depolarizing neuromuscular blocking agents, of which succinylcholine (Anectine) is the prototype and the only one in common clinical use. The competitive or nondepolarizing agents are divided into two main classes: the benzylisoquinolinium compounds and the aminosteroid compounds. The benzylisoquinolines, d-tubocurarine (Tubarine), metocurine (Dimethyltubocurarine), atracurium (Tracrium), cisatracurium (Nimbex), and mivacurium (Mivacron) share common properties, and the aminosteroids, vecuronium (Norcuron), pancuronium (Pavulon), and rocuronium (Zemuron) also share common attributes that are distinct from those of the benzylisoquinolines.

II. Depolarizing (noncompetitive) neuromuscular blocking agent: succinylcholine (Anectine)

The ideal muscle relaxant to facilitate tracheal intubation would have a rapid onset of action, rendering the patient paralyzed within seconds; a short duration of action, returning the patient's normal protective reflexes within 3 to 4 minutes; no significant adverse side effects; and metabolism and excretion independent of liver and kidney function. Unfortunately, such an agent does not exist. Succinylcholine (SCh) comes closest to meeting all these desirable goals. Despite the historic and well-known adverse effects of succinylcholine and the continuous advent of new competitive NMBAs, SCh remains the drug of choice for emergency RSI in both adults and in children.

A. Clinical pharmacology

SCh is actually two molecules of ACH linked back-to-back over an ester bridge and as such, is chemically similar to acetylcholine. It stimulates all of the nicotinic and muscarinic cholinergic receptors of the sympathetic and parasympathetic nervous system, not just those at the neuromuscular junction. Stimulation of cardiac muscarinic receptors can cause bradycardia, especially in children, but this effect can be blocked by the prior administration of atropine (see Chapters 16, 19, and 20). Although SCh can be a negative inotrope, this effect is so minimal as to have virtually no clinical relevance. SCh also releases histamine, but this effect also does not appear to be clinically significant. Once SCh reaches the neuromuscular junction, it binds tightly to the acetylcholine receptors, resulting in depolarization that manifests initially as fasciculations, then subsequent paralysis. The onset, activity, and duration of action of SCh are resistant to acetylcholinesterase and dependent on rapid hydrolysis by pseudocholinesterase, an enzyme of the liver and plasma not present at the neuromuscular junction. Therefore diffusion away from the neuromuscular junction motor end plate and back into the vascular compartment is ultimately responsible for SCh metabolism. This extremely important pharmacological concept explains why only a fraction of the initial intravenous dose of succinylcholine ever reaches the motor end plate to promote paralysis. More important, it is for this reason that larger, rather than smaller, doses of SCh should always be given in emergency RSI. Incomplete paralysis may jeopardize the patient by compromising respiration and may not provide adequate relaxation to facilitate otherwise easy endotracheal intubation. Succinylmonocholine, the initial metabolite of SCh, sensitizes the cardiac muscarinic receptors in the sinus node to repeat does of SCh, which may then cause bradycardia that will respond to atropine. At room temperature SCh retains 90% of its activity for up to three months. Refrigeration mitigates this degradation. Therefore, if SCh is stored at room temperature rather than being refrigerated in the emergency department, awareness of this degradation will be helpful in deciding when to exchange SCh to the operating room (OR) where it will be refrigerated and rapidly used.

B. Indications and contraindications

SCh remains the neuromuscular blocking agent of choice for emergency RSI because of its rapid onset and relatively brief duration of action. A personal or family history of malignant hyperthermia is an absolute contraindication to the use of SCh. Patients judged to be at risk for succinylcholine-related hyperkalemia represent absolute contraindications to its use and should receive a competitive, nondepolarizing NMBA. Relative contraindications to the use of SCh are dependent on the skill and proficiency of the intubator and the individual patient's clinical circumstance. A patient who is felt to represent a difficult intubation, and in whom ventilation with a bag and mask is also felt to be difficult or impossible, should not receive any NMBA except as part of a planned approach to the difficult airway (see Chapters 2 and 6).

C. Dosage and clinical use

In the normal-sized adult patient, the recommended dose of SCh for emergency RSI is 1.5 to 2 mg/kg IV. In a rare, life-threatening circumstance when SCh must be given IM because of inability to secure venous access, a dose of 3 to 4 mg/kg IM may be used. Absorption and delivery of drug will be dependent on the patient's circulatory status. This may result in a prolonged period of vulnerability for the patient, during which respiration will be compromised, but relaxation is not sufficient to permit intubation. Active bag/mask ventilation may be required before laryngoscopy in this circumstance.

Although length-based drug dosing will lead to the correct dose of SCh for children, adults continue to be dosed on an ideal body weight basis. It may be impossible in the emergency department to know the exact weight of a patient let alone the ideal body weight, and weight estimates, especially of supine patients, have been shown to be notoriously inaccurate. In those uncertain circumstances, it is better to err on the side of a higher dose of SCh to ensure adequate patient paralysis. One approach is to calculate the dose of SCh based on the estimated weight plus an additional 20%. For example, a 70-kg patient would require 105 mg of SCh (70 kg × 1.5 mg/kg) based on weight estimate alone, but to ensure paralysis in case of inadvertent underestimation of weight, 125 mg is recommended (105 mg plus 20% of 105 = 105 mg + 20 mg = 125 mg). The other option is to administer 2 mg/kg IV to all patients, thereby eliminating uncertainty or any miscalculation. The margin of safety in dosing SCh is up to a cumulative dose of 6 mg/kg. At doses greater than 6 mg/kg, the typical phase 1 depolarization block of SCh becomes a phase 2 block, which changes the pharmacokinetic displacement of SCh from the motor end plate, that is, becomes competitive rather than noncompetitive. This may prolong the duration of paralysis but otherwise is clinically irrelevant. The benefit of too much SCh far outweighs the risk of an inadequately paralyzed patient.

In obese patients pseudocholinesterase activity increases linearly with increasing weight as does the size of the extracellular fluid compartment. Both of these factors afford increasing doses of SCh in the obese patient. Because of the downside of inadequate paralysis (may promote a difficult or failed intubation), obese patients should be dosed based on actual body weight, not ideal body weight. The trade-off is perhaps a larger dose, which leads to a longer period of paralysis after intubation or a longer period of bag/mask ventilation should intubation fail. Again the benefit of complete paralysis outweighs the risk.

In children less than 10 years of age, length-based dosing is recommended, but if weight is used as the determinant, the recommended dose of SCh for emergency RSI is 2 mg/kg IV, and in the newborn (less than 12 months of age) the appropriate dose is 3 mg/kg IV. Because children have higher vagal tone than adults, atropine 0.02 mg/kg IV should be administered as a pretreatment agent to any child under 10 years of age who is receiving SCh (see Chapters 16, 19, and 20). Atropine will attenuate the bradycardia caused by both airway manipulation and SCh. This same vagotonic effect must be anticipated in adults when repeated doses of SCh are administered. In this case, it is not necessary to administer atropine prophylactically, but atropine should be readily at hand in case bradycardia ensues.

D. Adverse effects

The recognized side effects of SCh include fasciculations, hyperkalemia, bradycardia, prolonged neuromuscular blockade, malignant hyperthermia, and trismus-masseter muscle spasm. Each of these will be discussed separately.

1. Fasciculations

Fasciculations are thought to be produced by stimulation of the nicotinic ACH receptors. Fasciculations occur simultaneously with increases in intracranial pressure (ICP), intraocular pressure, and intragastric pressure, but these are not the result of concerted muscle activity. Of these, only the increase in ICP is clinically important.

The exact mechanisms by which these effects occur are not well elucidated. In patients suspected of having increased intracranial or intraocular pressure, it may be prudent to inhibit these fasciculations. This can be accomplished by giving a defasciculating dose (10% of the normal paralyzing dose) of a nondepolarizing NMBA such as vecuronium, pancuronium, or rocuronium. The recommended doses are 0.01 mg/kg of vecuronium or pancuronium, or 0.06 mg/kg of rocuronium.

The relationship between muscle fasciculation and subsequent postoperative muscle pain is controversial. Studies have been variable with respect to prevention of fasciculations in absence of muscle pain. Some studies have shown no difference between defasciculation and placebo with patients continuing to complain of muscle pain in the same proportions, raising further questions regarding cause, effect, and prevention. Clinically, inhibition of fasciculations is much more important with elevated ICP than with an open globe injury. The pathophysiologic concern in open globe injury is extrusion of vitreous, which has never been attributed to the administration of SCh. In fact, many anesthesiologists continue to use SCh as a muscle relaxant in cases of open globe injury, with or without an accompanying defasciculating agent. Similarly, the increase in intragastric pressure that has been measured has never been shown to be of any clinical significance, perhaps because it is offset by a corresponding increase in the distal esophageal sphincter pressure.

2. Hyperkalemia

Under normal circumstances, serum potassium increases minimally (0 to 0.5 mEq/L) when SCh is administered. A pathological response to SCh can occur, however, resulting in rapid and dramatic increases in serum potassium. These pathologic hyperkalemic responses occur by two distinct mechanisms: receptor upregulation and rhabdomyolysis. In either situation potassium increase may approach 5 to 10 mEq/L and result in hyperkalemic dysrhythmias or cardiac arrest.

Two forms of postjunctional receptors exist, mature (junctional) and immature (extrajunctional). Each receptor is composed of five proteins arranged in circular fashion around a common channel. Both types of receptors contain two alpha subunits. ACH must attach to both alpha subunits to open the channel and effect depolarization and muscle contraction. When receptor upregulation occurs, the mature receptors at and around the motor end plate are gradually converted over a 4- to 5-day period to immature receptors that propagate throughout the entire muscle membrane. Immature receptors are characterized by low conductance and prolonged channel opening times (four times longer than mature receptors), resulting in increasing levels of potassium, clinically significant dysrhythmias, and cardiac arrest. Most of the entities associated with hyperkalemia during emergency RSI are the result of receptor upregulation. Interestingly, these same extrajunctional nicotinic receptors are relatively refractory to nondepolarizing agents, so larger doses of vecuronium, pancuronium, or rocuronium will be required to produce paralysis.

Rhabdomyolysis is the other mechanism by which hyperkalemia may occur. It is most often associated with myopathies. In cardiac arrest situations related to rhabdomyolysis, resuscitation may be less successful than in receptor upregulation because of potentially coexisting myopathies (cardiac) yielding less physiologic reserve. SCh is a toxin to unstable membranes in any patient with a myopathy and should be avoided.

Receptor upregulation occurs in the following circumstances:

a. Burns

In burn victims, the extrajunctional receptor sensitization becomes clinically significant 5 days postburn. It lasts an indefinite period of time, at least until there is complete healing of the burned area. If the burn becomes infected or healing is delayed, the patient remains at risk for hyperkalemia. It is prudent not to administer SCh to burned patients if any question exists regarding the status of their burn. The percent of body surface area burned does not determine the magnitude of hyperkalemia; significant hyperkalemia has been reported in patients with as little as 8% total body surface area burn (less than the surface of one arm), but this is rare. Most emergency department intubations for burns are performed well within the safe 5-day window after the burn occurs, but if later intubation is required, rocuronium or vecuronium provide excellent alternatives for emergency RSI in these situations.

b. Denervation

The patient who suffers a denervation event, such as spinal cord injury or stroke, is at risk for hyperkalemia from the fifth day postevent until there is healing or total muscle fiber atrophy. Patients with neuromuscular disorders such as multiple sclerosis or amyotrophic lateral sclerosis are at risk for hyperkalemia indefinitely, depending on the dynamic state of their disease. As long as the neuromuscular disease is dynamic, there will be augmentation of the extrajunctional receptors and the risk for hyperkalemia. Unlike fasciculations, the hyperkalemic response cannot be attenuated by administering defasciculating doses of nondepolarizing NMBAs, and therefore, these specific clinical situations should be considered absolute contraindications to SCh during the designated time periods.

c. Crush injuries

The data regarding crush injuries are scant. The hyperkalemic response begins about 5 days postinjury similar to denervation and persists for several months after healing seems complete.

d. Intraabdominal infections

This entity seems to relate to the intensive care unit environment where total body disuse atrophy and chemical denervation of the ACH receptors can occur if muscle relaxants are chronically infused. Again the at-risk time period is 5 days after initiation of the illness and continues indefinitely as long as the disease process is dynamic.

e. Myopathies

SCh is absolutely contraindicated in patients with inherited myopathies. Myopathic hyperkalemia can be devastating because of the combined effects of receptor upregulation and rhabdomyolysis. As previously stated, these patients tend to be the most difficult to resuscitate following cardiac arrest. Any patient suspected of a myopathy should be paralyzed with nondepolarizing muscle relaxants rather than SCh.

f. Renal failure

There is a paucity of evidence supporting the notion that chronic renal failure presents a risk for hyperkalemia in patients receiving SCh. Indeed, the majority of renal failure patients are successfully intubated using SCh without adverse cardiovascular complications. SCh itself does not stimulate abnormal increases in potassium in renal failure. Rocuronium or vecuronium are safer choices for emergency RSI in renal failure patients presenting with known disease-related hyperkalemia (missed dialysis, necrotic muscle, etc.).

3. Bradycardia

Bradycardia following the administration of SCh is seen most commonly in children because of their heightened vagotonic state (Chapter 19). Bradycardia is attenuated or abolished by administering atropine 0.02 mg/kg IV as a pretreatment drug before administering SCh. In adults, repeated doses of SCh may produce the same vagotonic effects and administration of atropine may become necessary.

4. Prolonged neuromuscular blockade

Prolonged neuromuscular blockade may result from either an acquired reduction in pseudocholinesterase (PCHE) concentration, a congenital absence of PCHE, or the presence of an atypical form of PCHE, all three of which will delay the degradation of SCh and prolong paralysis. Reduced concentrations of PCHE may be a result of liver disease, pregnancy, burns, oral contraceptives, metoclopramide, bambuterol, or esmolol. Atypical or abnormal genetic variants of PCHE can be disclosed by testing the patient's PCHE against dibucaine. A 20% reduction in normal levels will increase apnea time about 3 to 9 minutes. The most severe variant (0.04% of population) will prolong paralysis for 4 to 8 hours.

5. Malignant hyperthermia

A personal or family history of malignant hyperthermia (MH) is an absolute contraindication to the use of SCh. MH is a myopathy characterized by a genetic skeletal muscle membrane abnormality of the Ry_1 ryanodine receptor. It can be triggered by halogenated anesthetics, SCh, vigorous exercise, and even emotional stress. Following the initiating event, its onset can be acute and progressive or delayed for hours. Generalized awareness of MH, earlier diagnosis, and the availability of dantrolene (Dantrium) have decreased the mortality from as high as 70% to less than 5%. Acute loss of intracellular calcium control results in a cascade of rapidly progressive events manifested primarily by increased metabolism as well as muscular rigidity, autonomic instability, hypoxia, hypotension, severe lactic acidosis, hyperkalemia, myoglobinemia, and disseminated intravascular coagulation. Elevations in temperature are a late manifestation. The presence of more than one of these clinical signs is suggestive of MH. Masseter spasm has been claimed to be the hallmark of MH. However, SCh can promote isolated masseter spasm as an exaggerated response at the neuromuscular junction, especially in children. Therefore, masseter spasm alone is not pathognomonic of MH.

The treatment for MH consists of discontinuing the known or suspected precipitant and the immediate administration of dantrolene sodium (Dantrium). Dantrolene is essential to successful resuscitation and should be given as soon as the diagnosis is seriously entertained. Dantrolene is a hydantoin derivative that acts directly on skeletal muscle to prevent calcium release from the sarcoplasmic reticulum without affecting calcium reuptake. The initial dose is 2.5 mg/kg IV and is repeated every five minutes until muscle relaxation occurs or the maximum dose of 10 mg/kg is administered. Dantrolene is free of any serious side effects. Additionally, measures to control body temperature, acid base balance, and renal function must be used. All cases of MH require constant monitoring of pH, arterial blood gases, and serum potassium. Immediate and aggressive management of hyperkalemia with the administration of calcium gluconate, glucose, insulin, and sodium bicarbonate may be necessary. Interestingly, full paralysis with nondepolarizing NMBAs will prevent SCh-triggered MH. MH has never been reported related to use of SCh in the emergency department. The 24/7 MH emergency hotline number is 1-800-MH-HYPER or 209-634-4917. Ask for "index zero." The e-mail address is *mhaus@norwich.net*. The Website is *www.mhaus.org*. MHAUS is the abbreviation for the Malignant Hyperthermia Association of the United States.

6. Trismus/masseter muscle spasm

SCh normally raises jaw muscle tone. This is not true spasm and laryngoscopy is usually unaffected. On occasion, SCh may cause transient trismus/masseter muscle spasm, especially in children. This is manifested as jaw muscle rigidity associated with limb muscle flaccidity. Pretreatment with defasciculating doses of nondepolarizing NMBAs will not prevent masseter spasm. If masseter spasm interferes with intubation, a full paralyzing dose of a competitive nondepolarizing agent (e.g., rocuronium 1 mg/kg or vecuronium 0.15 mg/kg) should be administered and will relax the involved muscles. The patient may require bag and mask ventilation until relaxation is complete and intubation is possible. In such circumstances, serious consideration should be given to the diagnosis of MH (see earlier discussion).

III. Nondepolarizing (competitive) neuromuscular blocking agents

A. Clinical pharmacology

The nondepolarizing NMBAs actually compete with and block the action of ACH transmission at the postjunctional cholinergic nicotinic receptors in the neuromuscular junction. The blockade is accomplished by competitively binding to one or both of the alpha subunits in the receptor, preventing ACH access to both alpha subunits, which is required for muscle contraction. This competitive blockade is characterized by the absence of fasciculations and the reversal of paralysis by acetylcholinesterase inhibitors that prevent metabolism of ACH and allow its reaccumulation and retransmission at the motor end plate, promoting a muscle contraction. These drugs are metabolized and eliminated by Hoffman degradation, liver metabolism, and renal excretion.

The nondepolarizing NMBAs are divided into two groups: the benzylisoquinolinum compounds (atracurium and mivacurium) and the aminosteroid compounds (vecuronium, pancuronium, and rocuronium). Of the two groups, the aminosteroid compounds are the only agents used commonly for emergency RSI and postintubation paralysis.

In general the aminosteroid compounds do not release histamine, they do not cause ganglionic blockade, they vary inversely regarding their potency and time to onset (more potent agents require longer time to onset), and they exhibit differences in their vagolytic effects (i.e., moderate in pancuronium, slight in rocuronium, and absent in vecuronium). These compounds are further subdivided based on their duration of action, which is determined by their metabolism and excretion. None has the brief duration of action afforded SCh. Pancuronium is longer lasting than vecuronium or rocuronium. Although pancuronium is excreted primarily by the kidney, 10% to 20% is metabolized in the liver. Vecuronium is more lipophilic, hence more easily absorbed. It is eliminated primarily in the bile and is very stable cardiovascularly. Rocuronium is lipophilic and excreted in the bile.

The nondepolarizing NMBAs can be reversed by administering acetylcholinesterase inhibitors such as neostigmine (Prostigmine) 0.06 to 0.08 mg/kg IV after significant (40%) spontaneous recovery has occurred. Atropine 0.02 mg/kg IV or glycopyrrolate (Robinul) 0.2 mg IV should be available to block excessive muscarinic stimulation. Reversal of blockade is rarely, if ever, indicated in the emergency department.

B. Indications and contraindications

The nondepolarizing NMBAs serve a multipurpose role in emergency airway management. They can be used as pretreatment agents to attenuate increases in ICP attributed to muscle fasciculations, they can serve as the muscle relaxant of choice if SCh is contraindicated or unavailable, or most commonly they can be used to maintain postintubation paralysis. There are no known contraindications to using nondepolarizing NMBAs.

	Intubating dose (mg/kg)	Pretreatment (mg/kg)	Onset (sec)	Duration (min)	Full recovery (hr)
pancuronium		0.01	100–150	120–150	3–5
vecuronium	0.15	0.01	90–120	60–75	1.5–2
rocuronium	1	0.06	55–70	30–60	1–2

C. Dosage and clinical use

1. For defasciculation when SCh is used in patients with elevated ICP. The appropriate dose is 10% of the paralyzing dose of any of the nondepolarizing agents (pancuronium 0.01 mg/kg, vecuronium 0.01 mg/kg, rocuronium 0.06 mg/kg). In this clinical circumstance, there is no preference for any one of these three agents over the other two.

2. For RSI when SCh is contraindicated (see Chapter 22) or not available. In these situations, nondepolarizing NMBAs can be used for emergency RSI. The drug of choice is rocuronium 1.0 mg/kg IV based on its time to onset. If rocuronium is not available, vecuronium 0.15 mg/kg is a reasonable alternative. Pancuronium 0.1 mg/kg could be used for this indication as well but would not be ideal, secondary to its long time to onset and its prolonged duration of action.

3. For postintubation management when continued neuromuscular blockade is desired, vecuronium 0.1 mg/kg IV or pancuronium 0.1 mg/kg IV is appropriate.

   Table 18-1 lists the dosage, onset, and duration of action of all the muscle relaxants.

D. Adverse effects

Of the three aminosteroid compounds, pancuronium is the least expensive but may be less desirable because it has a tendency to produce tachycardia. Vecuronium and rocuronium are more expensive but do not promote tachycardia. All of the competitive NMBAs are generally less desirable for intubation than SCh because of either delayed time to paralysis, prolonged duration of action, or both. Their onset can be shortened by administering an intubating dose, but this further prolongs the duration of action.

TABLE 18-1. *Onset and duration of action of neuromuscular blocking drugs*

Drug	Dose (mg/kg)	Time to maximal blockade (min)	Time to recovery (min) 25%	Time to recovery (min) 75%
Quarternary amine				
Succinylcholine	1.0	1.1	8	11 (90%)
Benzylisoquinolinium compounds				
Tubocurarine	0.5	3.4	—	130
Metocurine	0.4	4.1	107	—
Alcuronium	0.2	7.1	47 (20%)	90 (70%)
Atracurium	0.4	2.4	38	52
Doxacurium	0.05	5.9	83	116
Mivacurium	0.15	1.8	16	25
Cisatracirium	0.1	7.7	46	63
Aminosteroid compounds				
Pancuronium	0.08	2.9	86	—
Vecuronium	0.1	2.4	44	56
Pipecuronium	0.07	2.5	95	136
Rocuronium	0.6	1.0	43	66

From Hunter JM. Drug therapy: new neuromuscular blocking drugs. *N Engl J Med* 1995;332:1691–1699, with permission.

EVIDENCE

1. NMBA use in emergency rapid sequence intubation (RSI). RSI with a paralytic agent is the current standard of care for routine emergency intubation. NMBAs have been safely and successfully used in the emergency setting since the late 1970s to provide paralysis for intubation (1,2,3). Cicala and Westbrooke demonstrated an improved intubation success rate with neuromuscular blockade over deep-plane anesthesia without neuromuscular blockade (4). Syverud et al. found that the use of paralytics improved physician intubation success rates from 54% to 96% in the prehospital setting (5). Dronen et al. found that SCh-assisted oral intubation was far superior (96% success rate) to blind nasotracheal intubation (37% success rate) in the overdose patient (6). Multiple prospective studies confirm the high success rate of RSI with NMBAs when performed by experienced operators (7,8,9), with a lower rate of complications compared to sedatives alone (10,11).

2. Succinylcholine use compared to the nondepolarizing NMBAs. Multiple studies have compared SCh to rocuronium and vecuronium, for intubation, but only a few have approximated the conditions and circumstances of emergency department RSI (7,12,13). Three recent review articles compared intubation success rates and intubating conditions for SCh versus rocuronium, and all three concluded that the two drugs are similar but not identical (14,15,16). SCh produces slightly better intubating conditions and has a statistically significant reduced number of intubation attempts when compared to intubating doses of rocuronium (17). Importantly, the dose of rocuronium is critical to the success of intubation. This has been elegantly studied, and the correct dose of rocuronium for RSI is 1.0 to 1.2 mg/kg, not 0.6 mg/kg as is commonly recommended. The duration for 1.0 mg/kg dose is 46 minutes (16,18,19). SCh has been repeatedly shown to produce better intubating conditions at 45 to 60 seconds compared to pancuronium, vecuronium, and atracurium in well-designed prospective studies (20,21,22).

3. NMBAs and intramuscular administration. Intravenous administration of NMBAs is vastly preferred to other routes, but infrequently a situation arises in which IV or intraosseous access cannot be obtained. Intramuscular administration of NMBAs has been described, with multiple NMBAs (SCh, rocuronium, and mivacurium) studied. Invariably, the onset to paralysis is delayed. Schuh performed a prospective comparison of SCh via IM and IV routes and found that the IM dose required is 3.0 to 4.0 mg/kg and time to onset is 5 to 6 minutes (23). Sutherland et al. performed a prospective study that demonstrated obliteration of muscle twitch at 4.0 ± 0.6 minutes with an intramuscular dose of 4 mg/kg (24). Each of the studies assessing IM rocuronium combines it with prior halothane use, which is not applicable to the emergency department environment. Reynolds et al. prospectively demonstrated that deltoid injection of 1.0 mg/kg in infants and 1.8 mg/kg in children created adequate or good intubating conditions in 2.5 and 3.0 minutes, respectively (25,26). Kaplan et al., however, found that equivalent doses gave inadequate intubating conditions at 2.5 and 3.0 minutes, and only half of the children receiving these doses had adequate intubating conditions at 3.5 and 4 minutes (27). The majority of patients had adequate conditions only after 7 to 8 minutes. Although IM administration of NMBAs has been described, its use in the emergent situation should be limited to the rare situation when absolutely no intravenous or intraosseous access can be obtained.

4. Neuromuscular blockers and intubating conditions for RSI. SCh has been repeatedly demonstrated to produce the most optimal conditions for intubation in the shortest amount of time, compared to any of the nondepolarizing agents (see earlier discussion). The dose of paralytic agent used is critical to the success of intubation. Larger doses of paralytic consistently provide better intubating conditions than do smaller ones: 1.0 mg/kg SCh has been prospectively demonstrated to provide better intubating conditions than does placebo, 0.3 mg/kg or 0.5 mg/kg (28,29). Similarly, rocuronium doses of 0.6 mg/kg are inferior to doses of 0.9 to 1.2 mg/kg (13). Inadequate dosing of a NMBA can impair chances of successful intubation by causing insufficient paralysis.

5. Succinylcholine use in patients with open eye injuries. SCh has been linked with increases in intraocular pressure. Concern has been raised about its use in penetrating eye injuries (30). However, there has never been a case report of vitreous extrusion following the use of SCh in a patient with an open globe (31). The more pressing concern for the protection of the injured eye is the prevention of stimuli associated with laryngoscopy (32). Pretreatment with a nondepolarizing NMBA is recommended in patients with open globe injuries.

6. Timing of hyperkalemia after significant (>5% body surface area) burns. Schaner et al. and Gronert et al. found the greatest risk 18 to 66 days postburn in two studies in 1969 and 1975, and Viby-Mogensen et al. found dangerous rises in serum potassium as early as 9 days postburn (33–35). SCh can be safely used within the first week of a burn, but should be withheld after the first week through clinical healing of the burn wound.

7. SCh use in denervation injuries (stroke, Guillain-Barré syndrome, polio, spinal cord trauma, myasthenia gravis, etc.). Denervation injuries cause a change in the number and function of junctional and extrajunctional ACH receptors at 4 to 5 days postinjury (36,37). This can result in massive serum potassium increases that can cause cardiac arrest. SCh can be safely used up to 5 days postdenervation and not again until complete muscle atrophy has occurred or the event is no longer dynamic.

8. SCh use in myopathic patients (muscular dystrophy, rhabdomyolysis, crush injuries, etc.). Myopathies cause hyperkalemia by a similar mechanism as denervation, that is, changes in ACH receptor function and density (38). Congenital myopathies are considered an absolute contraindication to SCh; its use with the myopathies can result in rhabdomyolysis and resuscitation-resistant hyperkalemic arrest (39,40). Hyperkalemia and occult, undiagnosed myopathy must be considered in children who experience cardiac arrest after SCh (41,42). When a patient with known rhadomyolysis is encountered, SCh should be avoided.

9. SCh use in patients with renal failure. Hyperkalemia is a concern in patients on hemodialysis who require intubation. The long-term dogma is to avoid SCh in these patients

(43,44); some small studies have shown no instances of cardiac arrest when using it in the setting of renal failure (45,46). Insufficient data exist to declare it safe for routine use if a patient is suspected to have significant hyperkalemia.

10. SCh use in patients with severe (especially intraabdominal) infections. Intraabdominal infections lasting longer than 1 week are susceptible to SCh-induced hyperkalemia (47). SCh-induced hyperkalemia risk increases with increasing severity of infection (48).

11. Treatment for SCh-induced MH. Discontinue any anesthetic use. Dantrolene, 2 mg/kg IV, is the recommended therapy, and it can be repeated every 5 minutes to a total dose of 10 mg/kg (49). In a review of 21 patients with presumed MH, 11 patients immediately treated with dantrolene survived; and 3 of 4 patients who did not receive treatment until 24 hours later died (6 patients were excluded because of insufficient evidence that MH was the cause of decompensation) (50).

REFERENCES

1. Roberts DJ, Clinton JE, Ruiz E. Neuromuscular blockade for critical patients in the emergency department. *Ann Emerg Med* 1986;15:152–156.
2. Thompson JD, Fish S, Ruiz E. Succinylcholine for endotracheal intubation. *Ann Emerg Med* 1982;11:526–529.
3. Brown EM, Krishnaprasad D, Smiler BG. Pancuronium for rapid induction technique for tracheal intubation. *Can Anaesth Soc J* 1979;26:489–491.
4. Cicala R, Westbrook L. An alternative method of paralysis for rapid-sequence induction. *Anesthesiology* 1988;69:983–986.
5. Syverud SA, Borron SW, Storer DL, et al. Prehospital use of neuromuscular blocking agents in a helicopter ambulance program. *Ann Emerg Med* 1988;17:236–242.
6. Dronen SC, Merigian KS, Hedges JR, et al. A comparison of blind nasotracheal and succinylcholine-assisted intubation in the poisoned patient. *Ann Emerg Med* 1987;16:650–652.
7. Sagarin MJ, Chiang V, Sakles JC, et al. National Emergency Airway Registry (NEAR) investigators. Rapid sequence intubation for pediatric emergency airway management. *Pediatr Emerg Care* 2002;18:417–423.
8. Tayal VS, Riggs RW, Marx JA, et al. Rapid-sequence intubation at an emergency medicine residency: success rate and adverse events during a two-year period. *Acad Emerg Med* 1999;6(Jan):31–37.
9. Sakles JC, Laurin EG, Rantapaa AA, et al. Airway management in the emergency department: a one-year study of 610 tracheal intubations. *Ann Emerg Med* 1998;31:325–332.
10. Li J, Murphy-Lavoie H, Bugas C, et al. Complications of emergency intubation with and without paralysis. *Am J Emerg Med* 1999;17:141–143.
11. Gnauck K, Lungo JB, Scalzo A, et al. Emergency intubation of the pediatric medical patient: use of anesthetic agents in the emergency department. *Ann Emerg Med* 1994;23:1242–1247.
12. Vijayakumar E, Bosscher H, Renzi FP, et al. The use of neuromuscular blocking agents in the emergency department to facilitate tracheal intubation in the trauma patient: help or hindrance? *J Crit Care* 1998;13(Mar):1–6.
13. Magorian T, Flannery KB, Miller RD. Comparison of rocuronium, succinylcholine, and vecuronium for rapid-sequence induction of anesthesia in adult patients. *Anesthesiology* 1993;79:913–918.
14. Laurin EG, Sakles JC, Panacek EA, et al. A comparison of succinylcholine and rocuronium for rapid-sequence intubation of emergency department patients. *Acad Emerg Med* 2000;7:1362–1369.
15. Mazurek AJ, Rae B, Hann S, et al. Rocuronium versus succinylcholine: are they equally effective during rapid-sequence induction of anesthesia? *Anesth Analg* 1998;87:1259–1262.
16. Andrews JI, Kumar N, van den Brom RH, et al. A large simple randomized trial of rocuronium versus succinylcholine in rapid-sequence induction of anaesthesia along with propofol. *Acta Anaesthesiol Scand* 1999;43 (Jan):4–8.
17. Perry JJ, Lee J, Wells G. Are intubating conditions using rocuronium equivalent to those using succinylcholine? *Acad Emerg Med* 2002;9:813–823.
18. Cheng CA, Aun CS, Gin T. Comparison of rocuronium and suxamethonium for rapid tracheal intubation in children. *Paediatr Anaesth* 2002;12:140–145.
19. McCourt KC, Salmela L, Mirakhur RK, et al. Comparison of rocuronium and suxamethonium for use during rapid sequence induction of anaesthesia. *Anaesthesia* 1998;53:867–871.
20. Barr AM, Thornley BA. Thiopentone and pancuronium crash induction. A comparison with thiopentone and suxamethonium. *Anaesthesia* 1978;33(Jan):25–31.
21. Mehta MP, Sokoll MD, Gergis SD. Accelerated onset of non-depolarizing neuromuscular blocking drugs: pancuronium, atracurium and vecuronium. A comparison with succinylcholine. *Eur J Anaesthesiol* 1988;5(Jan):15–21.
22. Martin C, Bonneru JJ, Brun JP, et al. Vecuronium or suxamethonium for rapid sequence intubation: which is better? *Br J Anaesth* 1987;59:1240–1244.

23. Schuh FT. The neuromuscular blocking action of suxamethonium following intravenous and intramuscular administration. *Int J Clin Pharmacol Ther Toxicol* 1982;20:399–403.

24. Sutherland GA, Bevan JC, Bevan DR. Neuromuscular blockade in infants following intramuscular succinylcholine in two or five percent concentration. *Can Anaesth Soc J* 1983;30:342–346.

25. Reynolds LM, Lau M, Brown R, et al. Bioavailability of intramuscular rocuronium in infants and children. *Anesthesiology* 1997;87:1096–1105.

26. Reynolds LM, Lau M, Brown R, et al. Intramuscular rocuronium in infants and children. Dose-ranging and tracheal intubating conditions. *Anesthesiology* 1996;85:231–239.

27. Kaplan RF, Uejima T, Lobel G, et al. Intramuscular rocuronium in infants and children: a multicenter study to evaluate tracheal intubating conditions, onset, and duration of action. *Anesthesiology* 1999;91:633–638.

28. Donati F. The right dose of succinylcholine. *Anesthesiology* 2003;99:1037–1038.

29. Naguib M, Samarkandi A, Riad W, et al. Optimal dose of succinylcholine revisited. *Anesthesiology* 2003;99:1045–1049.

30. Cunningham AJ, Barry P. Intraocular pressure—physiology and implications for anesthetic management. *Can Anaesth Soc J* 1986;33:195–208.

31. Vachon CA, Warner DO, Bacon DR. Succinylcholine and the open globe: tracing the teaching. *Anesthesiology* 2003;99:220–224.

32. Miller RD. *Anesthesia,* 5th ed. Philadelphia: Churchill Livingstone, 2000:423, 2178.

33. Schaner PJ, Brown RL, Kirksey TD, et al. Succinylcholine-induced hyperkalemia in burned patients—Part I. *Anesth Analg* 1969;48:764–770.

34. Gronert GA, Dotin LN, Ritchey CR, et al. Succinylcholine-induced hyperkalemia in burned patients, Part II. *Anesth Analg* 1969;48:958–962.

35. Viby-Mogensen J, Hanel HK, Hansen E, et al. Serum cholinesterase activity in burned patients. II: anaesthesia, suxamethonium and hyperkalaemia. *Acta Anaesthesiol Scand* 1975;19:169–179.

36. Martyn JA, White DA, Gronert GA, et al. Up-and-down regulation of skeletal muscle acetylcholine receptors. Effects on neuromuscular blockers. *Anesthesiology* 1992;76:822–843.

37. Gronert GA, Lambert EH, Theye RA. The response of denervated skeletal muscle to succinylcholine. *Anesthesiology* 1973;39(Jul):13–22.

38. Gronert GA, Theye RA. Pathophysiology of hyperkalemia induced by succinylcholine. *Anesthesiology* 1975;43:89–99.

39. Gronert GA. Cardiac arrest after succinylcholine: mortality greater with rhabdomyolysis than receptor upregulation. *Anesthesiology* 2001;94:523–529.

40. Smith CL, Bush GH. Anaesthesia and progressive muscular dystrophy. *Br J Anaesth* 1985;57:1113–1118.

41. Larach MG, Rosenberg H, Gronert GA, et al. Hyperkalemic cardiac arrest during anesthesia in infants and children with occult myopathies. *Clin Pediatr (Phila)* 1997;36(Jan):9–16.

42. Pedrozzi NE, Ramelli GP, Tomasetti R, et al. Rhabdomyolysis and anesthesia: a report of two cases and review of the literature. *Pediatr Neurol* 1996;15:254–257.

43. Powell DR, Miller R. The effect of repeated doses of succinylcholine on serum potassium in patients with renal failure. *Anesth Analg* 1975;54:746–748.

44. Koide M, Waud BE. Serum potassium concentrations after succinylcholine in patients with renal failure. *Anesthesiology* 1972;36:142–145.

45. Thapa S, Brull SJ. Succinylcholine-induced hyperkalemia in patients with renal failure: an old question revisited. *Anesth Analg* 2000;91:237–241.

46. Kotani T, Nishio I, Kou H, et al. Effect of succinylcholine on serum potassium concentration in children with chronic renal failure. *Masui* 1993;42(Jan):20–24.

47. Kohlschutter B, Baur H, Roth F. Suxamethonium-induced hyperkalaemia in patients with severe intra-abdominal infections. *Br J Anaesth* 1976;48:557–562.

48. Khan TZ, Khan RM. Changes in serum potassium following succinylcholine in patients with infections. *Anesth Analg* 1983;62:327–331.

49. Gronert GA, Antognini JF, Pessah IN. Malignant hyperthermia. In: Miller *Anesthesia,* 5th ed., Churchill Livingstone, 2000:1033–1050.

50. Kolb ME, Horne ML, Martz R: Dantrolene in human malignant hyperthermia: a multicenter study. *Anesthesiology* 1982;56:254.

19

Approach to the Pediatric Airway

Robert C. Luten and Niranjan Kissoon

I. The clinical challenge

Airway management in the pediatric patient presents many potential challenges, including age-related differences in drug dosing and equipment sizes, anatomical variation that continuously evolves as development proceeds from infancy to adolescence, and the psychological stress that invariably accompanies the resuscitation of a critically ill child. Clinical competence in managing the airway of a critically ill or injured child requires mastery of age-related differences and familiarity and comfort with the fundamental approach to pediatric airway emergencies.

The principles of airway management in children and adults are the same. Medications used to facilitate intubation, the need for alternative airway management techniques, and many other aspects of airway management are generally the same in the child and adult. There are, however, a few important differences that must be considered in emergency airway management situations. These differences are most exaggerated in the first two years of life, after which the pediatric airway gradually evolves into the adult airway.

This discussion focuses on the main differences between adults and children and their significance in airway management.

II. Approach to the pediatric patient

A. General issues

A recent review of the pediatric resuscitation process attempted to define elements of the mental (cognitive) burden of providers when dealing with the unique aspects of critically ill children compared with adults. Age- and size-related variables unique to children introduce the need for more complex, nonautomatic, or knowledge-based mental activities, such as calculating drug doses and selecting equipment. The concentration required to undertake these activities may subtract from other important mental activity such as assessment, evaluation, prioritization, and synthesis of information, referred to in the resuscitative process as critical thinking activity. The cumulative effect of these difficulties leads to inevitable time delays and a corresponding increase in the potential for decision-making errors in the pediatric resuscitative process. This is in sharp contrast to adult resuscitation where drug doses, equipment sizing, and physiological parameters are usually familiar to the provider, and therefore, significantly more of the adult provider's attention is freed up for critical thinking. Decision making is prolonged in children secondary to the cognitive burden of age-related differences. In addition, calculations of drug doses are subject to error, particularly as doses are weight-related and the ultimate dose selected tends to vary significantly by age. The use of comprehensive resuscitation aids in pediatric resuscitation significantly reduces the cognitive load otherwise caused by obligatory calculations of dosage and equipment selection and relegates these activities to a lower order of mental function referred to as automatic or rule-based, thereby increasing critical thinking time. Table 19-1 is a length-based, color-coded equipment reference chart, used to eliminate age/weight-related differences in pediatric airway management. Both equipment and drug dosing information are included in the Broselow-Luten system and can be accessed by a single length measurement or patient weight.

B. Specific issues

1. Anatomical differences

The approach to the child with airway obstruction (the most common form of difficult airway encountered by the emergency physician) incorporates several unique features of the pediatric anatomy.

a. Children obstruct more easily than adults.

The pediatric patient is especially susceptible to airway obstruction from swelling, often from conditions that are less threatening to the adult. See Table 21-2 in Chapter 21, which outlines the effect of 1-mm edema on airway resistance in the infant (4-mm airway diameter) versus adult (8-mm airway diameter). Nebulized racemic epinephrine causes local vasoconstriction and can reduce mucosal swelling and edema to some extent. For diseases such as croup, where the anatomical site of swelling occurs in a very narrow portion of the airway, racemic epinephrine can have dramatic results. In other diseases, where the swelling affects the airway at a wide area, such as the supraglottic swelling of epiglottitis or the retropharyngeal swelling of an abscess in that area, the results are rarely clinically helpful. In these latter examples, especially in epiglottitis, efforts to force a nebulized medication on a child may actually exacerbate the obstruction.

b. Noxious interventions can exacerbate obstruction and precipitate respiratory arrest.

It should also be noted that the increased obstruction caused by the swelling in the previous example reflect the quietly breathing infant or adult. The crying child increases the work of breathing 32-fold, hence the principle of maintaining children in a quiet, comfortable environment during evaluation and management for potential airway obstruction.

Another very important factor particular to children is operative in airway obstruction. The extrathoracic airway is pliable, deforming with the negative pressure generated by inspiration. With obstruction, the airway distal to the obstruction collapses, effectively increasing the obstruction dynamically and creating a vicious cycle of increasing obstruction. Therefore all efforts need to be made to keep the child calm, hence another reason to "leave them alone" (see Fig. 19-1A,B,C).

c. Bag/mask ventilation (BMV) may still be of value in the patient who has arrested from airway obstruction.

Bag/mask ventilation is a proven technique. In emergencies, for providers who rarely encounter critically ill children, it may be as effective as endotracheal intubation as a short-term rescue/temporizing measure. It may still be effective in children with airway obstruction. Note in Fig. 19-1C that efforts

TABLE 19-1. *Equipment selection*

	Pink	Red	Purple	Yellow	White	Blue	Orange	Green
			Length (cm)-based pediatric equipment chart					
Weight (kg)	6–7	8–9	10–11	12–14	15–18	19–23	23–31	31–41
Length (cm)	60.75–67.75	67.75–75.25	75.25–85	85–98.25	98.25–110.75	110.75–122.5	122.5–137.5	137.5–155
ET tube size (mm)	3.5	3.5	4.0	4.5	5.0	5.5	6.0 cuff	6.5 cuff
Lip-tip length (mm)	10.5	10.5	12.0	13.5	15.0	16.5	18.0	19.5
Laryngoscope	1 Straight	1 Straight	1 Straight	2 Straight	2 Straight	2 Straight or curved	2 Straight or curved	3 Straight or curved
Suction catheter	8F	8F	8F	8–10F	10F	10F	10F	12F
Stylet	6F	6F	6F	6F	6F	14F	14F	14F
Oral airway	50 mm	50 mm	60 mm	60 mm	60 mm	70 mm	80 mm	80 mm
Nasopharyngeal airway	14F	14F	18F	20F	22F	24F	26F	30F
Bag/valve device	Infant	Infant	Child	Child	Child	Child	Child/adult	Adult
Oxygen mask	Newborn	Newborn	Pediatric	Pediatric	Pediatric	Pediatric	Adult	Adult
Vascular access	22–24/23–25 intraosseous	22–24/23–25 intraosseous	20–22/23–25 intraosseous	18–22/21–23 intraosseous	18–22/21–23 intraosseous	18–20/21–23 intraosseous	18–20/21–22	16–20/18–21
Catheter/butterfly	5–8F	5–8F	8–10F	10F	10–12F	12–14F	14–18F	18F
Nasogastric tube	5–8F	5–8F	8–10F	10F	10–12F	10–12F	12F	12F
Urinary catheter	5–8F	5–8F	8–10F	10F	10–12F	10–12F	12F	12F
Chest tube	10–12F	10–12F	16–20F	20–24F	20–24F	24–32F	24–32F	32–40F
Blood pressure cuff	Newborn/infant	Newborn/infant	Infant/child	Child	Child	Child	Child/adult	Adult
LMA[a]	1.5	1.5	2	2	2	2–2.5	2.5	3

Directions for use:
1. Measure patient length with centimeter tape or with a Broselow tape.
2. Using measured length in centimeters or Broselow tape measurement, access appropriate equipment column.
3. For endotracheal tubes, oral and nasopharyngeal airways, and LMAs, always select one size smaller, one size larger than the recommended size.

[a]Based on manufacturer's weight-based guidelines

Mask size	Patient size
1	up to 5 kg
1.5	5–10 kg
2	10–20 kg
2.5	20–30 kg
3	Over 30 kg

Permission to reproduce with modification from Luten RC, Wears RL, Broselow J, et al. *Ann Emerg Med* 1992;21:900–904.

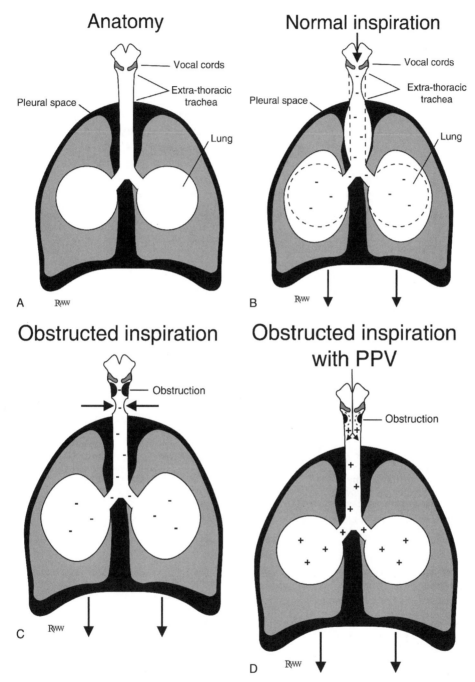

FIG. 19-1. Intra- and extrathoracic trachea and the dynamic changes that occur in the presence of upper airway obstruction. **A:** Normal anatomy. **B:** The changes that occur with normal inspiration; that is, dynamic collapsing of the upper airway associated with the negative pressure of inspiration on the extrathoracic trachea. **C:** Exaggeration of the collapse secondary to superimposed obstruction at the subglottic area. **D:** Positive pressure ventilation (PPV) stents the collapse/obstruction versus the patient's own inspiratory efforts, which increase the obstruction. (Adapted from Cote CJ, Ryan JF, Todres ID, et al., eds. *A practice of anesthesia for infants and children*, 2nd ed. Philadelphia: WB Saunders, 1993, with permission.)

by the patient to alleviate the obstruction actually cause worsening of the obstruction; that is, forced inspiration worsens obstruction as *negative* extrathoracic pressure is generated, collapsing the airway. When arrest occurs, usually a respiratory arrest secondary to fatigue from increased work of breathing (note, *not* from total obstruction, as the obstruction is partly fixed, and in children partly dynamic and reversible), application of *positive* pressure via BMV causes the opposite effect, actually stenting or relieving the dynamic component of obstruction. This mechanism explains the recommendation to try BMV as a temporizing measure even if the patient arrests from obstruction. Case reports of successful resuscitation status post (S/P) arrest from epiglottitis have borne this out (Fig. 19-1C and D).

Apart from differences related to size, there are certain anatomic peculiarities of the pediatric airway. The glottic opening of the trachea is at the level of C-1 in infancy. This transitions to the level of C-3 to C4 by age 7 and to the level of C-4 to C5 in the adult. These anatomic differences translate into a high anterior position of the glottic opening in children compared with adults. In addition, children, especially infants, possess a large tongue that occupies a relatively large portion of the oral cavity. During intubation of children under 3 years old, the high anterior airway position and the large tongue argue for use of a straight laryngoscope blade to elevate this distensible anatomy and enhance visibility of the glottic aperature (Table 19-2).

Children have large tonsils and adenoids that cause significant bleeding when traumatized. The angle between the epiglottis and the laryngeal opening is also more acute than that in the adult. Because of these considerations, blind nasotracheal intubation is difficult and relatively contraindicated in children under 10 years of age. Children also possess a small cricothyroid

TABLE 19-2. *Anatomic differences between adults and children*

Anatomy	Clinical significance
Large intraoral tongue occupying relatively large portion of the oral cavity	• High anterior airway position of the glottic opening compared with that in adults
High tracheal opening: C-1 in infancy versus C-3 to C-4 at age 7, C-4 to C-5 in the adult	• Straight blade preferred over curved to push distensible anatomy out of the way to visualize the larynx
Large occiput that may cause flexion of the airway, large tongue that easily collapses against the posterior pharynx	Sniffing position is preferred. The larger occiput actually elevates the head into the sniffing position in most infants and children. A towel may be required under shoulders to elevate torso relative to head in small infants
Cricoid ring is the narrowest portion of the trachea as compared with the vocal cords in the adult	• Uncuffed tubes provide adequate seal as they fit snugly at the level of the cricoid ring. • Correct tube size essential because variable expansion cuffed tubes not used
Consistent anatomic variations with age with fewer abnormal variations related to body habitus, arthritis, chronic disease	<2 years, high anterior 2 to 8, transition >8, small adult
Large tonsils and adenoids may bleed. More acute angle between epiglottis and laryngeal opening results in nasotracheal intubation attempt failures.	Blind nasotracheal intubation not indicated in children Nasotracheal intubation failure
Small cricothyroid membrane	Needle cricothyrotomy difficult, surgical cricothyrotomy impossible in infants and small children

membrane. Below 3 to 4 years of age it is virtually nonexistent. For this reason needle cricothyrotomy may be difficult, and surgical cricothyrotomy is virtually impossible and contraindicated in infants and small children up to the age of 10 years.

Although younger children possess a relatively high anterior airway with the attendant difficulties in visualization of the glottic aperature, this anatomical pattern is fortunately rather consistent from one child to another, so this difficulty can be anticipated. Adults may have difficult airways related to body habitus, arthritis, or chronic disease, modified by variations in individual underlying anatomy, and so are less consistent from one person to another. In summary, children below the age of 2 years have higher anterior airways. Above 8 years of age the airway tends to be similar to the adult; years 2 to 8 represent a transition period. Fig. 19-2 demonstrates anatomic differences particular to children.

2. Physiological differences

There are many physiological differences between children and adults, but one is of particular significance in emergency airway management (Box 19-1). Children have a basal oxygen consumption that is about twice that of adults. Coupled with a

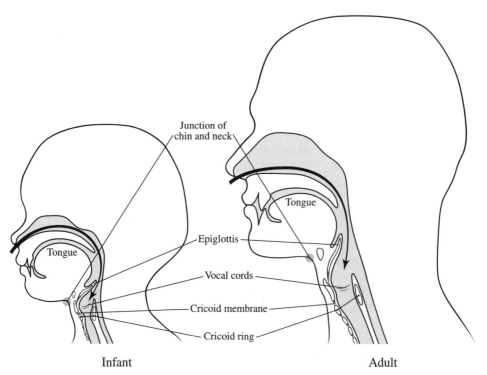

Junction of chin and neck

Tongue

Tongue

Epiglottis

Vocal cords

Cricoid membrane

Cricoid ring

Infant   Adult

FIG. 19-2. The anatomic differences particular to children are these: 1. Higher, more anterior position of the glottic opening. (Note the relationship of the vocal cords to the chin/neck junction.) 2. Relatively larger tongue in the infant, which lies between the mouth and glottic opening. 3. Relatively larger and more floppy epiglottis in the child. 4. The cricoid ring is the narrowest portion of the pediatric airway versus the vocal cords in the adult. 5. Position and size of the cricothyroid membrane in the infant. 6. Sharper, more difficult angle for blind nasotracheal intubation. 7. Larger relative size of the occiput in the infant.

Box 19-1. Physiologic Differences

Physiologic difference	**Significance**
Basal O_2 consumption is twice adult values (>6 mL/kg/min). Proportionally small FRC as compared with adults.	Shortened period of protection from hypoxia for equivalent adult preoxygenation time as compared with adults. Infants and small children often require BMV while maintaining cricoid pressure to avoid hypoxia.

---

decrease in functional residual capacity (FRC) particular to children, they are thus prone to desaturate much more rapidly than adults given an equivalent duration of preoxygenation. The clinician must anticipate and communicate this possibility to the staff and be prepared to provide supplemental oxygen by BMV if the patient's oxygen saturation drops below 90%.

3. **Drug dosage and selection**

A significant problem in the management of pediatric emergencies is the timely and accurate delivery of medications. The use of the color-coded resuscitation aids, as described earlier, for drug dosing in children precludes many of these problems, including having to estimate weight and to remember and calculate drug doses. The dose of succinylcholine in children is different from that in adults. Succinylcholine is rapidly distributed into extracellular water. Children have a larger relative volume of extracellular fluid than adults: At birth 45% of the weight is extracellular fluid water (EFW); at age 2 months, approximately 30%; at age 6 years, 20%; and at adulthood, 16% to 18%. The recommended dose of succinylcholine therefore is higher in children. In 1993 the Food and Drug Administration, in conjunction with pharmaceutical companies, revised the package labeling of succinylcholine because of reports of hyperkalemic cardiac arrests due to its administration to patients with previously undiagnosed neuromuscular disease. The warning went as far as saying that the drug was contraindicated for elective anesthesia in pediatric patients because of this concern. The wording of the warning has since been softened to a more cautionary tone. However, both the initial advisory warning and the revised warning continue to recommend succinylcholine for emergency or full-stomach intubation in children. Pediatric drug doses are provided in Box 19-2 and Table 19-3.

4. **Equipment selection**

Table 19-1 references emergency equipment needed for pediatric patients based on length. Appropriate equipment can be chosen with a centimeter length measurement or with a Broselow tape. Despite best efforts (such as equipment lists or periodic checks), it is not uncommon for newborn equipment to be mixed in with or placed in proximity to the smallest pediatric equipment—the pink zone. This equipment not only does not function properly in older children its use may also be detrimental. Examples include the 0 laryngoscope blade, which is not long enough to allow visualization of the airway, the 250 cc newborn BMV, which provides inadequate volume, and various other equipment like oral airways that can create, not alleviate, obstruction; or the curved no. 1 laryngoscope blade, which may be difficult to use as it may not pick up the relatively large epiglottis or effectively remove the large tongue from the laryngoscopic view of the airway. A few pieces of equipment deserve special mention.

Box 19-2. Pediatric Airway Management: Drug Dosage, Metabolism, and Selection

Succinylcholine dose is higher in children: 2 mg/kg. Succinylcholine is the drug of choice for neuromuscular blockade for emergency rapid sequence intubation (RSI) in children.

A defasciculating dose of a nondepolarizer before using succinylcholine is not indicated in children <10 years of age. Beyond 10 years of age, indications are the same as those for adults.

Always use atropine for any child under 5 years of age undergoing airway manipulation and for *all* children aged ten years or less receiving succinylcholine.

Fentanyl should be used with extreme caution, as infants and small children are very sensitive to the respiratory depressant effect of the drug. The sympathetic blockade effect can also be detrimental if the patient is in a situation that depends on sympathetic discharge to maintain perfusion.

Lidocaine may also be effective in reactive airway disease but is not universally used in children.

The use of the Broselow tape for drug dosing children in emergencies precludes having to estimate weight or to remember and calculate drug doses.

---

a. Endotracheal tubes

The correct-sized tube for the patient can be determined by a length measurement and referring to the equipment selection chart. The formula:

$$(16 + \text{age in years})/4$$

is also a reasonably accurate method of determining the correct tube size. However, the formula cannot be used below one year of age and is only useful if an accurate age is known, which is not always the case in an emergency. Uncuffed endotracheal tubes are recommended in the younger pediatric age groups, and

TABLE 19-3. *Drugs—pediatric considerations*

Drug	Dosage	Pediatric-specific comments
Premedications		
Atropine	0.02 mg/kg IV	Prevents bradycardia 2° to airway maneuvers or succinylcholine.
Lidocaine	1.5 mg/kg IV	Head injury, asthma as for adults.
Defasciculating agent (pan/vecuronium)	0.01 mg/kg IV	Never <5 yr/20 kg. Above 5 yr/20 kg, use for head injury.
Fentanyl	1 to 3 mcg/kg IV	In head injury. Use with extreme caution.
Induction agents		
Midazolam	0.3 mg/kg IV	Use 0.1 mg/kg if hypotensive.
Thiopental	3 to 5 mg/kg IV	Lower dose to 1 mg/kg or delete if perfusion poor.
Etomidate	0.3 mg/kg IV	
Ketamine	1 to 2 mg/kg IV 4 mg/kg IM	
Propofol	1 to 2 mg/kg IV	
Paralytics		
Succinylcholine	2 mg/kg IV	Always precede with atropine.
Pan/Vecuronium		
Defasciculation	0.01 mg/kg IV	
Paralysis	0.1 mg/kg IV	May increase to 0.3 mg/kg of vecuronium for RSI.
Rocuronium	1.0 mg/kg IV for RSI	

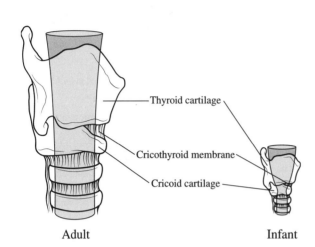

Thyroid cartilage

Cricothyroid membrane

Cricoid cartilage

Adult   Infant

FIG. 19-3. Airway shape. Note the position of the narrowest portion of the pediatric airway, which is at the cricoid ring, creating a funnel shape, versus a straight pipe as seen in the adult, where the vocal cords form the narrowest portion. This is the rationale for using the uncuffed tube in the child; it fits snugly, unlike the cuffed tube used in the adult, which is inflated once the tube passes the cords to produce a snug fit. (Modified with permission from Cote CJ, Todres ID. The pediatric airway. In: Cote CJ, Ryan JF, Todres ID, et al., eds. *A practice of anesthesia for infants and children,* 2nd ed. Philadelphia: WB Saunders, 1993.)

cuffed tubes are used for size 5.5 mm and up (see Fig. 19-3). When intubating a young child, there is a tendency to push the tube too far down, usually into the right mainstem bronchus. Insertion of the tube to a predetermined, appropriate distance will avoid this. Various formulas have been proffered as aids to accomplish correct insertion length. One is the internal diameter (ID) of the tube times 3. For example, for a 3.5-mm, ID tube, internal diameter $3.5 \times 3 = 10.5$ cm insertion depth. Alternatively, the length-based chart gives tube insertion depth that can be determined directly from the one initial length measurement.

b. Oxygen mask

The simple rebreather mask used for most patients provides a maximum of 35% to 60% oxygen and requires a flow of 6 to 10 L/min. A nonrebreather mask can provide approximately 75% oxygen in children if a flow rate of 10 to 12 L/min is used. For emergency airway management, and particularly for preoxygenation for RSI, the pediatric nonrebreather mask is preferable. The adult nonrebreather mask can be used for older children but is too large to be used for infants and small children. Alternatively, a properly configured bag and mask system may be capable of delivering oxygen at greater than 75%, if correctly used.

c. Oral airways

Oral airways should only be used in patients who are unconscious. In the conscious or semiconscious patient, these airways can cause vomiting. Oral airways can be selected based on the Broselow tape measurement or can be approximated by selecting an oral airway that fits the distance from the angle of the mouth to the tragus of the ear.

d. Nasopharyngeal airways

Nasopharyngeal airways are helpful in the obtunded but responsive pediatric patient. The correct nasopharyngeal airway to use is the largest one that comfortably fits in the naris but does not produce blanching of the nasal skin. The correct length is from the tip of the nose to the tragus of the ear, and usually corresponds to the nasopharyngeal airway with the correct diameter. Care must be taken to suction these airways regularly to avoid blockage.

e. Nasogastric tubes

Nasogastric (NG) tubes are a critical aspect of airway management in children. With BMV, the stomach often becomes distended with air, hindering full diaphragmatic excursion, thus preventing effective ventilation. An NG tube should be placed soon after intubation to decompress the stomach in any patient who has undergone BMV and requires ongoing ventilation by endotracheal tube. Often in such patients, the abdomen is distended or tense, making the problem obvious, but other times it is difficult to identify the difference between this and the normally protuberant abdomen of the young child. If there is any difficulty in ventilation, particularly related to apparently high resistance, an NG tube should be placed. NG tube size may also be selected using length criteria.

f. Bag/mask ventilation equipment

For emergency airway management, the self-inflating bag is preferred over the anesthesia ventilation bag. The BMV should have an oxygen reservoir so that when giving 10–15 L oxygen flow, one can obtain 90% to 95% F_iO_2. The smallest bag that should be used is 450-mL. Neonatal bags that are smaller (250 mL) do not provide effective tidal volume even for small infants. Many of the BMV devices have a pop-off valve. The pop-off valve is usually set around 35 to 45 cm of water pressure (CWP) and is used to prevent barotrauma by providing a release of excessive pressure generated during routine BMV. In many emergent airway situations a higher inspiratory pressure is needed to ventilate a patient, so the bag should either be configured without a pop-off valve or the pop-off valve should be adjusted or occluded. From a practical point, it is probably a good practice to store the BMV device with the pop-off valve occluded so that initial attempts to ventilate the patient can use maximal pressures for ventilation if needed. It is not uncommon for personnel that only infrequently treat critically ill children not to notice that air is escaping from the pop-off valve during initial attempts to ventilate the child. Valuable time may be lost in the process of recognizing that this is indeed occurring and the patient is not being adequately ventilated.

g. End-tidal CO_2 detectors

Colorimetric end-tidal carbon dioxide (CO_2) detectors are equally useful in children as in adults. A pediatric size exists for children below 15 kg. The adult model should be used for children weighing greater than approximately 15 kg. Although the pediatric model will function correctly to detect end-tidal CO_2 when used with larger children, the amount of resistance created when ventilating through the smaller model may make it difficult to ventilate the larger patient.

h. Airway alternatives

Orotracheal intubation is the procedure of choice for emergency airway management of the pediatric patient, including those patients with potential cervical spine injury, in whom RSI with in-line manual stabilization provides rapid definitive control while minimizing the risk of aspiration and preventing movement. Nasotracheal intubation is relatively contraindicated in children for the reasons previously discussed.

The usual surgical alternative airway technique in adults is surgical cricothyrotomy. Because of the minuscule size of the cricothyroid membrane in children, this procedure is extremely difficult in a child the size of a 10-year-old, and should definitely be considered to be contraindicated in children under

TABLE 19-4. *Alternatives for airway support*

Bag/mask ventilation	May be the most reliable temporizing measure in children. Equipment selection, adjuncts, and good technique essential.
Orotracheal intubation (usually with RSI)	Still the procedure of choice for emergent airway in potential cervical spine injury and most other circumstances.
Needle cricothyrotomy	Recommended as last resort in infants and children, but data lacking.
Laryngeal mask	Possible alternative but requires further evaluation.
Blind nasotracheal intubation	Not indicated for children younger than 10 years of age.

6 to 8 years of age. Needle cricothyrotomy is the recommended procedure in the small child, although there are minimal data as to its effectiveness in children. The laryngeal mask airway (LMA) includes sizes small enough for young infants and newborns, and, as a temporizing measure, might be useful when intubation cannot be done or fails. The Combitube is easy to insert, but currently there are no models for pediatric patients less than 48 inches tall (Table 19-4). These and other adjuncts are discussed in chapter 20.

III. Initiation of mechanical ventilation

In pediatrics, two modes of ventilation are used for emergency ventilation. For newborns and small infants, pressure-limited ventilators are traditionally used. For larger infants and older children, volume-limited ventilators are used, as in adults. One can arbitrarily set 10 kg as the weight below which pressure-limited ventilators should be used, although volume ventilators have been used effectively in smaller children. When using pressure ventilators, the respiratory rate is initially 20 to 25 because of the small size of the infant or newborn. Inhale/exhale (I/E) ratios are set at 1:2. Begin with a tidal volume of 8 to 12 mL/kg. Adjust according to subsequent clinical evaluation and chest rise. Positive end-expiratory pressure (PEEP) should also be set at 3 to 5 cm of water and F_iO_2 at 1.0. Once initial settings have been established, it is critical that the patient be quickly reevaluated and adjustments made, because compliance and leaks can preclude adequate ventilation with initial settings. Clinical determinations of ventilatory adequacy are more important than formulae or guidelines for initial ventilation. Once the adjustments are made and the patient appears clinically to be ventilated and oxygenating, blood gas determinations or continuous pulse oximetry and end tidal carbon dioxide ($ETCO_2$) monitoring should be used for confirmation and further adjustments (Table 19-5 and Box 19-3).

IV. Recommended RSI techniques for children

The procedure of rapid sequence intubation (RSI) in children is essentially the same procedure as in adults with a few important differences outlined below.

   A. Preparation

      • Use resuscitation aids that facilitate age/size-related issues in drug dosing and equipment selection.

   B. Preoxygenation

      • Be meticulous. Children desaturate more rapidly than adults.

   C. Pretreatment

      • Atropine 0.02 mg/kg IV for children under 10 who will receive succinylcholine for neuromuscular blockade

      • Other pretreatment agents follow same indications as for adults with few exceptions, but are given in pediatric doses. Exceptions: Lidocaine is not used for pretreatment

TABLE 19-5. *Initiation of mechanical ventilation*

I. Initial settings		
Ventilator type	Pressure-limited	Volume-limited
Respiratory rate	20–25/minute	12–20, by age
PEEP	3–5 cm H_2O	3–5 cm H_2O
F_iO_2	1.0 (100%)	1.0 (100%)
Inspiratory time	$\geq$0.6 sec.	$\geq$0.6 sec.
I/E ratio	1:2	1:2
Pressure/volume settings	For pressure ventilation start with peak inspiratory pressure (PIP) of 15–20 cm H_2O. Assess chest rise and adjust to higher pressures as needed. For volume ventilation start with tidal volumes of 8–12 mL/kg. Start at lower volumes and increase to a PIP of 20–30 cm H_2O. ***These are initial setting guidelines only. Assess chest rise and adjust accordingly.***	
II. Evaluate clinically and make adjustments	Most patients will be ventilated with volume-cycled ventilators. Poor chest rise, poor color, decreased breath sounds require *higher* tidal volume. Check for pneumo, blocked tube. Ensure that tube size and position are optimal and leaks are not present. For patients ventilated with pressure-cycled ventilators, these findings may indicate the need to increase the peak inspiratory pressure.	
III. Laboratory information	ABG should be performed approximately 10–15 minutes after settings are stabilized. Additional samples may be necessary after each ventilator adjustment, unless ventilatory status is monitored by end-tidal CO_2 and SpO_2.	

of bronchospasm in children, opioids must be used with extreme caution in children to avoid complications, and defasciculating agents are not used below ten years of age.

D. Paralysis with induction
- Induction agent selection as for adult: dose by length or weight.
- Succinylcholine 2 mg/kg IV

Box 19-3. Emergency Pediatric Airway Management—Practical Considerations

Anatomic
- Anticipate high anterior glottic opening.
- Do not hyperextend the neck.
- Uncuffed tubes are used in children less than 8 years old.
- Use straight blades in young children.

Physiologic
- Anticipate possible desaturation.

Drug dosage and equipment selection
- *Always* use atropine (under 10 years of age).
- Use length-based system. Do *not* use memory or do calculations.
- NG tube is an important airway adjunct in infants.
- Stock pediatric nonrebreather masks.

Airway alternatives for failed or difficult airway
- Surgical cricothyrotomy—contraindicated until age 10 years
- Blind NT intubation—contraindicated until age 10 years
- Combitube—only if >4 feet tall
- Needle cricothyrotomy—acceptable

    E. Protection and positioning
      • Apply Sellick's maneuver
    F. Placement with proof
      • Anticipate desaturation, bag ventilate if oxygen saturation (SpO_2) is less than 90%
      • Confirm tube placement with $ETCO_2$ as for adult
    G. Postintubation management

      Mechanical ventilation in the child can be accomplished using either pressure-controlled or volume-controlled techniques. Regardless of the technique used one should ensure that the chest rise is adequate. Further manipulation of the pressure or volumes should be guided by blood gas analysis or measurement of SpO_2 and capnography. The Broselow-Luten length-based system gives guidelines for approximate starting tidal volumes and ventilator rates. In almost all cases children who are intubated and mechanically ventilated should be paralyzed and sedated in the emergency department to prevent deleterious rises in intracranial or intrathoracic pressures.

EVIDENCE

1. Pediatric emergency airway management involves a lack of familiarity and degree of complexity for the emergency physician that may translate into errors and time delay. The mental burden or cognitive load involved in treating children can be lessened by the use of resuscitation adjuncts and simplification of the process with resultant time savings and error reduction. Time delay and error are associated with managing children in emergency situations (1). Pediatric emergencies are complicated by the fact that children vary in size, which creates logistical difficulties, especially in the area of drug dosing and equipment selection. A recent review analyzed the effect of these variables on the mental burden in the resuscitative process and demonstrated how resuscitation aids can help mitigate their effect (2). Simulated patient emergency encounters have confirmed that the Broselow-Luten color-coded emergency system reduces time delay and errors by eliminating the cognitive burden associated with these situations (3).

Other factors also contribute to an increased cognitive load in managing children. To the extent that the process can be simplified, reducing the complexity and number of decisions required, time is freed up for critical thinking that can then be dedicated to the priorities of airway management. An example of simplification is the use a *single age cutoff* for various interventions. For example, recommending *all* children below 10 years of age receiving succinylcholine be pretreated with atropine even though maximum benefit is in the smaller child (eliminating a decision) and recommending that *no* child below 10 years paralyzed with succinylcholine receive pretreatment with a defasiculating agent (eliminating a step). See details of evidence later.

2. RSI in pediatrics. RSI has now been recommended for use in children by all of the major pediatric life support courses (4). Although there are no randomized prospective studies, large series from multiple centers support the use of RSI in children and document its safety (5) and apparent superiority to other methods used in children (6).

The drugs of RSI

a. *Atropine.* Atopine is recommended in pediatric emergency airway management, not for its antisialogue effect, but rather to prevent the bradycardia associated with vagal stimulation from instrumenting the airway and from the administration of succinylcholine. Younger children (less than 2 years old) are especially prone to develop bradycardia because of well-developed parasympathetic vagal responses. The optimal dose of atropine has been debated, with recommendations ranging from 0.01 to 0.02 mg/kg. Detractors to the use of the higher dose site the deleterious side effects in the very young (7), whereas others point out the need for the higher dose to achieve consistent vagolysis, especially in the presence of succinylcholine (8). On balance, there seems to be a valid argument for using the larger (0.02 mg/kg) dose of atropine and little potential downside to this dose, when compared to 0.01 mg/kg. The higher dose may be particularly important in the unlikely circumstance that a second dose of succinylcholine is required. Although the excessive influence of the parasympathetic system is greatest in the very young child, and the transition to the adult sympathetic/parasympathetic balance occurs on a continuum of time, an empirical approach based on an age cutoff and other associated factors seems reasonable. Therefore, based on the available literature and clinical experience, the risk of the treatment, and to avoid the cognitive burden of adding an additional decision to an already complex process, we recommend a dose of 0.02 mg/kg of atropine intravenously in the pretreatment phase of RSI for *all children* under 10 years of age who will be receiving succinylcholine.

b. *Lidocaine.* Lidocaine is recommended in children with presumed elevation of ICP (usually due to head trauma) to prevent further rises in ICP related to laryngoscopy and intubation (9). Most of the data for this recommendation is extrapolated from adult studies and nontraumatic elevated ICP situations (see Chapter 16).

There are no data to support or refute the use of lidocaine in children to prevent or mitigate the reflex bronchospasm related to airway manipulation. Studies related to the use of lidocaine in children to blunt the sympathetic response to intubation are inconsistent (10,11).

c. *Defasiculation.* The role of a defasiculating dose of a nondepolarizing NMBA before succinylcholine in patients with elevated ICP is discussed in Chapters 16, 18, and 24. Equivalent studies have not been done in children. Fasiculations are minimal in infants and small children (12). Small children are also potentially at more risk from incorrect dosage of a defasiculating nondepolarizing NMBA because of their small body mass. Therefore, until evidence is available of beneficial effect, in an effort to minimize the cognitive burden of adding an additional medication, and to be consistent in age cutoff criteria, a defasiculating dose of a nondepolarizing NMBA before succinylcholine is not recommended until children are *greater than 10 years old,* after which age the adult recommendations apply.

d. *Etomidate.* The package insert for etomidate contains no recommendations for patients below 10 years of age. Although not as extensively studied in children, the issue of inhibition of steroid synthesis (13) has also been evaluated in children and has been shown to have no significant clinical implications (14). There is also mounting evidence (15) attesting to its safety in children to go with a wealth of clinical experience.

e. *Rocuronium.* With the removal of rapacuronium from the market, there is no available nondepolarizing agent that can match the performance characteristics of succinylcholine. Rocuronium presents the best alternative for RSI in pediatric patients when succinylcholine is contraindicated. Although the duration of action of rocuronium far exceeds succinylcholine (45 minutes versus 5 to 10 minutes), studies in children have now demonstrated equivalent time to adequate intubating conditions in doses of 0.9 (16) to 1.2 (17,18) mg/kg. The recommended dose of rocuronium for pediatric RSI is therefore the same as for adults, 1 mg/kg IV.

f. *Succinylcholine.* As mentioned earlier, despite controversy surrounding the FDA warning/cautions concerning its use in elective pediatric patients, succinylcholine remains the recommended choice for emergency full-stomach intubations (19,20). Although rocuronuim is the preferred paralytic in pediatrics by some practicioners, for simplicity's sake we recommend succinylcholine as first line for adults and children.

3. Uncuffed endotracheal tubes are recommended in pediatric advanced emergency airway management. The issue of whether cuffed endotracheal tubes are needed in children has been debated for some time. Because of the physiological seal afforded by the narrow subglottic area, the cuffed tube may not be necessary in most children under 8 to 10 years of age. Two studies have addressed this issue (21,22). Deakers and colleagues (21) studied 282 patients intubated either in the OR, ED, or ICU. In their observational prospective, nonrandomized study, they found no difference in post extubation stridor, the need for reintubation, or long-term upper-airway symptomatology. Khine and colleagues (22) compared the incidence of postextubation croup, inadequate ventilation, and anesthetic gases in the environment and the requirement for second laryngoscopy secondary to the tube being too large. In this study, which looked at children less than 8 years of age only, the authors found no difference in croup, more attempts at intubation with uncuffed tubes, less gas flow required with cuffed tubes, and less gas leakage into the environment.

It would seem, therefore, that the use of cuffed tubes in younger children may not result in any postextubation sequelae; however, these studies note the need to monitor inflation pressures. When this is not done reliably, as is often the case in emergency intubations, the uncuffed tube is recommended to avoid excessive tracheal mucosal pressure with the potential sequelae of scarring and stenosis. Placement of a cuffed endotracheal tube especially in children less than 8 to 10 years of age will result in placement of a tube with a smaller internal diameter and hence may increase airflow resistance. On the other hand, in some patients in whom high mean airway pressures are expected such as those with acute respiratory diseases and asthma, the placement with a cuffed tube with the cuff initially deflated and inflated only when necessary may be appropriate.

4. Children desaturate more quickly than adults with comparable degrees of preoxygenation. The infant metabolizes at least 6 mL of oxygen per kilogram per minute as compared with adult values of approximately 3 mL per kilogram per minute. The measured FRC in children and adults is similar on a per kilogram basis at all ages; however, the decrease in FRC in an apneic child is far greater than in the apneic adult. This is due to the differences in the elastic forces of the chest wall and the lung. In children the chest wall is more compliant and the lung elastic recoil is less than in adults. An analysis of these forces reveals that if they are brought into equilibrium as in the apneic patient, a value of FRC around 10% of TLC is predicted instead of the observed value of slightly less than 40%.

These same factors also reduce the FRC in the spontaneously breathing patient, albeit to a lesser degree. FRC is further reduced with the induction of anesthesia and by the supine position. The clinical implication of the decreased effective FRC combined with increased oxygen consumption is that the preoxygenated paralyzed infant has a disproportionately smaller store of intrapulmonary oxygen to draw on as compared to the adult. Pulmonary pathology in critically ill patients may further reduce the ability to hyperoxygenate. It is therefore critical that these factors be considered when preoxygenating and intervening in pediatric patients. Bag/mask ventilations with cricoid pressure may be required to maintain oxygen saturation above 90% during RSI, especially if multiple attempts are required or the child is injured in a way that compromises preoxygenation (23,24).

REFERENCES

1. Oakley P. Inaccuracy and delay in decision making in pediatric resuscitation, and a proposed reference chart to reduce error. *Brit Med J* 1988;297:817–819.
2. Luten R, Wears R, Broselow J, et al. Managing the unique size related issues of pediatric resuscitation: reducing cognitive load with resuscitation aids. *Acad Emerg Med* 2002;9:840–847.

3. Shah AN, Frush KS. *Reduction in error severity associated with use of a pediatric medication dosing system: a crossover trial.* Accepted for presentation at the AAP 2001 National Conference and Exhibition, Section on Critical Care, October 23, 2001.
4. Gerardi MJ, Sacchetti AD, Cantor RM, et al. Rapid-sequence intubation of the pediatric patient. Pediatric Emergency Medicine Committee of the American College of Emergency Physicians. *Ann Emerg Med* 1996;28:55–74.
5. Gnauck K, Lungo J, Scalzo A, et al. Emergency intubation of the pediatric medical patient: use of anesthetic agents in the emergency department. *Ann Emerg Med* 1994;23:1242–1247.
6. Sagarin MJ, et al. Rapid sequence intubation for pediatric emergency airway management. *Pediatr Emerg Care* 2002;18:417–23.
7. Shorten GD, Bissonnette B, Hartley E, et al. It is not necessary to administer more than 10 μg · kg^{-1} of atropine to older children before succinylcholine. *Can J Anaesth* 1995;42:1:8–11.
8. Guyton DC, Scharf SM. Should atropine be routine in children? *Can J Anaesth* 1996;43:7:754–756.
9. Zaritsky AL, Nadkarni VM, Hickey RW, et al. *PALS provider manual.* Dallas, TX: American Heart Association, 2002.
10. Splinter WM. Intraenous lidocaine does not attenuate the haemodynamic response of children to laryngoscopy and tracheal intubation. *Can J Anaesth* 1990;37(Pt 1):440–443.
11. Tanaka K. Effects of intravenous injections of lidocaine on hemodynamics and catecholamine levels during endotracheal intubation in infants and children. *Aichi Gakuin Daigaku Shigakkai Shi.* 1989;27:345–358. Japanese.
12. Salem MR, Wong AY, Lin YH. The effect of suxamethonium on the intragastric pressure in infants and children. *Br J Anaesth* 1972;44:166–170.
13. Guldner G, et al. Etomidate for rapid sequence intubation in young children: hemodynamic effects and adverse events. *Acad Emerg Med* 2003;10(Feb):134–139.
14. Sokolove PE, Price DD, Okada P. The safety of etomidate for emergency rapid sequence intubation of pediatric patients. *Pediatr Emerg Care* 2000;16(Feb)8–21.
15. Donmez A, Kaya H, Haberal A, et al. The effect of etomidate induction on plasma cortisol levels in children undergoing cardiac surgery. *J Cardiothorac Vasc Anesth* 1998;12:182–185.
16. Cheng CA, Aun CS, Gin T. Comparison of rocuronium and suxamethonium for rapid tracheal intubation in children. *Paediatr Anaesth* 2002;12:140–145.
17. Mazurek AJ, Rae B, Ham S, et al. Rocuronium versus succinylcholine: are they equally effective during rapid-sequence induction of anesthesia? *Anesth Analg* 1998;87:1259–1262.
18. Woolf RL, Crawford MW, Choo SM. Dose-response of rocuronium bromide in children anesthetized with propofol: a comparison with succinylcholine. *Anesthesiology* 1997;87:1368–1372.
19. Robinson AL, Jerwood DC, Stokes MA. Routine suxamethonium in children. A regional survey of current usage. *Anaesthesia* 1996;51:874–878.
20. Weir PS. Anaesthesia for appendicectomy in childhood: a survey of practice in Northern Ireland. *Ulster Med J* 1997;66(May):34–37.
21. Deakers TW, Reynolds G, Stretton M, et al. Cuffed endotracheal tubes in pediatric intensive care. *J Pediatr* 1994;125(J):57–62.
22. Khine HH, Corddry DH, Kettrick RG, et al. Comparison of cuffed and uncuffed endotracheal tubes in young children during general anesthesia. *Anesthesiology* 1997;86:627–631.
23. Angostoni E, Mead J. Statics of the respiratory system. In: Fenn WO, Rahn H, eds.: *Handbook of physiology.* Washington, DC: American Physiologic Society, 1964.
24. Lumb, A. Elastic forces and lung volumes. In: Nunn's applied respiratory physiology, 5th ed. Oxford, England: Butterworth-Heineman, 2000:51–53.

20

Pediatric Airway Techniques

Robert C. Luten and Stephen A. Godwin

In general, the same airway techniques are used in older children and adolescents as are used in adults. A different approach is required, however, for small children (less than 3 years) and infants (less than 1 year). The following discussion will describe the appropriate use of the various airway modalities in pediatrics, with emphasis on age appropriateness.

I. Airway techniques used in all children

A. Bag/mask ventilation (BMV) and endotracheal intubation

Please see Chapter 5 for a detailed description of bag/mask ventilation (BMV) and endotracheal intubation. As in adults, oral and nasopharyngeal airways are important adjuncts to BMV. The rationale for the use of specific equipment (curved or straight blades, cuffed versus uncuffed tubes) is described in Chapter 19. In pediatric airway management, identification and use of size-appropriate equipment is crucial, because without properly sized equipment, the procedure will be doomed to failure, even in the most experienced hands. Proper BMV technique is particularly important in pediatric patients, whose crisis is often driven by a primary respiratory problem. Pediatric patients are more frequently hypoxemic than their adult counterparts, and are subject to more rapid oxyhemoglobin desaturation (see Chapter 3), so bag/mask ventilation with cricoid pressure (Sellick's maneuver) is frequently required during the preoxygenation and paralysis phases of rapid sequence intubation (RSI) to achieve and maintain adequate oxygen saturation. Pediatric ventilation requires smaller tidal volumes, higher rates, and size-specific equipment. The pediatric airway is particularly amenable to positive pressure ventilation, even in the presence of upper airway obstruction (Chapter 19).

1. Tips for successful BMV and endotracheal intubation in infants and children

a. Positioning

Children have a relatively large occiput compared with adults. In the supine position, the occiput of the unsupported, relaxed patient may cause flexion of the head and neck and resultant airway obstruction. Proper positioning of the patient therefore is key to prevent obstruction and provide optimal alignment of the axes of the airway (Chapter 19). Optimal alignment of the laryngeal, pharyngeal, and oral axes in adults usually requires elevation of the occiput to flex the neck on the torso and hyperextend the head at the atlantooccipital joint. Because of the larger relative size of the occiput in small children, elevation of the occiput is usually unnecessary, and hyperextension of the head may actually cause obstruction.

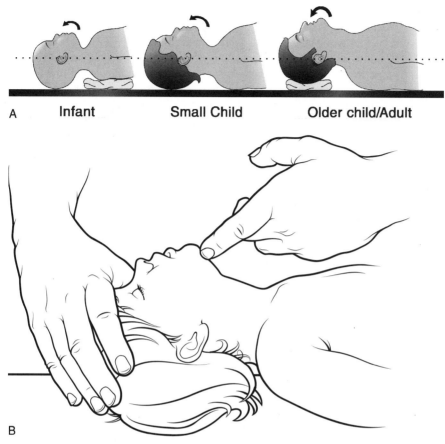

A **Infant**   **Small Child**   **Older child/Adult**

B

FIG. 20-1. A: Clinical determination of optimal airway alignment. Using a line passing through the external auditory canal and anterior to the shoulder (see text for details). **B:** Application of the line to determine optimal position. In this small child the occiput obviates the need for head support, yet the occiput is not so large as to require support of the shoulders. Note that the line traversing the external auditory canal passes anterior to the shoulders. With only slight extension of the head on the atlantooccipital joint, the sniffing position is achieved.

Slight anterior displacement of the atlantooccipital junction is all that is needed (pulling up on the chin to create the sniffing position). In small infants, elevation of the shoulders with a towel may be needed to counteract the effect of the large occiput that causes the head to flex forward to the chest. As a general rule, once correctly positioned the external auditory canal should lie just anterior to the shoulders. Whether this position requires support beneath the occiput (older child/adult), the shoulders (small infant), or no support (small child) can be determined using this rule of thumb (Fig. 20-1A). These are guidelines only. Each individual patient is different. A quick trial to find the optimal position for your patient may be warranted. Figure 20-1B demonstrates the most common position for intubating the small child, the so-called sniffing position, and how this is achieved in this size child.

b. Bag/mask ventilation (BMV)

Always place an oral airway in the unconscious patient before ventilating a child with a bag and mask. The identical principles apply as in the adult, but the pediatric tongue is even larger relative to the size of the oropharynx and is more prone to obstruct the upper airway. The positioning described in the previous paragraph is usually obtained simultaneously while applying the one-handed C-grip technique. The thumb and forefinger place and support the mask from the bridge of the nose to the cleft of the chin, avoiding the eyes. The bony prominences of the chin are lifted up by the rest of the fingers, placing the head in mild extension to form the sniffing position. Care is taken to avoid pressure on the airway anteriorly to prevent collapsing and obstructing the pliable trachea. The cadence for bagging can be facilitated by the mnemonic "squeeze, release, release," which will allow adequate time for exhalation during the cycle. If ventilation is not immediately obtained with these maneuvers, positioning should be reassessed and a nasopharyngeal airway be placed to supplement the oropharyngeal airway.

c. Endotracheal intubation

Even with optimal positioning, external manipulation of the airway (e.g. BURP maneuver, Chapter 5) may increase visualization of the glottis. This may be especially helpful in small children who have anterior airways and trauma patients who cannot be optimally aligned.

d. BMV and cricoid pressure

Studies in children have shown that cricoid pressure not only prevents passive regurgitation, but also prevents gastric insufflation, even with ventilation pressures greater than 40 cm H_2O. This is especially important in infants, in whom gastric distention may lead to decreased respiratory excursion, and increases the chances of aspiration.

e. Pop-off valves: the good and the bad

A pop-off valve is designed to prevent the delivery of excessive pressure, and therefore excessive volume, to the lungs. At a preset level, an escape valve opens and keeps the pressure below a predetermined level, usually 35–45 CWP. However, certain conditions require higher pressures to overcome upper-airway obstruction or to open noncompliant lungs. In these situations, the operator should occlude the valve manually or with the built-in occluding device. Before concluding that ventilatory difficulty is caused by intrinsic lung resistance, however, one must exclude inadequate airway patency as the cause; that is, manipulate the airway position to optimize patency.

B. Laryngeal mask airway (LMA)

The laryngeal mask airway (LMA) is a safe and effective airway management device for children undergoing general anesthesia and is considered a rescue option in the event of a failed airway in children and infants. Placement of the LMA in children requires some training but is a relatively easily learned skill, particularly if the correct size of mask is chosen. The LMA has also been used successfully in difficult pediatric airways and should be considered as an alternative device for emergency airway management in these patients. As in the adult, difficult pediatric intubations have also been facilitated by the use of the LMA in combination with such devices as the bronchoscope.

The LMA has a few important associated complications, which are especially prevalent in smaller infants, including partial airway obstruction by the epiglottis, loss of adequate seal with patient movement, and air leakage with positive pressure ventilation. To avoid obstruction with the epiglottis in these younger children and infants, some authors have suggested a rotational placement technique where the mask is placed in a back-to-front manner and then rotated 180 degrees as it is advanced into the hypopharynx. The LMA is also contraindicated in the pediatric patient or adult with intact protective airway reflexes and therefore is not suitable for awake airway management unless the patient is adequately sedated and the airway is topically anesthetized. The LMA is contraindicated if foreign body aspiration is present or suspected, as it would most likely fail to provide adequate ventilation and oxygenation because of the distal obstruction. The LMA comes in multiple sizes to accommodate children from neonate to adolescent. (See also Chapter 9.)

C. Pediatric lighted stylet

The lighted stylet is discussed in detail in Chapter 11. One device (Trachlight) has pediatric and infant stylets that mount to the same handle as is used for adults. These pediatric stylets accommodate intubation in children as young as neonates. Although some training and experience with these devices is required, the relative anterior airway of the young child is particularly suited to lighted stylet intubation, which does not require direct visualization of the glottis. Ease of use and a low complication rate make the lighted stylet a viable airway alternative in the relatively stable patient (i.e., the can't intubate, *can* oxygenate scenario.)

D. Needle cricothyrotomy

Although virtually every textbook chapter, article, or lecture on pediatric airway management refers to the technique of needle cricothyrotomy as the recommended last-resort rescue procedure, there is little literature to support its use and safety. Few of the "experts" who write about needle cricothyrotomy have significant experience performing the procedure on a live human patient. Newer devices, such as the LMA and the lighted stylet, may further reduce the very infrequent need for needle cricothyrotomy, but nevertheless, any clinician who manages pediatric emergencies as part of his or her practice must be familiar with the procedure and its indications and have the appropriate equipment readily accessible in the emergency department.

Needle cricothyrotomy is indicated as a life-saving, last-resort procedure in patients who present or progress to the can't intubate, can't ventilate scenario and whose obstruction is proximal to glottic opening. The classic indication is epiglottitis where BMV and intubation are judged to have failed, although true failure of BMV is rare in epiglottitis, and failure is more often caused by a failure of technique than by a truly insurmountable obstruction. Other indications include facial trauma, angioedema, and other conditions that preclude proximal access to the glottic opening. Needle cricothyrotomy is rarely helpful in patients who have aspirated a foreign body that cannot be visualized by direct laryngoscope, as it is unlikely that the obstruction is located proximal to the cricothyroid membrane. It also would be of questionable value in the patient with croup, as the obstruction is subglottic and more likely to be bypassed by an endotracheal tube (ETT) introduced orally into the trachea with a stylet, rather than blindly by needle cricothyrotomy.

Various premade kits have been recommended for percutaneous needle cricothyrotomy. The simplest equipment, appropriate for use in infants, consists of the following:

14-gauge over-the-needle catheter
3.0-mm ETT adapter
3 mL or 5 mL syringe

It is a good practice to preassemble the kit, place it in a clear bag, seal the bag, and tape it in an accessible position in the resuscitation area.

1. Procedure

Place the child in the supine position with the head extended with a towel under the shoulder to further exaggerate the extension. This forces the trachea anteriorly so that it becomes easily palpable and can be stabilized with two fingers of one hand. The following statement appears in many textbooks describing this procedure: "Carefully palpate the cricothyroid membrane." In reality it is very difficult to do this in an infant and not essential. Indeed in smaller children it may be impossible to precisely locate the cricothyroid membrane, so often the proximal trachea is accessed; the key to success is strict immobilization of the trachea throughout the procedure. The priority is an airway and provision of oxygen. Complications from inserting the catheter elsewhere into the trachea besides the cricothyroid membrane can be addressed later. Consider the trachea as a large vein, and cannulate it with the catheter directed caudad at a 30-degree angle. Aspirate air to ensure tracheal entry, then slide the catheter gently off the needle, removing the needle. Attach the 3.0-mm ETT adapter to the catheter and commence bag ventilation. The provider will note exaggerated resistance to bagging. This is normal and is related to the turbulence created by using a 14-gauge catheter as an airway; it is not the result of a misplaced catheter or poor lung compliance secondary to pneumothorax. It is helpful to practice BMV through a catheter to experience the feel of the significantly increased resistance. The required pressures are well above the limits of the pop-off valve. Therefore it must be occluded in order to permit gas flow through the catheter. Jet ventilation has also been advocated in this situation. Extreme caution, however, must be exercised to avoid the complications of excessive flow and resultant barotrauma. Jet ventilation should be considered only by those familiar with its use and in children more than 5 to 6 years old. Even in a child of 6 or older, if adequate oxygen saturation can be maintained with the bag technique described previously, this is preferable to jet ventilation. If jet ventilation is used, the ventilator must have a pressure control valve system on it. Start with low pressure (20 PSI) and titrate to adequate chest rise and fall and oxygen saturation, using a one-half to one second burst of ventilation, followed by 3 to 4 seconds of exhalation time.

II. Airway techniques used in adolescents and adults but not in small children

A. Blind nasotracheal intubation

Nasotracheal intubation in children is uniformly discouraged and is frequently considered contraindicated. This recommendation is based on the fact that the sharp angle of the nasopharynx and pharyngotracheal axis in children precludes a high likelihood of success with this technique when performed blindly. A second reason is that children are at increased risk for hemorrhage because of the preponderance of highly vascular and delicate adenoidal tissue. The direct-visualization technique is, however, commonly used in small infants and children for chronic ventilator management in the intensive care unit setting. Using direct visualization with a laryngoscope once the ETT has passed into the oro- and hypopharynx, tracheal placement is aided with Magill forceps. However, this technique is not helpful in emergency airway management. In general, the technique of blind nasotracheal intubation, which is essentially the same as that described for adults in Chapter 8, has few, if any, primary indications in pediatric emergency airway management, and in any case is not recommended for patients less than 10 years of age.

B. Combitube

The Combitube represents an excellent, easily learned rescue airway device that is available only for patients of height greater than 48 inches, so is of limited application

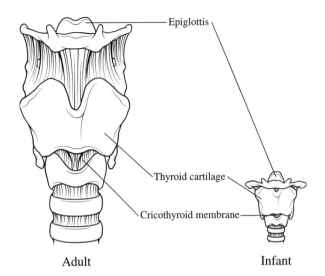

Adult   Infant

FIG. 20-2. Cricothyroid membrane. Comparative size of the adult (***left***) versus pediatric (***right***) cricothyroid membrane. Note that not only is the larynx smaller, but the actual membrane is smaller proportionately in comparison involving 1/4 to 1/3 the anterior tracheal circumference versus 2/3 to 3/4 in the adult. This pediatric drawing is that of a toddler, which accommodates a 4.5-mm ETT.

in pediatric emergency airway management. The use of the Combitube is identical to that described in Chapter 10.

C. Surgical cricothyrotomy

The cricothyroid membrane in small infants and children is minimally developed (Fig. 20-2). Identification of the key landmarks is at best extremely difficult, even in the non-crisis situation. The low likelihood of success, combined with the high anticipated complication rate from attempts to perform this procedure in an emergency, make it contraindicated in small children and infants. Surgical or cricothyrotome-based cricothyrotomy should not be attempted in children under 10, except in extraordinary circumstances. In children under 10 years of age, needle cricothyrotomy with bag or jet ventilation is preferable. As with adults, adolescents may have easily identifiable and accessible anatomy, and therefore cricothyrotomy may be a reasonable rescue technique in this age group. Transtracheal jet ventilation (TTJV) continues to be an option, as for adults. Cricothyrotomy using a commercially available kit (Pedi-trake) has not been shown to be successful or even safe. Box 20-1 summarizes recommendations for invasive airway procedures in children.

Box 20-1. Summary Recommendations for Invasive Airway Procedures in Children

< 5 years old
Needle cricothyrotomy and bag ventilation
5 to 10 years old
Needle cricothyrotomy and bag ventilation
If oxygen saturation is inadequate: transtracheal jet ventilation regulated to low PSI
>10 years
Operator preference
Needle cricothyrotomy with TTJV
or
Surgical cricothyrotomy

EVIDENCE

1. Does a needle cricothyrotomy in children provide sufficient oxygenation and ventilation to avoid hypoxia and hypercarbia? The evidence surrounding pediatric needle cricothyrotomies is based on an animal study by Cote et al. using an approximately 30-kg dog model. Cote was able to demonstrate that dogs representative in size of an approximate 9 to 10 year old could be oxygenated through a 12-gauge catheter and 3.0 ETT adapter with a bag for at least 1 hour (the study duration). Rises in P_aCO_2 levels were noted but were not felt to be significant as children normally tolerate mild degrees of hypercarbia well (1).

One adult retrospective study reported that 48 patients were successfully oxygenated and ventilated utilizing transtracheal ventilation through a 13-gauge intratracheal catheter for up to 360 minutes. TTJV was used primarily in 47 of these patients although 6 patients did receive conventional bagging measures until TTJV circuits could be initiated. During manual transtracheal ventilation, each of these patients demonstrated increases in P_aCO_2 on blood gases but maintained P_aO_2 values greater than 100 mm Hg (2).

2. The LMA should be considered as both a rescue device and an alternative airway in the management of difficult emergency pediatric airways. Most of the literature regarding the use of LMAs in children has been compiled from the anesthesia experience in the operating room. Therefore, little information is available for the use of the LMA in the acute emergency setting. However, an observational study by M. Lopez-Gil et al. has demonstrated that the skill for placement of the LMA could be rapidly learned by anesthesia residents with a low complication rate (3,4). Published case reports have demonstrated success of the LMA in the pediatric patient with difficult airways including isolated severe retrognathia, Dandy-Walker syndrome, and Pierre Robin syndrome (5,6).

At least one prospective study reports a higher incidence of airway obstruction, higher ventilatory pressures, larger inspiratory leaks, and more complications in smaller children (less than 10 kg) with LMA use than in the older child. These authors recommend that the risk/benefit should be carefully weighed in younger children before using the LMA with paralysis and positive pressure ventilation. Importantly, the success rate for placement of the LMA in this study that was performed in elective cases undergoing prolonged ventilation was high at 98% (7). Although physicians should be aware of these potential complications, this study is not generalizable to the emergency setting and should not deter providers from implementing this as a *rescue device* in infants or young children with failed airways, or as a planned approach to an infant or young child with an identified difficult airway. In the failed airway situation, the LMA may be a life-saving bridge, providing effective oxygenation and ventilation until a definitive airway may be obtained.

REFERENCES

1. Cote CJ, Eavey RD, Todres ID, et al. Cricothyroid membrane puncture: oxygenation and ventilation in a dog model using an intravenous catheter. *Crit Care Med* 1988;16:615–619.
2. Ravussin P, Freeman J. A new transtracheal catheter for ventilation and resuscitation. *Can Aneaesth Soc J* 1985;32:60–64.
3. Lopez-Gil, Brimacombe J, Alvarez M. Safety and efficacy of the laryngeal mask airway: a prospective survey of 1400 children. *Anaesthesia* 1996;51:969–972.
4. Lopez-Gil, Brimacombe J, Cebrian J, Arranz J. Laryneal mask airway in pediatric practice: a prospective study of skill acquisition by anesthesia residents. *Anesthesiology* 1996;84:807–811.

5. Selim M, Mowafi H, Al-Ghamdi A, et al. Intubation via LMA in pediatric patients with difficult airways. *Can J Anaesth* 1999;46:891–893.
6. Stocks RM, Egerman R, Thompson JW, et al. Airway management of the severely retrognathic child: use of the laryngeal mask airway. *Ear Nose Throat J* 2002;81:223–226.
7. Park C, Bahk JH, Ahn WS, et al. The laryngeal mask airway in infants and children. *Can J Anaes* 2001;48:413–417.

21

The Difficult Pediatric Airway

Robert C. Luten and Niranjan Kissoon

Securing an airway in a patient, adult or child, is made more challenging or difficult for two principal reasons:

1. The patient's normal airway anatomy is modified because of an acute insult or
2. The patient with an abnormal airway (e.g., a congenital anomaly) requires airway management for an unrelated cause, such as respiratory failure due to an asthma exacerbation.

The approach to the emergent difficult adult airways is described in Chapter 6, which should be read before this chapter. Pediatric difficult airways, especially those encountered in emergency situations, are far less common, not well studied, and not extensively covered in any textbook. For purposes of this discussion, difficult pediatric airways will be divided functionally into difficult airways secondary to:

1. Acute infectious disease
2. Acute noninfectious disease
3. Congenital anomalies, most commonly with a superimposed indication for emergency airway management unrelated to the airway abnormality (e.g., respiratory failure secondary to asthma or pneumonia).

I. Difficult airways secondary to acute infectious disease
1. Epiglottitis
2. Croup (usually not a difficult intubation; see Table 21-1)
3. Retropharyngeal abscess
4. Bacterial tracheitis
5. Ludwig's angina

Most of the entities in this and the next section present because the normal anatomy is altered, usually by swelling, which leads to varying degrees of airway obstruction. The pediatric patient is especially susceptible to airway obstruction from swelling, often from conditions that are less threatening to the adult. This is illustrated in Table 21-2, which outlines the effect of 1-mm edema on airway resistance in the infant (4-mm airway diameter) versus adult (8-mm airway diameter). These figures reflect the quietly breathing infant or adult. If the child cries, the work of breathing is increased 32-fold, hence the principle of maintaining children in a quiet, comfortable environment during evaluation and management for potential airway obstruction.

TABLE 21-1. Management of the "most-feared" pediatrics airway problems

Disease	Pathology and deterioration	Approach	FB removal maneuvers	BMV two-person techniques	Intubation	Needle cricothyrotomy
Epiglottitis	Rapidly progressing disease process affecting the supraglottic structures (epiglottis, aryepiglottic folds). Patients usually present in minimal distress. Decompensation rarely occurs unless the patient is overstimulated or manipulated, leading to increasing airway resistance or functional obstruction. Otherwise, decompensation is the result of progressive deterioration over time secondary to fatigue although the respiratory arrest may occur precipitously.	Stable → observe → transfer to OR for definitive airway Decompensation BMV ↓ Intubation ↓ Needle cric	Not indicated	Effective *in most* patients who deteriorate. Technique: 2-handed seal with another rescuer providing sufficient pressure to overcome the obstruction	Usually successful. Use tube size 1 mm smaller. Use stylet. Suction, visualize, press on chest, and look for bubble.	Probably one of the few indications for needle cric *if* BMV *and* intubation unsuccessful
Croup	Slowly progressive (hours to days) disease process affecting the subglottic trachea, causing dynamic inspiratory augmented obstruction. Deterioration is usually progressive rather than sudden and related to respiratory muscle fatigue, and as in the case of epiglottis, the arrest may also occur precipitously.	Racemic epi Steroids Stable → ICU Decompensation BMV ↓ Intubation	Not indicated	Effective. Positive pressure overcomes obstruction by acting as a stent. Will also probably require higher pressures.	Proximal airway normal; therefore should not be problematic. Consider ETT 1 size smaller and use stylet.	Not indicated since obstruction is distal
FB aspiration	Patients with aspirated foreign bodies continuously have the potential for decompensation secondary to acute airway obstruction. The level of obstruction may vary from the hypopharynx, above or below the glottis, to the mainstem bronchus.	Stable → observe → transfer for removal Decompensation: FB removal maneuvers ↓ Direct visualization and removal with Magill ↓ Intubation to force FB distally into mainstem bronchus	indicated if *appropriate* i.e., patient totally obstructs	Should not be used before attempts to remove FB. May be obviated by intubation.	Last resort in an effort to push FB distally.	Usually not indicated since FB will be distal to the obstruction if other efforts have failed.

Abbreviations: BMV, bag/mask ventilation; epi, epinephrine; ETT, endotracheal tube; FB, foreign body; ICU, intensive care unit; OR, operating room.

TABLE 21-2. *Effect of 1-mm edema on airway resistance*

	Change in cross-sectional area	Change in resistance
Infant	44% decrease	200% increase
Adult	25% decrease	40% increase

Table 21-1 outlines the two most well known infectious diseases involving the upper airway with potential for obstruction in children (epiglottitis and croup). Epiglottitis is rarely seen in the western world since the introduction of the *Hemophilus* influenza vaccine, and croup, commonly referred to in the differential diagnosis of epiglottitis, is usually a clinically distinct entity and is even more rarely a difficult intubation, as the obstruction is subglottic. It is of value still to discuss epiglottitis because it represents the prototype indication for needle cricothyrotomy (Chapter 20) for obstruction proximal to the glottic opening when bag/mask ventilation (BMV) and intubation fail. Other, non-infectious, problems causing obstruction proximal to the glottic opening include facial trauma, angioedema, and caustic ingestions and burns involving the hypopharynx. To put these "most-feared" diseases in perspective, the following points should be kept in mind:

A. All these problems have in common the fact that airway intervention in the emergency department (ED) should never be attempted unless deterioration occurs or is imminent. If one adheres to this principle and then follows a stepwise approach as outlined in Table 21-1, results will be optimal and complications, especially iatrogenic complications, will be avoided.

B. Epiglottitis and croup are clinically very distinct entities, rarely, if ever, requiring an x-ray to distinguish the two. The fact that textbooks group them together in the differential diagnosis of acute life-threatening upper-airway obstruction is misleading, as the differentiation is usually clinically obvious.

C. Croup, as opposed to epiglottitis or foreign-body aspiration, will respond to medical intervention (inhaled epinephrine), which may obviate the need for intubation.

D. Retropharyngeal abscess in children usually presents without airway compromise, although it is virtually always found in textbooks in the differential diagnosis of acute life-threatening airway obstruction. The same is true of Lugwig's angina, an even less common disease. The term *paraairway diagnoses* is used to describe conditions involving the airway above the level of the glottis. These conditions rarely require emergency airway intervention for the pediatric patient in the ED. A retropharyngeal abscess most commonly presents with odynophagia and neck stiffness. Lateral neck films reveal thickening of the retropharyngeal space. Most of these patients have retropharyngeal cellulitis and respond to antibiotics. If an abscess is present, incision and drainage is required, but rarely, if ever, is it necessary to actively manage the airway in the ED.

II. **Difficult airways secondary to noninfectious causes**
  1. Foreign body
  2. Burns
  3. Anaphylaxis
  4. Caustic ingestion
  5. Trauma
  6. Other swellings (angioneurotic edema, Quinke's disease, etc.)

  Foreign-body aspiration is probably the most feared pediatric airway problem. The procedure for removal of a foreign body in the partially obstructed airway is described elsewhere (Chapter 32) for adults and is the same procedure for children with one important exception. Younger children may not cooperate, in which case sedation is important. Ketamine 1 to 2 mg/kg IV or 4 mg/kg IM produce dependable deep sedation/anesthesia while maintaining respiratory drive and reflexes. In both adults and children, if the foreign body becomes lodged causing complete obstruction and cannot be retrieved or expelled by blind maneuvers, BMV, followed by advancement of the foreign body into a mainstem bronchus as described later should be immediately initiated.

With complete obstruction of the airway, oxygen desaturation, which renders the patient unconscious, occurs within one minute or so. A stepwise approach should be followed.

A. The conscious child

Although controversy exists regarding the ideal emergency procedure for relief of choking, the Heimlich manuever is suggested by the American Heart Association for children above 1 year of age. For children below 1 year of age, a series of five back blows followed by five chest thrusts is recommended.

If the patient is conscious, the correct initial treatment is the application of the maneuvers, which should be repeated until the foreign body is expelled or the patient loses consciousness. To summarize:

- Children aged less than 1 year: Five back blows followed by five chest thrusts
- Children aged more than 1 year: Repetitive abdominal thrusts
- Attempt ventilation
- Continue this sequence as long as the child is conscious.

Attempting instrumentation to remove the foreign body of a completely obstructed upper airway while the patient is still conscious is not wise. If the maneuvers are successful in removing the foreign body and the patient can phonate and breathe normally, then observation for 12 to 24 hours is advised.

B. *The unconscious child*

If the maneuvers are unsuccessful in removing the foreign body and the patient loses consciousness, or if the patient presents unconscious with an upper-airway foreign body, then direct laryngoscopy should be attempted. In most cases, an unconscious child will be flaccid and it will be unnecessary to administer neuromuscular agents. However, occasionally the child may present with clenched teeth; this presentation may be similar to the crash airway, and hence the judicious use of succinylcholine to achieve relaxation to identify and remove the foreign body may be necessary. If under direct laryngoscopy the foreign body can be identified, it should be removed.

Occasionally, BMV using high pressure (usually a two-person–two-handed technique) is required to achieve an adequate seal and to try to inflate the lung. If ventilation is successful in these cases, it is usually because the foreign body has been forced into the subglottic region and then into one of the mainstem bronchi. If this occurs, BMV may be continued if breathing is ineffective. If BMV is unsuccessful, the child should be intubated.

The child should be intubated and an attempt be made to advance the foreign body further down the airway. Usually it will be possible to push the foreign body into a mainstem bronchus (usually in the right). The tube should then be withdrawn above the carina and ventilation of the unobstructed lung attempted. Practical point: The lip-to-tip distance provides an objective guide to positioning of the endotracheal tube (ETT) in the trachea of a child. When the tube is positioned at the correct cm lip marker, the distal opening of the ETT is halfway between the vocal cords and the carina. The position can, and should, be clinically verified. Occasionally if the foreign body is soft such as foodstuff, it may lodge within the ETT, which will need to

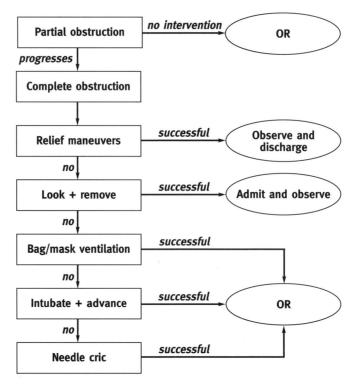

FIG. 21-1. Stepwise approach for the management of an aspirated foreign body.

be withdrawn out of the airway. The patient may then breathe spontaneously and be successfully ventilated using BMV, or another ETT can be reintroduced. If the foreign body cannot be be removed, then immediate cricothyrotomy may be indicated. However, cricothyrotomy will be successful only if the foreign body is lodged in the airway above the entrance of the needle into the airway. A more distal lodgment of a foreign body cannot be bypassed with this procedure. If the child is breathing spontaneously or there is need for further ventilatory assistance, a second direct laryngoscopy should be done to ensure that no additional foreign bodies are in the upper airway before starting positive pressure ventilation with BMV. An overview of the sequence is presented in Table 21-1, and detail is provided in Fig. 21-1.

As is the case for adults, the anticipated clinical course of the presenting condition becomes a key determinant in the decision whether to intubate or to observe the patient for possible deterioration. Table 21-3 groups entities from both infectious and non-infectious causes according to timing of intervention based on anticipated clinical course.

The *expectant intervention group* represents patients in whom the intervention itself may be more hazardous than a period of close observation during which preparation is rapidly undertaken for definitive management. In these children, the airway should be actively managed in the ED only if deterioration occurs. The rationale in these cases is that intervention is best done in controlled circumstances by a multidisciplinary team with expertise in the management of difficult airways. Treatment in less than ideal conditions may lead to untoward outcomes.

TABLE 21-3. *Timing of intervention according to anticipated clinical course*

Expectant intervention group: Intervene *only* if deterioration occurs:
1. Assemble subspecialty multidisciplinary team for definitive management:
   Foreign body
   Epiglottitis
2. Obtain subspecialty assistance if deterioration appears likely
   Paraairway diagnoses (diseases such as retropharyngeal or peritonsillar abscess or Ludwig's angina
     that are usually stable on presentation and deterioration is uncommon)

Early intervention group: Intervene *early* (preventively):
   Burns
   Anaphylaxis (usually responds to medical treatment)
   Caustic ingestions
   Trauma

The signs and symptoms of impending airway obstruction in children are important indicators to guide the approach to the *early intervention group*. These entities, if left to expectant treatment, have a greater potential for deterioration. An example is the burn or caustic ingestion patient who is beginning to develop a raspy voice. The initial symptoms herald the potential for deterioration, and the extent of the progression cannot be predicted. It must be assumed to be progressive to the point of obstruction, which will compromise the patient's breathing and also render intubation extremely difficult. Patients with anaphylaxis and airway involvement who do not respond to immediate medical treatment similarly require early intervention to prevent a more difficult, unmanageable problem later. As outlined previously, children are less capable anatomically of accommodating swelling in the airway and can deteriorate precipitously.

III. Difficult airways secondary to congenital anomalies

Patients with difficult airways secondary to congenital anomalies receive the most attention in discussions of difficult airways in pediatrics. However, they are encountered only rarely in the ED, much less frequently than groups 1 and 2. Also, the literature concerning these patients usually discusses elective situations, managed by experienced pediatric anesthesiology subspecialists in well-equipped operating rooms with the intubation done under controlled conditions. Little of the information provided in theses discussions is relevant, therefore, to the emergency physician presented with an acute indication for airway management in one of these patients.

Most patients with congenital anomalies presenting to the ED require intubation for reasons unrelated to their difficult airway (e.g., a child with Pierre Robin syndrome with respiratory failure secondary to asthma). The best approach for these patients is to obtain expert subspecialty assistance as early as possible and to aggressively manage the medical condition to try to obviate the need for intubation. Unlike the conditions discussed earlier in this chapter, there is some luxury of time here, because the airway difficulty is not increasing. Delay in managing the airway may result in some deterioration of the patient, but will not make the airway itself any more difficult, except possibly by limiting the time available to achieve intubation in a severely hypoxemic patient.

A common feature of many anomalies complicating endotracheal (ET) intubation is the micrognathic mandible. The small mandible reduces the space into which the tongue and mandibular tissue must be compressed with the laryngoscope blade to visualize the glottic opening. A significantly recessed (micrognathic) mandible can be recognized by

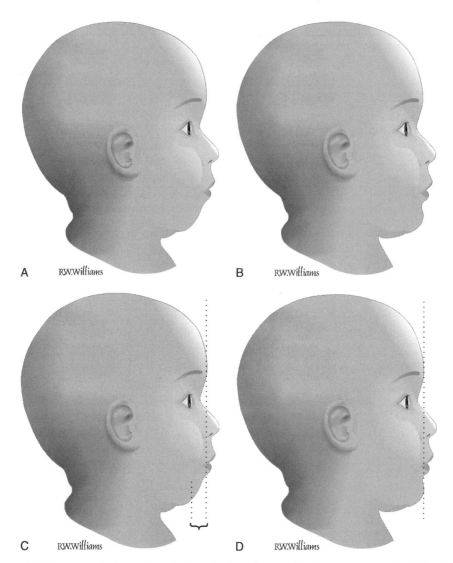

FIG. 21-2. It may not always be obvious that a given patient possesses a difficult airway (**A**). When compared with a normal child, the differences may be more striking (**A** vs. **B**). In the individual patient, however, a line drawn inferiorly from the forehead, touching the maxilla, will also touch the mandible (**D**). The failure to do so demonstrates a certain degree of micrognathia (**C**), which must be correlated with the clinical picture. (Extrapolated from Frankville D. In: *ASA refresher course*, Parkridge, IL: American Society of Anesthesiologists. 2001:126).

drawing a line that touches the forehead and maxilla and continues inferiorly. In a patient with grossly normal anatomy, the line also touches the mandible. In the micrognathic patient, an obvious distance between the line and the mandible is observed (see Fig. 21-2). In such patients a quick look to assess compressibility of the anatomy in the potentially reduced submandibular space may be an option before opting for rapid sequence intubation (RSI).

TABLE 21-4. *Therapeutic options for the difficult airway*

The difficult airway algorithm applies to children as well as adults with few exceptions; most notably the use of blind nasotracheal intubation is contraindicated below 10 years of age, as is surgical cricothyrotomy. Combitubes, a useful adjunct in adults, are not manufactured for patients less than 48 inches tall. Otherwise, the same approach and options are recommended for both children and adults, the only difference being that they are required less often.

There are a variety of airway devices for use in the pediatric patient. However, because of lack of frequency of use except in elective subspecialty situations, only a few have been used in emergencies and even fewer by emergency physicians. It is probably best to limit the number of options in an effort to gain the maximum experience with them. The following devices and procedures are listed according to appropriateness in different levels of clinical acuity.

Crash situation
  Noninvasive
    ET intubation (infancy to adulthood)
    LMA (infancy to adulthood)
    Combitube (>48 in. tall)
  Invasive
    Needle cricothyrotomy[a]
    Seldinger cricothyrotomy (>5 yr)[a]
    Surgical or Seldinger cricothyrotomy (>10 yr)
  Stable situation
    ET intubation (awake) (infancy to adulthood)
    ET intubation (RSI) (infancy to adulthood)
    Combitube (>48 in. in height; patient must be obtunded)
    LMA (infancy to adulthood)
    Lightwand (infancy to adulthood)
    Blind nasotracheal intubation (>10 yr)
Stable Expectant Management Patients
All emergency departments should have in place a plan for managing these patients, which includes foreign body aspiration, epiglottitis, etc. This usually requires prior agreement of consultants willing to respond immediately to those emergencies.

[a]Below age 5 yr BMV is recommended with these options. From 5–10 yr TTJV has been recommended, but requires an adjustable pressure regulator. There is very little literature to support TTJV recommendation for pediatric emergency airway management, just as there is little literature to support needle cricothyrotomy and BMV. However, the risk of complications with the former is very high. TTJV should used with extreme caution in children and is best reserved for use by clinicians familiar with TTJV.

For patients *in extremis* or in crash situations, the clinician is left with no other options than those used in other patients. Often such simple procedures as BMV or ET intubation are successful in these patients and should remain as the mainstay of therapy. Therapeutic options for the pediatric difficult airway are outlined in Table 21-4.

EVIDENCE

Unfortunately, there is minimal evidence on the recognition and management of emergent difficult pediatric airways. Most of the descriptions of difficult pediatric airways deal with children with congenital anomalies. The literature on the systematic prediction of which airways will present difficulty, specifically which bedside evaluations might be helpful, is confined to adult series and is not necessarily applicable to children (1; see Table 21-5). With the establishment of the National Emergency Airway Registry project, it is hoped that new information will emerge regarding the scope of this problem and its solutions.

1. Heimlich maneuver. There is a controversy in the literature as to the ideal emergency procedure for relief of choking due to foreign body aspiration (2,3). However, the Heimlich

TABLE 21-5. *Comparison of pediatric and adult risk factors*

A. *Risk factors for adult difficult airway usually not present in infants and young children:*
 1. Obesity
 2. Decreased neck mobility
 3. Teeth abnormalities
 4. Temporomandibular joint problems
B. *Risk Factors for pediatric difficult airway not present in adults:*
 1. Small airway caliber susceptible to obstruction from infection
 2. Discomfort secondary to dealing with age/size-related variables
 3. Discomfort secondary to infrequency of patient encounters

maneuver is suggested by the American Heart Association as the maneuver to be tried initially for children over 1 year of age. In children less than 1 year of age, the danger of intraabdominal injury precludes its use, and a combination of back blows and chest thrusts is recommended (4). While little evidence exists, it is recommended that if obstruction is incomplete and the patient is phonating, then no intervention should be tried. This approach is based on the fact that the force of a cough generates five to six times the airflow velocity of any maneuvers and is more likely to expel the foreign body. Moreover, there is concern that these interventions may have the potential to convert a partial obstruction to a total obstruction.

REFERENCES

1. Kopp VJ, Bailey A, Calhoun PE, et al. Utility of the Mallampati classification for predicting difficult intubation in pediatric patients. *Anesthesiology* 1995;83:3A1147.
2. Redding JS. The choking controversy: critique of evidence on the Heimlich maneuver. *Crit Care Med* 1979;7:475–479.
3. Heimlich HJ. First aid for choking children: back blows and chest thrusts cause complications and death. *Pediatrics* 1982;70:120–125.
4. Zaritsky A, Nadkarni V, Hickey R, et al., eds. *PALS provider manual.* Dallas, TX: American Heart Association, 2002.

22

RSI Using Nondepolarizing Agents

John C. Sakles and Ron M. Walls

I. The clinical challenge

Succinylcholine is the preferred agent for rapid sequence intubation (RSI) in the emergency department (ED), but certain patients have contraindications to its use, principally related to hyperkalemia risk or, rarely, to known prior adverse reactions. These are discussed in detail in Chapter 18. This chapter addresses the approach to patients for whom an alternative neuromuscular blocking agent (NMBA) is required for RSI.

II. Approach to the airway

Of the nondepolarizing NMBAs, two have pharmacokinetic properties that support use during RSI: rocuronium (Zemuron) and vecuronium (Norcuron). Of these, rocuronium is superior for ED use because of its consistently rapid onset; it has been shown to produce intubating conditions almost comparable to succinylcholine 60 seconds after administration. Rocuronium does not release histamine, is not a ganglionic blocking agent, and is devoid of cardiac muscarinic blocking effects, so it is virtually free of adverse effects. The biggest drawback to rocuronium is its relatively longer duration, which averages 46 minutes when used in the 1 mg/kg RSI dose. If rocuronium is not available to the clinician, then vecuronium may be used. Vecuronium is also devoid of any clinically significant side effects, but its onset is somewhat delayed (at least 90 seconds) even when the priming technique is used (see later.)

III. Technique

When a nondepolarizing agent is used for RSI, the time to adequate relaxation for laryngoscopy and intubation is slightly prolonged when compared to that for succinylcholine. In general, succinylcholine achieves intubation-level paralysis in 45 seconds, rocuronium in 60 seconds, and vecuronium in 75 to 90 seconds. One method to shorten the apparent time to paralysis for vecuronium is to reverse the order of administration of the induction agent and the NMBA, giving the vecuronium first, followed immediately by the induction agent. This approach is not necessary or recommended with rocuronium.

Alternatively, and preferably, the priming principle can be used to hasten the onset of paralysis with vecuronium. The priming principle requires the administration of a small, or priming, dose of vecuronium (0.01 mg/kg) as a pretreatment drug 3 minutes before the administration of an increased paralyzing dose (0.15 mg/kg). The small priming dose serves to bind a small percentage of the motor end plate acetycholine (ACh) receptors, such that clinical weakness is not experienced by the patient, yet the onset of action of the subsequent full paralytic dose is hastened. Using the priming principle, intubation-level paralysis can be achieved with vecuronium in 75 to 90 seconds. When using the priming principle, it is recommended that the full paralytic dose be increased from the typical dose of 0.1 mg/kg (two times the effective dose that results in paralysis of 95% of the population, or ED_{95}) to 0.15 mg/kg (three times the ED_{95}).

Another method that has been advocated is that of the timing principle, in which the vecuronium is administered first, but the induction agent is withheld until the first sign of clinical weakness (ptosis) is observed, at which time the induction agent is then rapidly pushed. This timing principle is advocated on the basis that it facilitates the simultaneous onset of paralysis and hypnosis, minimizing the period that the patient is unconscious (but not intubatable) and at risk of aspiration. The timing principle also has the potential for severe discomfort for the patient, who becomes paralyzed while still awake, and requires a level of patient observation and timing of drugs not used in any other RSI, so seems prone to error. Use of the timing principle is not recommended for routing use the ED.

IV. Drug dosage and administration

Much research has been done on rocuronium to determine the appropriate dose for the fastest onset of paralysis for RSI. The ED_{95} of rocuronium is 0.3 mg/kg. Consequently, the most commonly studied dosages in the literature are multiples of that, namely 0.6 mg/kg, 0.9 mg/kg, and 1.2 mg/kg. Pharmacokinetic studies have identified 1.0 mg/kg as the best intubation dose for RSI. This dose allows for laryngoscopy and intubation to occur 45 to 60 seconds after administration and results in approximately 45 minutes of motor paralysis. Rocuronium is distributed as a solution in 50-mg and 100-mg vials, at a concentration of 10 mg/mL. Using the larger vial (100 mg) allows the dose for the average adult patient (70 mg) to be obtained from a single vial. Because reconstitution is not necessary, the drug can be drawn up and administered quickly during the RSI protocol. The shelf life of rocuronium at room temperature is only a month and thus refrigeration or active inventory control is required to avoid spontaneous degradation of the drug. A sample RSI using rocuronium is shown in Box 22-1.

Vecuronium is supplied as a lyophilized powder in 10-mg vials that must be reconstituted with normal saline before use. When the vial is mixed with 10 cc of saline, a solution

---

Box 22-1. RSI Using Rocuronium

Time zero minus 10 minutes: Preparation
Time zero minus 5 minutes: Preoxygenation
Time zero minus 3 minutes: Pretreatment
  LOA—no defasciculation required
Time zero: Paralysis with induction
  Induction agent IV push
  Rocuronium 1 mg/kg IV push
Time zero plus 30 seconds: Protection (Sellick's maneuver)
Time zero plus 60 seconds: Placement with proof
Time zero plus 90 seconds: Postintubation management
  Administer longer-acting sedation (e.g., lorazepam 0.05 mg/kg) to supplement long-acting paralysis of rocuronium.

Box 22-2. RSI Using Vecuronium with the Priming Principle

Time zero minus 10 minutes: Preparation
Time zero minus 5 minutes: Preoxygenation
Time zero minus 3 minutes: Pretreatment
    LOA—as with succinylcholine
    Vecuronium 0.01 mg/kg (priming dose—given to all patients)
Time zero: Paralysis with induction
    Induction agent IV push
    Vecuronium 0.15 mg/kg IV push
Time zero plus 30 seconds: Protection (Sellick's maneuver)
Time zero plus 90 seconds: Placement with proof
Time zero plus 120 seconds: Postintubation management
    Administer longer-acting sedation (e.g., lorazepam 0.05 mg/kg) to supplement long-acting
    paralysis of vecuronium.

---

of 1 mg/mL vecuronium is produced. When performing RSI using vecuronium, the priming principle should be used, so the patient should receive 0.01 mg/kg (usually rounded to a full 1 mg in most adult patients of average weight), during the pretreatment phase of RSI, followed 3 minutes later by 0.15 mg/kg of vecuronium, given by rapid IV administration. This treatment should be accompanied by the appropriate dose of the induction agent selected. In most circumstances laryngoscopy can be initiated in 75 to 90 seconds. Paralysis will likely last for 30 to 40 minutes. When using the priming principle, the operator must be extremely vigilant of the patient, as a severely debilitated patient or a patient with severe respiratory failure may experience very significant motor paralysis after the priming dose alone and require bag/mask ventilation and accelerated movement to the paralysis/induction step of RSI. A sample RSI using vecuronium with the priming principle is shown in Box 22-2. See Box 22-3 for a summary of various methods for RSI with non-depolarizing agents.

V. Postintubation management

Postintubation management after RSI with a nondepolarizing NMBA is comparable to that of conventional RSI with succinylcholine, with an obvious exception. The duration of action of succinylcholine is so short that an intermediate-acting NMBA must be given immediately after intubation if the operator wishes to maintain the patient in a paralyzed state. After performing RSI with rocuronium or vecuronium, motor paralysis will continue for approximately 45 minutes. The patient must therefore be given adequate sedation and analgesia to accompany the long-acting paralytic.

VI. Tips and pearls

When succinylcholine is contraindicated, rocuronium is the preferable NMBA for RSI, as it provides an earlier onset of paralysis and a shorter duration of action than vecuronium. Rocuronium substitutes easily for succinylcholine in the RSI protocol and it is supplied in solution, like succinylcholine, so it does not need to be reconstituted. Also, the additional step of priming is not necessary. It is strongly recommended that the priming principle *not* be used with rocuronium as its rapid onset of action may allow the patient to experience the dreadful feeling of the onset of paralysis before the induction agent has taken effect. Additionally, concerns regarding hypoxia and aspiration of gastric contents have been raised when using the priming principle with ROC.

Box 22-3. Protocols

1. Rocuronium
    a. Preparation
    b. Preoxygenation
    c. Pretreatment
       • As indicated by patient condition
       • Defasciculation *not* required
    d. Paralysis with induction
       • Etomidate 0.3 mg/kg IV
       • Rocuronium 1.0 mg/kg IV
    e. Protection and positioning
    f. Placement with proof
       • At 45 seconds
    g. Postintubation management
2. Vecuronium, using "High Dose VEC"
    a. Preparation
    b. Preoxygenation
    c. Pretreatment
       • As indicated by patient condition
       • Defasciculation *not* required
    d. Paralysis with induction
       • Etomidate 0.3 mg/kg IV
       • Vecuronium 0.3 mg/kg IV
    e. Protection and positioning
    f. Placement with proof
       • At 60 seconds
    g. Postintubation management
3. Vecuronium, using the priming principle
    a. Preparation
    b. Preoxygenation
    c. Pretreatment
       • As indicated by patient condition
       • Vecuronium 0.01 mg/kg IV
    d. Paralysis with induction
       • Etomidate 0.3 mg/kg IV
       • Vecuronium 0.15 mg/kg IV
    e. Protection and positioning
    f. Placement with proof
       • At 60 seconds
    g. Postintubation management

Although the timing principle with rocuronium has been described, it is unnecessary and potentially hazardous, and is not recommended for the ED. Protocols for using rocuronium and vecuronium are summarized in Box 22-3.

EVIDENCE

1. Time to achieve intubating conditions with rocuronium. Many studies performed in the operating room have shown that rocuronium can produce excellent intubating conditions within 60 seconds. The best analysis is that of Kirkegaard-Nielsen et al. who were able to use pharmacokinetic measurements to calculate the optimal intubating dose of rocuronium for RSI at 1.04 mg/kg (1). This dose provided for intubation at 60 seconds in 95% of patients with a duration of action of 46 minutes. This result strongly supports the use of 1.0 mg/kg of rocuronium for RSI, rather than the frequently recommended 0.6 mg/kg.

Perry et al. performed a detailed metaanalysis of 26 randomized clinical trials including 1,606 patients undergoing RSI with succinylcholine versus rocuronium and found that there was a statistically significant relative risk (0.87) of less favorable intubating conditions with rocuronium (2). In a subgroup analysis, when propofol was used as the induction agent, intubation conditions were found to be the same between succinylcholine and rocuronium. These data support the widely held notion that using a very potent induction agent can significantly improve the intubation conditions during RSI. This is likely because when intubation is attempted, the NMBA has not reached its peak effect, and the additional muscle relaxation produced by the induction agent thus further optimizes the intubation conditions. The differences between succinylcholine and rocuronium depend on the definitions and outcomes used, however, and much of the apparent superiority of succinylcholine over rocuronium depends on narrow definitions of "excellent" intubating conditions. Success rates were comparable in the two groups.

2. Emergency department use of rocuronium. Unfortunately, few ED-based studies exist because of the practical difficulties involved in carrying out pharmacological intubation studies in an uncontrolled setting on unstable patients with unplanned intubations. Over a 6-month period, Sakles et al. studied 58 patients who received rocuronium for RSI in the ED and found that a mean dose of 1.0 ± 0.2 mg/kg of rocuronium was used for intubation and that etomidate was the most frequently used induction agent (3). The time from rocuronium administration to the initiation of laryngoscopy was able to be timed in 34 patients and averaged 45 ± 15 seconds (range 20 to 90 seconds). Laurin et al. studied 520 ED intubations in which succinylcholine or rocuronium was used for RSI over a one-year period (4). In the 382 patients receiving succinylcholine, the mean onset time of paralysis was 39 ± 13 seconds, and in the 138 patients receiving rocuronium the onset time was 44 ± 20 seconds. This difference has no statistical or clinical significance.

REFERENCES

1. Kirkegaard-Nielsen H, Caldwell JE, Berry PD. Rapid tracheal intubation with rocuronium: a probability approach to determining dose. *Anesthesiology* 1999;91(Jul):131–136.
2. Perry JJ, Lee J, Wells G. Are intubation conditions using rocuronium equivalent to those using succinylcholine? *Acad Emerg Med* 2002;9:813–823.
3. Sakles JC, Laurin EG, Rantapaa AA, et al. Rocuronium for rapid sequence intubation of emergency department patients. *J Emerg Med* 1999;17:611–616.
4. Laurin EG, Sakles JC, Panacek EA, et al. A comparison of succinylcholine and rocuronium for rapid sequence intubation of emergency department patients. *Acad Emerg Med* 2000;7:1362–1369.

ADDITIONAL READING

Agoston S. Onset time and evaluation of intubating conditions: rocuronium in perspective. *Eur J Anaesthesiol* 1995;11[Suppl]:31–37.
Alastair JJ, Wood MD. New neuromuscular blocking drugs. *N Engl J Med* 1995;332:1691–1699.
Andrews JI, Kumar N, Van den Brom RHG, et al. A large simple randomized trial of rocuronium versus succinylcholine in rapid-sequence induction of anaesthesia along with propofol. *Acta Anaesthesiol Scand* 1999;43:4–8.
Baillard C, Korinek AM, Galanton V, et al. Anaphylaxis to rocuronium. *Br J Anaesth* 2002;88:600–602.
Book WJ, Abel M, Eisenkraft JB. Adverse effects of depolarizing neuromuscular blocking agents. *Drug Safety* 1994;10:331–349.

Culling RC, Middaugh RE, Menk EJ. Rapid tracheal intubation with vecuronium: the timing principle. *J Clin Anesth* 1989;1:422–425.

Dobson AP, McCluskey A, Meakin G, et al. Effective time to satisfactory intubation conditions after administration of rocuronium in adults. *Anaesthesia* 1999;54:172–177.

Gronert GA, Theye RA. Pathophysiology of hyperkalemia induced by succinylcholine. *Anesthesiology* 1975; 943(Jan):89–99.

Kierzek G, Audibert J, Pourriat JL. Anaphylaxis after rocuronium. *Eur J Anaesthesiol* 2003;20:169–170.

Larach MG, Rosenberg H, Gronert GA, et al. Hyperkalemic cardiac arrest during anesthesia in infants and children with occult myopathies. *Clin Pediatr* 1997;36:9–16.

Mazurek AJ, Rae B, Hann S, et al. Rocuronium versus succinylcholine: are they equally effective during rapid-sequence induction of anasthesia? *Anesthesia* 1998;87:1259–1262.

Orebaugh SL. Succinylcholine: Adverse effects and alternatives in emergency medicine. *Am J Emerg Med* 1999;17:715–721.

Perry J, Lee J, Wells G. Rocuronium versus succinylcholine for rapid sequence induction intubation. *Cochrane Database Syst Rev* 2003;1:CD002788.

Rubin MA, Sadovnikoff N. Neuromuscular blocking agents in the emergency department. *J Emerg Med* 1996;14:193–199.

Schwarz SI, Ilias W, Lackner F, et al. Rapid tracheal intubation with vecuronium: the priming principle. *Anesthesiology* 1985;62:388–391.

Sieber TJ, Zbinden, Curatalo M, et al. Tracheal intubation with rocurinium using the timing principle. *Anesth Analg* 1998;86:1137–1140.

Skinner HJ, Biswas A, Mahajan RP. Evaluation of intubating conditions with rocuronium and either propofol or etomidate for rapid sequence induction. *Anaesthesia* 1998;53:702–706.

Weiss JH, Gratz I, Goldberg ME, et al. Double-blind comparison of two doses of rocuronium and succinylcholine for rapid-sequence intubation. *J Clin Anesth* 1997;9:379–382.

Yavascaoglu B, Cebelli V, Kelebek N, et al. Comparison of different priming techniques on the onset time and intubating conditions of rocuronium. *Eur J Anaesthesiol* 2002;19:517–521.

23

Trauma

Michael A. Gibbs

THE CLINICAL CHALLENGE

Airway management is the most critical intervention in acute trauma care. Early intubation has been shown to improve outcome in the severely injured patient. Conversely, failure to adequately manage the airway is the number one cause of preventable early morbidity and mortality in trauma.

Airway management in the trauma patient poses several unique challenges. Often the nature of the injuries, the fact that multiple organ systems or body areas may be injured simultaneously, and the need for airway management to assume its position amongst many often conflicting priorities presents a series of challenges with respect to technical skills, knowledge, judgment, and team management. Success demands excellent assessment skills, an understanding of the physiology of injury, a thorough knowledge of airway pharmacology, and strong leadership. Fundamentally, though, the principles of trauma airway management are no different than those applied to management of the airway in other complex medical situations. A consistent approach and the ability to apply a reproducible thought process help to demystify the process and provide the ingredients necessary for success.

APPROACH TO THE AIRWAY

By definition, all intubations performed in the injured patient should be considered at least *potentially difficult*. During the primary survey, the treating clinician should immediately assess the patient for:

1. Injury to the face, mouth, or neck that may distort anatomy or limit access, making the process of intubation difficult or impossible.
2. The potential for cervical spine injury and the need for in-line cervical immobilization.
3. Chest injury, oxygen saturation, and preexisting medical conditions [e.g., chronic obstructive pulmonary disease (COPD), asthma, congestive heart failure (CHF)] that may limit the patients' respiratory reserve and tolerance of hypoventilation.
4. Signs of obvious or occult hemodynamic instability that can be worsened or unmasked by some of the pharmacologic agents used for rapid sequence intubation (RSI).
5. The presence of traumatic brain injury (TBI) that may alter airway management decision-making and drug selection.

Some of the essentials can be rapidly determined at the bedside during the first 10 to 20 seconds of the resuscitation. As soon as the patient is moved to the stretcher in the trauma room, ask the following four questions:

"What is your name?"
"Are you having trouble breathing?"
"Can you move your toes?"
"Where do you hurt?"

Answers to these questions will immediately help you establish the patient's level of consciousness and Glasgow Coma Score (GCS), elicit signs of upper airway obstruction or labored breathing, assess the integrity of the spinal cord, and focus on the predominant anatomic sites of injury.

Next, the airway should be examined for intraoral bleeding, edema, or foreign body. It is important to approach the airway consistently, evaluating the patient's airway maintenance and protection, oxygenation and ventilation, and then interpreting these findings in the context of the anticipated clinical course to begin to form a judgment as to whether early intubation is indicated. The anterior neck should be inspected and palpated for signs of injury and the external anatomy of the anterior airway (laryngeal prominence, cricoid cartilage, cricothyroid membrane) should be briefly ascertained. Significant airway injury may exist with minimal or no external findings, and any abnormalities (e.g., subcutaneous air, swelling or distortion, tenderness) should be considered to be signs of potentially serious airway injury. Delaying definitive airway management in this situation can have predictably perilous results.

An assessment of the patient's hemodynamic status and physical examination of the torso will provide additional information crucial to the airway management plan. Perform and document a brief neurological examination (GCS, pupillary response and symmetry, and the presence or absence of lateralizing motor findings) *before* neuromuscular blocking agents are given. This information will assist with the subsequent management of the patient with traumatic brain injury.

Although this entire evaluation occurs within the "A" (airway) of the ABCDE approach to multiple trauma, one can also think of the **ABCs** of trauma airway management to help to identify the key parameters that will influence choices of drugs and approach, as shown in Box 23-1.

In tandem with the primary and secondary survey of significantly injured patients, preparations for airway management should be ongoing:

1. Establish adequate monitoring [heart rate (HR), blood pressure (BP), (SpO_2)].
2. Secure at least two large-bore intravenous catheters.
3. Assemble airway equipment.
4. Perform the LEMON assessment to ascertain whether there are particular difficult airway issues aside from the need for cervical spine immobilization (see Chapter 6).

Box 23-1. ABCs

A = **A**irway Injury?
B = **B**rain Injury?
C = **C**hest or Cervical Spine Injury?
S = **S**hock?

---

5. Use the difficult airway algorithm approach to determine whether the patient is suitable for RSI or if another method will be used. Formulate a backup airway rescue plan.
6. Assign specific tasks to all team members (i.e., Who will give drugs? Who will stabilize the spine? Who will hold cricoid pressure? Who will assist the intubator?) This plan will help you organize your thoughts and maintain control of the room.

CLINICAL ISSUES IN TRAUMA AIRWAY MANAGEMENT

Disrupted Airway Anatomy

The patient who presents with distorted airway anatomy secondary to maxillofacial trauma presents a significant challenge. The very condition that may mandate intubation will also render it much more difficult and prone to failure. Direct airway injury may be the result of :

1. Maxillofacial trauma
2. Blunt or penetrating anterior neck trauma
3. Smoke inhalation
4. Caustic ingestion

In cases of distorted anatomy, the approach must be one that minimizes the potential for catastrophic deterioration. Although some argue in favor of a period of expectant observation, waiting for the nearly obstructed airway to become completely obstructed can be disastrous. In many cases expansion of a deep hematoma may not be clinically obvious.

A careful approach must be planned, taking into account the expertise of the physician(s) in the department and in the hospital, the equipment at hand, the need for transfer, the urgency of the need for surgery, the need for diagnostic studies, and a myriad of other factors. If there is a theme that unifies the approach to this type of airway problem, it is "plan ahead." The optimal approach for airway management will vary, depending on the clinical scenario, but a consistent approach is guided by the difficult airway algorithm. In patients with signs of significant airway compromise (e.g., stridor, drooling, respiratory distress, neck hematoma) the urgency of the intubation is high, but the risk of using neuromuscular blockade is also high. Application of the difficult airway algorithm will lead the clinician through the evaluation of the patient's oxygenation (i.e., "Is there time?"), and then whether RSI may be advisable, possibly under a double setup, even though the airway is difficult, depending on the clinician's confidence about the likelihood of success of bag ventilation and intubation by direct laryngoscopy (Chapters 2 and 6). It may be most appropriate to attempt awake intubation by direct or fiberoptic laryngoscopy with sedation and topical anesthesia, or to proceed directly to a surgical airway. When symptoms are modest, but intubation is still indicated (e.g., before interfacility transport or in anticipation of possible deterioration), there is usually more time for evaluation and planning, and more options may be available, but the approach is the same.

Traumatic Brain Injury

The principles of management of the patient with TBI fall within those discussed in Chapter 24 for patients with elevated intracranial pressure (ICP). Maintenance of cerebral oxygenation and perfusion are fundamental goals during the initial resuscitation. Hypoxemia and hypotension should be avoided at all costs, as either will worsen the outcome. It has been demonstrated that a single episode of hypoxia (Po_2 less than 60 mm Hg) or hypotension (BP less than 90 mm Hg) increases mortality in the brain-injured patient by 150%. Provision of a stable airway and aggressive hemodynamic resuscitation should be the priorities of initial care. The technique should be focused on methods to attenuate the potential rise in ICP that accompanies laryngoscopy and intubation. Several drugs may be used to attenuate this physiologic response. Pretreatment with lidocaine will block the *direct* response, and it should be used in all patients with brain injury. Pretreatment with fentanyl attentuates the catecholamine-mediated response, but its use in trauma is reserved for patients who are hemodynamically stable.

Cerebroprotective induction agents, such as thiopental, propofol, or etomidate are all reasonable, but etomidate is often the best choice because of its superior hemodynamic characteristics. Although thiopental provides excellent cerebroprotection, it is also a potent myocardial depressant and vasodilator, and must be used with great caution. Because of concerns about elevations of ICP, ketamine is usually reserved for hemodynamically unstable patients *without* severe head injury (e.g., GCS of 12 or higher).

Chest Trauma

Chest injury, such as pneumothorax, hemothorax, flail chest, pulmonary contusion, or open chest wound, impairs ventilation and oxygenation. Preoxygenation may be difficult or impossible in these patients, and rapid desaturation following paralysis is the rule. In addition, the positive pressure delivered via the endotracheal tube may convert a simple pneumothorax to a tension pneumothorax. A clinical dilemma often ensues when a patient presents with multiple injuries including obvious chest injuries, is hypoxemic and hemodynamically compromised, and is in need of prompt intubation. The difficulty revolves around the decision whether to intubate first, then perform a tube thoracostomy, or whether to perform the tube thoracostomy first, then intubate.

The likelihood that the patient's pneumothorax will worsen with positive pressure ventilation and that placement of the chest tube will likely improve oxygenation, desaturation time, and hemodynamic status argues strongly for the sequence chest tube, then intubate. If, however, the patient is combative, and chest tube placement will likely not be possible until the patient is controlled, it may be tempting to intubate first, with a plan for chest tube placement immediately after the trachea is intubated. The patient's combative behavior, however, may be caused or exacerbated by shock and the hypoxia of the chest injury, and the temptation to intubate first to permit more controlled placement of the chest tube must be tempered by the very real possibility that the severely compromised patient often experiences vascular collapse following the administration of the induction agent and initiation of positive pressure ventilation. In almost all cases, the best approach is to deal with the compromising chest injury first, then intubate the patient. In circumstances where multiple clinicians are present, such as the trauma team in a level one trauma center, the intubation and thoracostomy can occur virtually simultaneously. When only a single clinician is available, however, the situation is more complicated, and a temporizing needle thoracostomy may be used to relieve or prevent tension pneumothorax, and the patient may then be intubated, followed rapidly by a tube thoracostomy. In general, the best approach is to deal with the chest compromise first (i.e., place the chest tube), then intubate, but this approach has to be customized, depending on patient, provider, and facility attributes.

Cervical Spine Injury

All severely injured blunt trauma patients have cervical injury until proven otherwise. In the vast majority of cases, the patient will be immobilized by prehospital providers in the field. While this step is essential to prevent further spinal injury, it can create several problems as well. Intoxicated or head injured patients typically become agitated and difficult to control when strapped down on a backboard. Physical and chemical restraint may be required. Aspiration is a significant risk in the supine patient with traumatic brain injury or vomiting. In this position ventilation may be impaired, especially in the presence of chest injury. High-flow oxygen should be provided to all patients, and suction must be immediately available.

If urgent airway management is needed, there is no purpose served by obtaining a cross-table-lateral cervical spine x-ray before intubation. This single view is inadequate to exclude injury, with a sensitivity of 80% at best, even with a technically perfect film. Waiting for the x-ray will expend precious time and give the operator a false sense of security when the film is interpreted as "normal." Instead, all patients must be assumed to have cervical injury and in-line stabilization must be maintained at all times. The preintubation neurological status of the patient and the use of in-line manual immobilization of the cervical spine during intubation should be clearly documented in the medical record.

Much debate has centered around the safety of oral intubation in the presence of cervical spine injury. Practitioners and scholars alike have been deeply divided on this issue. Those who supported one theory argued that blunt injury could create an instability in the cervical spine and that manipulation of the airway during direct laryngoscopy might cause movement of the unstable elements, thus resulting in spinal cord injury. This argument, although largely theoretical, was widely accepted and one of the principal factors in the historical adoption of blind nasotracheal intubation as the airway maneuver of choice in the multiply injured blunt trauma patient. If nasotracheal intubation was not possible, surgical cricothyrotomy was recommended. The countervailing position was that oral endotracheal intubation could be safely performed even in the presence of cervical spine injury, provided that proper technique was used and strict attention was paid to meticulous immobilization of the cervical spine throughout the process of intubation. Although no definitive study has demonstrated the safety of oral intubation in the presence of cervical spine injury, there is an increasing body of literature that would argue in favor of the safety of this maneuver.

Several large case-series show no evidence that properly performed RSI with in-line cervical stabilization presents any hazard to the patient, even in the presence of proven cervical spine injury. This approach is safe, provided that:

1. Laryngoscopy and intubation are performed in a gentle, atraumatic manner. RSI is the preferred technique, as that will allow for immediate airway control and eliminate the risk of patient movement during laryngoscopy.
2. Precise cervical immobilization is maintained throughout the intubation sequence. This will require the presence of a second individual, whose sole responsibility is manual immobilization of the spine. Ideally, this person should stand on the side of the bed rather than at the head of the bed to give the intubator unimpeded access to the airway.

When the assessment indicates that intubation will be difficult or impossible, an alternative technique should be considered. The technique used in this situation (e.g., laryngoscopy with sedation, fiberoptic intubation, blind nasotracheal intubation, cricothyrotomy) will depend on the clinical scenario and the experience of the operator.

Shock

Patients suffering significant injury may have obvious or occult hypotension from many different sources. Victims of blunt multisystem trauma are especially vulnerable. Shock in this patient population can be broadly classified as *hemorrhagic* (e.g., external, intrathoracic, intraabdominal, retroperitoneal, long-bone), or *nonhemorrhagic* (e.g., tension pneumothorax, pericardial tamponade, myocardial contusion, spinal shock). A diligent search for the primary source(s) of hypotension must begin at the earliest opportunity. Clinical signs can be misleading. For example: Patients on the verge of cardiovascular collapse often maintain a "normal" blood pressure, especially if they are young; and tension pneumothorax rarely, if ever, causes clinically evident tracheal deviation in a nonarrested patient.

Several of the agents used for RSI may cause significant myocardial depression and vasodilatation that will cause or worsen shock in the hypovolemic patient. This is especially true for the barbiturates (e.g., thiopental) and the opioids (e.g., fentanyl). Both drugs are contraindicated in the hemodynamically unstable patient and should be used with great caution in "normotensive" patients who are felt to be at risk for significant hypovolemia. If RSI is planned, etomidate, which possesses a favorable hemodynamic profile, is the preferred induction agent. Ketamine is also an excellent choice, provided there is no evidence of intracranial hypertension.

TECHNIQUE

Paralysis versus Rapid Tranquilization of the Combative Trauma Patient

The combative trauma patient presents a series of conflicting problems. The causes of combative behavior in the trauma patient are numerous and include head injury, drug or ethanol intoxication, preexisting medical conditions (diabetes in particular), hypoxemia, shock, anxiety, personality disorder, and others. The priority is to rapidly control the patient so that potentially life-threatening causes can be identified and corrected. Controversy exists as to whether such patients ought to undergo rapid tranquilization with a neuroleptic agent or sedative, or whether immediate intubation with neuromuscular blockade is appropriate. Rapid tranquilization using haloperidol is well established as a safe and effective means for gaining control of the combative trauma patient who cannot be settled by other means. Haloperidol can be used intravenously in 5 to 10 mg increments every 3 to 5 minutes until a clinical response is achieved. There is extensive literature supporting the safety of this approach. Opioids, such as morphine or fentanyl, should not be used because of their profound respiratory depressant effects.

The decision to use rapid tranquilization rather than RSI with neuromuscular blockade should rest on the nature of the patient's presentation and injuries. If intubation is indicated on the basis of injuries identified, and if the patient is in need of control, then immediate intubation is indicated. If the patient is presenting primarily with control problems and does not appear to be seriously injured, rapid tranquilization is appropriate. In many situations the decision will not be clear-cut. When a diagnostic dilemma exists, it is most prudent to assume the worst and not dismiss profoundly altered mentation as merely the consequence of inebriation. If there is no clear explanation of the combative behavior and trauma, especially head trauma, is present, it may be best to assume that the behavior is a result of injury, or multiple injuries, and if intubation is necessary to control and properly assess the patient, it should be planned and executed.

The Airway Management Plan

The process of choosing the most appropriate airway management technique is a complex one, based on multiple variables. In the injured patient, the steps taken to develop an airway management plan should follow the same fundamental principles thoughtfully outlined throughout this text.

Contemporary studies have demonstrated that RSI provides the highest success rate and lowest complication rate in patients requiring emergency airway management. The same holds true for victims of injury, and RSI is the procedure of choice in the vast majority of these patients. In the face of significant face, mouth, or neck injury, another approach may be required, as described by the difficult airway algorithm. Understanding that "significant" is in the eye of the beholder and that the spectrum of injury is vast, using either a double setup, an awake technique, a surgical approach, or airway adjunct may be necessary.

Failed Airway Rescue

When a failed airway situation develops in the trauma patient, the failed airway algorithm is followed, just as for the nontrauma patient. The trauma patient has a higher incidence of upper-airway distortion that may render oral approaches impossible, necessitating cricothyrotomy, and cricothyrotomy is necessary much more often in trauma than in medical cases. When planning the backup options for intubation of a patient with upper-airway, face, or oral trauma, an infraglottic rescue option, that is, surgical or percutaneous cricothyrotomy, must be prepared for.

DRUG DOSAGE AND ADMINISTRATION

Use of Neuromuscular Blocking Agents in the Trauma Patient

Advantages of RSI in the trauma patient include:

1. The most rapid attainment of a definitive airway
2. Ability to perform gentle controlled laryngoscopy in cases of head injury or suspected cervical spine injury
3. Control of the combative severely injured patient
4. Facilitation of specific diagnostic and therapeutic procedures
5. A higher success rate and lower complication rate than other available methods.

Succinylcholine has been the mainstay of RSI in the emergency department. The advantages of succinylcholine include its rapid onset and brief duration of action. Concerns about causing hyperkalemia in patients with burns or crush injury are not relevant in the acute setting, as this risk does not become clinically significant until 5 days postinjury (see Chapter 18).

Succinylcholine has also been implicated in the elevation of ICP in the patient with traumatic brain injury. This effect can be mitigated by appropriate use of a competitive neuromuscular blocking agent in a defasciculating dose before administration of succinylcholine. Rocuronium has been advocated for use in RSI; however, the onset of rocuronium is not as rapid as succinylcholine, and its duration of action is significantly longer. The brief duration of action (clinical duration 8–10 minutes) of succinylcholine is also desirable to permit ongoing assessment of neurological status and evaluation of level of functioning in the context of computed tomography (CT) scan findings to determine whether neurosurgical intervention is indicated.

Choosing an Induction Agent

Table 23-1 provides a summary of recommendations for RSI sedative selection based on the particular clinical situation. It is no accident that etomidate occupies the first choice column for all the scenarios outlined, as this agent offers the ideal balance of hemodynamic stability and cerebroprotection.

TABLE 23-1. *RSI induction agent selection in the injured patient*

Clinical scenario	First choice	Alternatives
No shock; no brain injury	Etomidate	Thiopental, Propofol, Midazolam
Brain injury; no shock	Etomidate	Thiopental, Propofol
Shock; no brain injury	Etomidate[a]	Ketamine[a]
Shock; brain injury	Etomidate[a]	Ketamine[a,b]
Profound shock	None	None

[a]In the presence of shock, reduce the dose by 25% to 50%.
[b]Prospect for worsening elevated ICP with ketamine is offset by ketamine prime.

TIPS AND PEARLS

There is nothing exotic about the trauma airway; it is just a type of difficult airway and the same, reasoned approach can be applied, modified by the need for cervical spine immobilization.

A very rapid, focused physical examination should elicit clinical evidence of spinal injury, traumatic brain injury, occult hypovolemia, direct airway trauma, and pulmonary dysfunction.

All blunt trauma patients are assumed to have injury to the cervical spine until proven otherwise. In-line stabilization should be performed and documented.

The priority in the initial management of the patient with traumatic brain injury is to maintain adequate CNS perfusion and oxygenation at all costs.

In the patient with direct injury to the airway, the clinician must always have an immediate plan (and the equipment for) airway rescue, particularly cricothyrotomy, should RSI fail.

Many of the drugs used for RSI (the opioids and barbiturates in particular) may precipitate hypotension in the hypovolemic patient. This is exacerbated by the effects of positive pressure ventilation.

Etomidate is the preferred induction agent in the injured patient, offering the attractive balance of hemodynamic stability and cerebroprotection.

SUMMARY

Oral endotracheal intubation using RSI is the airway maneuver of choice in the majority of trauma patients. A well-thought-out management plan, taking into account the patient's known or suspected injuries and hemodynamic status, will help the clinician rapidly develop and orchestrate an individualized airway management plan, guided by the difficult airway algorithm. During the often chaotic environment of a trauma resuscitation, effective reasoning, communication, and leadership are the ingredients for success.

EVIDENCE

1. Intubation of trauma patients. In a recent evidence-based literature review, Dunham et al. provided a comprehensive overview (demographics, airway management techniques, success rates) of trauma patients requiring emergency airway management (1). Although most of these patients were critically ill, the degree of injury was highly variable; the mean Injury Severity Score (ISS) was 29 (range 17 to 54), and the mean GCS was 6.5 (range 3 to 15). On average, 41% of patients died (range 2% to 100%), and this was much more common when airway management was delayed, difficult, or unsuccessful. Table 23-2 provides a summary of data looking at the frequency of intubation in trauma patients, based on treatment setting.

TABLE 23-2. *Frequency of trauma patient intubation based on treatment setting*

	Percent intubated (mean)	Range
Air-Medical	18.5%	6%–51%
Ground EMS	4%	2%–37
Ground EMS to Trauma Center	13.6%	11%–30%
Trauma Center	24.5%	9%–28%

2. Effect of intubation on head injury. The outcome of 717 patients with severe brain injury (GCS less than 8) was prospectively studied to evaluate the impact on outcome of hypotension (systolic BP less than 90 mm Hg) and hypoxemia (P_aO_2 less than 60 mm Hg or apnea or cyanosis in the field) as secondary brain insults. Both variables were independently associated with significant increases in morbidity and mortality. Hypotension was profoundly detrimental, occurring in 35% of patients and associated with a 150% increase in mortality (2).

3. Role of airway management in preventable trauma deaths. When 629 trauma deaths in the state of Montana were reviewed to determine the rate and cause of preventable mortality and "inappropriate" care by a panel of physicians and prehospital care providers, the overall preventable death rate was judged to be 13%. The most common cause of inappropriate care was inadequate management of the airway in either the prehospital setting (6.8% of cases) or emergency department (5.4% of cases) (3).

4. Hemodynamic effects of induction agents. The hemodynamic effects of three different agents used for RSI were compared in a double-blind study of 86 ED patients undergoing RSI with thiopental (5 mg/kg), fentanyl (5 mcg/kg), or midazolam (0.1 mg/kg). Of the patients who received thiopental, 93% were intubated within 2 minutes of paralysis ($p = 0.037$), but systolic blood pressure fell an average of 38 mm Hg in this group ($p = 0.045$). The midazolam group had a greater number of delayed intubations (31%) and an average heart rate increase of 17 beats per minute (bpm) ($p = 0.008$). Fentanyl provided the most neutral hemodynamic profile during RSI. Mortality was not affected by drug assignment (4).

5. Ability of fentanyl to blunt circulatory responses to intubation. When 60 patients were randomized to receive either placebo, esmolol (500 mcg/kg per minute for 6 minutes, followed by 300 mcg/kg per minute for 9 minutes), or fentanyl (0.8 mcg/kg per minute for 10 minutes) before intubation, fentanyl decreased HR and BP below baseline despite laryngoscopy. Esmolol blunted the HR response, but BP was slightly elevated (5). Many other studies of fentanyl for this purpose have shown similar effects.

6. Lidocaine before intubation: intravenous or topical? In 22 patients with brain tumors and elevated ICP under thiopental and succinylcholine general anesthesia, administration of intravenous lidocaine (1.5 mg/kg) decreased the ICP and ICP did not increase after intubation, in contrast to patients receiving laryngotracheal topical lidocaine (4 cc of 4%) who developed a significant increase in ICP after intubation, with three of these patients sustaining ICPs in excess of 40 torr. Some ICP effect was observed in response to the topical lidocaine administration itself (6).

7. Safety of oral endotracheal intubation in cervical spine injury. A prospective study of airway management practice and associated neurological outcome in 150 patients subsequently diagnosed with cervical spine injury used a standardized neurologic examination that was performed before and after intubation, which was performed using in-line stabilization. Twenty-six (32%) of 81 patients without a neurological deficit required intubation on presentation, and none manifested a subsequent neurological deficit. Twenty-nine (42%) of 69 additional patients with high cervical injury required intubation, and no patient exhibited neurological deterioration (7). A retrospective review was conducted of 150 patients with known cervical spine injuries who were electively intubated: 50 patients (33%) had preoperative neurological deficit, 83 patients (55%) were intubated after induction of general anesthesia, and 67 patients (45%) were intubated awake. Cervical immobilization with in-line stabilization was documented in 86 patients (57%). Two patients (1.3%) developed new neurological deficits. The study size was insufficient to determine whether awake intubation versus general anesthesia conferred any potential benefit (8). A retrospective study of 73 out of 393 patients with traumatic cervical spine injuries who underwent RSI with in-line stabilization within 30 minutes of presentation (36 patients) or between 30 minutes and 24 hours (37 patients) found no neurological sequellae as a result of the intubation (9).

A retrospective analysis of patients undergoing tracheal intubation for surgical fixation of cervical spine injuries compared results when awake fiberoptic intubation was used with those obtained using general anesthesia and neuromuscular blockade. Sixteen of the 45 patients had preoperative neurological deficit. Cervical traction was used to stabilize the spine for all intubations. None of the 45 patients sustained a new or worsened neurological injury (10). A similar retrospective review of 113 patients with cervical spine fractures requiring operative repair, of whom 33 (30%) had a partial neurologic deficit, found no new neurological deficits among the 86 (76%) who underwent nasal intubation or the 27 (24%) who underwent oral intubation with in-line stabilization (11).

8. Use of the intubating LMA or Combitube in cervical spine injury. A prospective study of radiographs taken before, during, and after intubation using the intubating LMA (ILMA) versus direct laryngoscopy in patients with normal cervical spines found that the ILMA intubation took about twice as long (39 seconds versus 21 seconds) but that the cervical spine movement was significantly less with the ILMA ($p < 0.008$) (12).

Although the Combitube (CT) airway has been recommended as a device for airway rescue when RSI fails, it may be more difficult to place in patients with immobilized cervical spines. When CT placement was attempted in 15 patients with Philadelphia collars on (mean age, 32 years) during anesthesia for elective surgery, blind insertion was possible in only five patients; in the remaining ten the investigators were unable to advance the device through the mouth into the hypopharynx and required laryngoscopy. Once placed, the CT functioned effectively. These results cast doubt on the use of the Combitube in the immobilized trauma patient (13).

REFERENCES

1. Dunham MC, et al. Guidelines for emergency tracheal intubation immediately after traumatic injury. *J Trauma* 2003;55:162–179.
2. Chesnut RM, et al. The role of secondary brain injury in determining outcome from severe head injury. *J Trauma* 1993;34:216–222.
3. Esposito TJ, et al. Analysis of preventable trauma deaths and inappropriate trauma care in a rural state. *J Trauma* 1995;39:955–962.
4. Sivilotti MLA, et al. Randomized double-blind study on sedatives and hemodynamics during rapid-sequence intubation in the emergency department: the SHRED study. *Ann Emerg Med* 1998;31:313–324.
5. Ebert JP, Pearson JD, Gelman S, et al. Circulatory response to laryngoscopy: the comparative effects of placebo, fentanyl, and esmolol. *Can J Anaesth* 1989;36:301–306.
6. Hamill JF, et al. Lidocaine before endotracheal intubation: intravenous or laryngotracheal? *Anesthesiology* 1981;55:578–591.
7. Shatney CH, Brunner RD, Nguyen TQ. The safety of orotracheal intubation in patients with unstable cervical spine fracture or high spinal cord injury. *Am J Surg* 1995;179:676–679.
8. Suderman VS, Crosby ET, Lui A. Elective oral tracheal intubation in cervical spine-injured adults. *Can J Anaesth* 1992;39:516–517.
9. Criswell JC, et al. Emergency airway management in patients with cervical spine injuries. *Anaesthesia* 1994;49:900–903.
10. McCrory C, Blunnie WP, Moriarty DC. Elective tracheal intubation in cervical spine injuries. *Irish Med J* 1997;90(Oct):234–235.

11. Holly J, Jorden R. Airway management in patients with unstable cervical spine fractures. *Ann Emerg Med* 1988;18:1237–1239.
12. Walt B, et al. Tracheal intubation and cervical spine excursion: direct laryngoscopy vs. intubating laryngeal mask. *Anaesthesia* 2001;56:221–226.
13. Mercer MH, et al. Insertion of the Combitube airway with the cervical spine immobilized in a rigid cervical collar. *Anaesthesia* 1998;53:971–974.

24

Increased Intracranial Pressure

Andy S. Jagoda and John J. Bruns, Jr.

I. The clinical challenge

Elevated intracranial pressure (ICP) poses a direct threat to the viability and function of the brain. In head trauma, elevated ICP has been clearly associated with worse outcomes. The problems associated with elevated ICP may be compounded by many of the techniques and drugs used in airway management because they may cause further elevations of intracranial pressure. In addition, victims of multiple trauma may present with hypotension, thus limiting the choice of agents and techniques available. This chapter provides the basis for an understanding of the problems of increased ICP and the optimal methods of airway management in this patient group.

When increased ICP occurs as a result of an injury or medical catastrophe, the brain's ability to regulate blood flow (autoregulation) over a range of blood pressures is often lost. In general, the ICP is maintained through a mean arterial blood pressure range of 80 to 180 mm Hg. When the ICP becomes elevated, autoregulation often, but not always, has been lost. In this setting, excessively high or excessively low blood pressure could aggravate brain injury by promoting cerebral edema or ischemia. Hypotension, even for a very brief period, is especially harmful, and along with hypoxia, has been shown to be an independent predictor of mortality and morbidity in patients with traumatic brain injury (TBI).

Cerebral perfusion pressure (CPP) is the driving force for blood flow to the brain. It is measured by the difference between the mean arterial blood pressure (MAP) and the ICP. Expressed as a formula,

$$CPP = MAP - ICP$$

It is clear from this formula that excessive decreases in MAP, as might occur during rapid sequence intubation (RSI), would decrease CPP and contribute to cerebral ischemia. Conversely, increases in MAP, if not accompanied by equivalent increases in ICP, may be beneficial because of the increase in the driving pressure for oxygenation of brain tissue. It is generally recommended that the ICP be maintained below 20 mm Hg, the MAP between 100 to 110 mm Hg, and the CPP near 70 mm Hg. There are a number of confounding elements that may increase ICP during airway management.

A. Reflex sympathetic response to laryngoscopy

The reflex sympathetic response to laryngoscopy (RSRL) is stimulated by the rich sensory innervation of the supraglottic larynx. Use of the laryngoscope and particularly the attempted placement of an endotracheal tube results in a significant afferent discharge that increases sympathetic activity to the cardiovascular system mediated through direct neuronal activity and release of catecholamines. Longer and more aggressive attempts at laryngoscopy and intubation result in greater and more prolonged sympathetic nervous system stimulation. This catecholamine surge leads to increased heart rate and blood pressure, which significantly enhances cerebral blood flow at the apparent expense of the systemic circulation through redistribution. These hemodynamic changes may contribute to increased ICP, particularly if autoregulation is impaired; therefore, it is desirable to mitigate this RSRL. Intubation techniques that minimize airway stimulation (e.g., lighted stylets) and pharmacologic adjuncts (e.g., beta blockade, lidocaine, synthetic opioids) have been studied to accomplish this mitigation.

There is some evidence that supports the use of lidocaine, 1.5 mg/kg intravenously, to blunt the hemodynamic response to laryngoscopy when given 2 to 3 minutes before endotracheal tube intubation (ETI). However, studies in patients without cardiovascular disease have failed to show this hemodynamic protection, and other studies have shown mixed results with respect to hemodynamic stability, with some appearing to demonstrate benefit and others showing none. As a result, lidocaine cannot be recommended at the present time as a sole agent for mitigation of the RSRL associated with emergency intubation.

The short-acting beta blocker esmolol, on the other hand, has consistently demonstrated the ability to control both heart rate and blood pressure responses to intubation. A dose of 2 mg/kg given 3 minutes before intubation has been shown to be effective. Unfortunately, in the emergency situation, the administration of a beta-blocking agent, even one that is short acting, may be problematic by causing or exacerbating hypotension in a trauma patient, or by confounding interpretation of a decrease in the blood pressure changes immediately following intubation. For these reasons, although esmolol is consistent and reliable for mitigation of RSRL in elective anesthesia, it is generally not used for this purpoe in the emergency department (ED).

Fentanyl at doses of 2 to 3 mcg/kg has also been shown to attenuate the RSRL associated with intubation. Although a full sympathetic blocking dose of fentanyl is 9 to 13 mcg/kg, the recommended dose of fentanyl for RSI in emergency department patients is 3 mcg/kg and should be administered as a single pretreatment dose over 30 to 60 seconds. This technique permits effective mitigation of the RSRL with greatly reduced chances of apnea or hypoventilation before sedation and paralysis. Although it is not known for certain whether fentanyl is superior to lidocaine, or whether the addition of fentanyl provides a significant advantage if lidocaine was used, fentanyl, like esmolol, is more predictable and consistent in its ability to mitigate RSRL.

Several studies have investigated the potential advantages of fiberoptic or lighted stylet intubation over direct laryngoscopy, working on the premise that these techniques minimize tracheal irritation and thus the RSRL. At this time the results are mixed and do not permit any conclusions regarding one technique over the other, and it appears that, at least in a controlled operating room setting, the insertion of the endotracheal tube into the trachea is more stimulating than a routine laryngoscopy. At present, it seems advisable to administer 3 mcg/kg of fentanyl intravenously as a pretreatment agent 3 minutes before administration of the induction and neuromuscular blocking agents to mitigate the RSRL. Fentanyl should not be administered to patients with incipient or actual hypotension or to those who are dependent on sympathetic drive to maintain an adequate blood pressure for cerebral perfusion. In such cases, the ensuing hypotension may cause further central nervous system (CNS) injury. In addition to pharmacological maneuvers to reduce RSRL, intubation should be performed in the most gentle manner possible, limiting both the time and intensity of laryngoscopy.

B. Reflex ICP response to laryngoscopy

Laryngoscopy may also increase the ICP by a direct reflex mechanism not mediated by sympathetic stimulation of the blood pressure or heart rate. The details of this reflex are poorly elucidated. Insertion of the laryngoscope or endotracheal tube may, therefore, further elevate ICP, even if the RSRL is blunted. It would seem desirable to blunt this ICP response to laryngoscopy in patients at risk for having elevated ICP. Although there have been no direct studies of lidocaine with respect to blunting the ICP response to laryngoscopy and intubation of patients with elevated ICP, it has been shown that the administration of lidocaine in a dose of 1.5 mg/kg intravenously effectively blunts the ICP response to endotracheal suctioning and laryngeal stimulation. Lidocaine appears also to (briefly) reduce ICP absolutely. Therefore, in patients with elevated ICP, lidocaine should be administered as a pretreatment drug in the dose of 1.5 mg/kg intravenously 3 minutes before succinylcholine (SCh) to mitigate the ICP response to laryngoscopy and intubation.

C. Choice of neuromuscular blocking agent

1. ICP response to succinylcholine (SCh)

SCh itself appears capable of causing an increase in ICP. Studies have shown that this increase is temporally related to the presence of fasciculations in the patient, but is not the result of synchronized muscular activity leading to increased venous pressure. Rather, there appears to be a complex reflex mechanism originating in the muscle spindle and ultimately resulting in an elevation of ICP. One recent study challenged the claim that SCh causes an elevation of ICP, and SCh remains the drug of choice for management of patients with elevated ICP because of its rapid onset and short duration. Studies have shown that administration of a full paralyzing dose of a competitive neuromuscular blocker, before administering the SCh, completely abolishes the ICP rise associated with SCh. It has also been shown that the administration of a small defasciculating dose of a competitive neuromuscular blocker, approximately one-tenth of the paralyzing dose, effectively blunts this intracranial response to SCh. Therefore, when SCh is used to intubate patients with suspected ICP increase, a defasciculating dose of a competitive neuromuscular blocker, such as 0.01 mg/kg of pancuronium or vecuronium, may be beneficial. An alternative is to use a competitive neuromuscular blocking agent, such as rocuronium or vecuronium, for RSI in cases where the patient has elevated ICP (see later), but SCh is reliable and familiar, and there is not compelling evidence arguing against its use. Fasciculation can also be reduced by administration of a small dose of SCh (0.2 mg/kg) 3 minutes before the full dose, but the effect of this additional dose on ICP, if any, is not known, and this treatment should not be considered a substitute for administration of a defasciculating dose of a competitive neuromuscular blocking agent.

2. Alternatives to SCh

Unlike SCh, nondepolarizing (competitive) neuromuscular blocking agents do not cause elevation of ICP, although ICP increase will still be stimulated by the act of intubation. Therefore, some practitioners may prefer to use these agents instead of SCh for intubation in patients with raised ICP. Rocuronium is the competitive agent most suited to this strategy because of its rapid onset and consistent achievement of intubating conditions. In addition, when rocuronium is used, a defasciculating dose is not needed, thus simplifying the intubation sequence. Rocuronium has a rapid onset, but one potential drawback may be the duration of paralysis, particularly if the airway cannot be secured. The competitive neuromuscular blocking agents and their reversal are discussed in Chapter 18, and use of these agents for RSI is in Chapter 22.

D. Choice of induction agent

When managing the patient with potential brain injury, it is important to choose an induction agent that will not adversely affect CPP. Ideally, one would like to choose an induction agent that is capable of improving or maintaining CPP and providing some cerebral protective effect. Sodium thiopental is an ultra short-acting barbiturate induction agent. Thiopental confers some cerebroprotective effect because it decreases the basal metabolic rate of oxygen utilization of the brain ($CMRO_2$). This effect can be likened to decreasing myocardial oxygen demand in the ischemic heart. In addition, sodium thiopental decreases cerebral blood flow, thus decreasing ICP. This combination of characteristics, the decrease in ICP and the decrease in $CMRO_2$, make thiopental a desirable agent for use in patients with elevated ICP and a normal or high blood pressure. However, thiopental is a potent venodilator and negative inotrope. Therefore, it has a tendency to cause significant hypotension and thus reduce CPP, even in relatively hemodynamically stable patients. In the hemodynamically unstable patient, this hypotensive effect can be profound. A single episode of hypotension significantly increases mortality in acute, severe head injury. Therefore, although thiopental is a desirable agent for management of patients with elevated ICP, its hemodynamic instability relegates it to an alternative role, with etomidate being the agent of choice. When the circulating blood volume is known to be normal, and hemodynamic stability is preserved, however, thiopental remains an appropriate choice as the induction agent.

Etomidate is a short-acting imidazole derivative that has a similar profile of activity to thiopental, but without the tendency to cause hemodynamic compromise. In fact, etomidate is the most hemodynamically stable of all commonly used induction agents (see Chapter 17). Its ability to decrease $CMRO_2$ and ICP in a manner analogous to that of sodium thiopental and its remarkable hemodynamic stability make it the drug of choice for patients with elevated ICP.

Ketamine, in general, is avoided in patients with known elevations in ICP because it may elevate the ICP further. However, in hypotensive patients, ketamine's superior hemodynamic stability may argue for its use.

II. Approach to airway management

RSI is the preferred method for patients with suspected elevated ICP because it provides protection against the reflex responses to laryngoscopy and rises in ICP. The presence of coma should not be interpreted as an indication to proceed without pharmacological agents, or to administer only a neuromuscular blocking agent without a sedative/induction drug. Although the patient may seem unresponsive, laryngoscopy and intubation will provoke the reflexes described earlier, if appropriate pretreatment and induction agents are not used. Following appropriate assessment and preparation as described in Chapter 3, the sequence in Box 24-1 is recommended for patients with elevated ICP.

III. Initiating mechanical ventilation

Mechanical ventilation in the patient with elevated ICP should be predicated on two principles: 1) optimal oxygenation, and 2) avoidance of ventilation mechanics [e.g., positive end-expiratory pressure (PEEP), high peak inspiratory pressure (PIP)] that would increase venous congestion in the brain.

Box 24-1. RSI Sequence for Patients with Elevated ICP

Time   **Action** (seven Ps)
Zero minus 10 minutes   Preparation
Zero minus 5 minutes   Preoxygenation
Zero minus 3 minutes   Pretreatment:
        Lidocaine 1.5 mg/kg IV
      and
        Vecuronium 0.01 mg/kg IV (if succinylcholine is used)
      and either
        Fentanyl 3 mcg/kg (over one minute) (if hemodynamically stable)
      or
        Esmolol 2 mcg/kg (if hemodynamically stable)
Zero   Paralysis with induction:
        Etomidate 0.3 mg/kg IV
        SCh 1.5 mg/kg IV
Zero plus 30 seconds   Protection and positioning
Zero plus 45 seconds   Placement with proof: intubate, confirm placement
Zero plus 60 seconds   Postintubation management

Controlled hyperventilation to a P_aCO_2 of approximately 30 mm Hg was formerly recommended for the early management of elevated ICP. It was believed that reduction in P_aCO_2 tensions in the brain leads to vasoconstriction, decreased cerebral blood flow, and therefore decreased ICP. Further declines in partial arterial pressure (P_aCO_2) below 30 mm Hg were not recommended because it was felt the vasoconstriction may become so severe as to compromise cerebral circulation. There is no scientific basis for the use of prophylactic hyperventilation, with good evidence that it promotes worse outcomes rather than better. The Brain Trauma Foundation Guidelines for the Management of Severe Traumatic Brain Injury (TBI) recommend that prophylactic hyperventilation be avoided, and that patients with severe TBI be ventilated in such a way as to target the lower limits of normocapnia (P_aCO_2 of 35 to 40 mm Hg). A similar approach seems prudent in patients with medically induced elevations of ICP (e.g., cerebral hemorrhage).

Hyperventilation to a P_aCO_2 of 30 mm Hg should be used only as a temporizing measure in patients demonstrating clinical signs of herniation (blown pupil or decerebrate posturing) or when osmotic agents and cerebrospinal fluid (CSF) drainage are not effective in managing an acute rise in ICP accompanied by patient deterioration. Normal initial ventilation parameters include a ventilatory rate of approximately 10 to 12 breaths per minute with a tidal volume of approximately 10 cc/kg. This rate would result in an approximately physiologic P_aCO_2 level in the normal patient. Therefore, the initial ventilator settings should maintain tidal volume at 10 to 12 cc/kg and the ventilatory rate at 10 breaths per minute. Initial inspired fraction of oxygen (F_iO_2) should be 1.0 (100%). F_iO_2 can later be decreased according to pulse oximetry, as long as 100% oxygen saturation is maintained. Carbon dioxide tension can be followed with arterial blood gases or capnography, the first assessment of which should occur approximately 10 minutes after initiation of steady state mechanical ventilation. Unless early and frequent neurological examinations are required (e.g., by a neurosurgeon to decide whether there is sufficient persisting neurological functioning to warrant an attempt at surgical evacuation of a massive subdural hematoma), long-term sedation and paralysis are recommended to permit effective controlled mechanical ventilation and other necessary interventions, while mitigating the stimulating effects of the tube in the trachea and eliminating any possibility of the patient coughing or bucking. A full paralyzing dose of a competitive neuromuscular blocking agent, such as vecuronium 0.1 mg/kg should be given, along with an initial dose of 0.05 mg/kg of lorazepam. Subsequently, doses of approximately one-third of the initial dose of both agents should be given if the patient shows evidence of regaining consciousness, increased sympathetic activity, or initiating motor movement.

IV. **Tips and pearls**

RSI is clearly the desired method for tracheal intubation in patients with suspected elevation of ICP. The technique allows control of various adverse effects and optimal control of ventilation after intubation. However, the use of neuromuscular blockade in patients with potential neurologic deficit carries the responsibility of performing a detailed neurological evaluation on the patient before initiation of neuromuscular blockade. The patient's ability to interact with the surroundings, spontaneous motor movement, response to deep pain, response to voice, localization, pupillary reflexes, and other pertinent neurological details must be assessed carefully before administration of neuromuscular blockade. The careful recording of these findings will be invaluable for the ongoing evaluation of the patient.

If the patient's ventilatory status is severely compromised by the head injury or by concommitant injuries, positive pressure ventilation with bag and mask may be required throughout the intubation sequence. In such circumstances, one is trading off the increased risk of aspiration against the hazard of inadequate oxygenation and rising P_aCO_2 during the intubation sequence. When such a trade-off arises, it should be resolved in favor of oxygenation over the risk of aspiration.

EVIDENCE

Evidence-based recommendations depend on a careful analysis of the methodology used in the studies reviewed and an understanding of the outcome measure, which must be found to make the study clinically relevant. In this light, it becomes challenging to make evidence-based recommendations regarding airway management in the patient with a brain injury. Regarding methodology, most of the studies of the effect of interventions discussed in this chapter were performed on stable patients in the operating room setting; others were performed on deeply anesthetized patients in the intensive care unit during tracheal suctioning. It is difficult to extrapolate the findings in these patient groups to critical patients being emergently managed in the ED. In addition, the timing and dosing of pharmacologic interventions varied significantly, making it difficult to compare one study with another. For example, in one study lidocaine was found effective when given 3 minutes before intubation and ineffective if given at 4, 2, or 1 minute before (1). There was only one randomized double-blind interventional study identified that was performed in the ED on patients with head injury (2). This prospective double-blind study found that esmolol and lidocaine had similar efficacies in attenuating the hemodynamic response to intubation of patients with isolated head injury.

Regarding outcome, there is no study in the literature that compares airway interventions with a functional outcome measure, that is, disability or death. Rises in heart rate, blood pressure, and ICP are the commonly measured parameters comparing one technique or pharmacological intervention with the other because these affect CPP. However, there is no evidence that these are valid surrogates for more meaningful outcome measures such as disability; nor is there evidence that transient rises in any of the previously mentioned measures has any meaningful impact on morbidity or mortality. That said, there is no evidence that the interventions presented in this chapter do harm, and pending more direct evidence, it does seem intuitive that minimizing changes in ICP, blood pressure, and heart rate can only contribute to maximizing good outcomes.

Regarding lidocaine, there is evidence that supports using 1.5 mg/kg intravenously to blunt the hemodynamic response and suppress dysrhythmias when administered to patients with cardiovascular disease 2 to 3 minutes before laryngoscopy and ETI (1,3) and when administered to noncardiovascular disease patients at 3 minutes before intubation. Contradictory results have been obtained in other studies in patients with and without cardiovascular disease where this hemodynamic protection was lacking (4,5). Additional investigations have revealed mixed or inconsistent attenuation of the blood pressure and pulse response to intubation (6,7,8).

It has been shown that the administration of 1.5 mg/kg lidocaine intravenously effectively blunts the direct ICP response in hypocarbic patients to endotracheal suctioning and laryngeal stimulation (9,10). However, no study to date has associated the use of lidocaine in the TBI patient undergoing ETI to an improved neurological outcome, and it may not be possible to design and conduct such a study.

Regarding fentanyl, a dose of 2 to 3 mcg/kg has been shown to attenuate the RSRL associated with DL/ETI (7); however, in that study fentanyl did not appear to offer an advantage over lidocaine nor was it clear that a group receiving both drugs had a better response (11). In other studies, fentanyl failed to control the tachycardia response although hypertension, which is more relevant to ICP issues, was avoided (6). In other investigations alfentanyl has exhibited superior hemodynamic attenuation to fentanyl and lidocaine, but this drug is rarely used in the ED and is unfamiliar to most emergency physicians (12).

Regarding esmolol, one randomized double-blind, placebo-controlled study demonstrated that a esmolol dose of 2 to 3 mg/kg intravenously provided better control of heart rate and blood pressure than either lidocaine or fentanyl (6). Of note, fixed doses of drugs were used, and the lidocaine and fentanyl were given only 2 minutes before intubation. Similar results were reported in another randomized double-blind study using 1.4 mg/kg (13) and 2 mg/kg (14). In a randomized double-blind study comparing the hemodynamic response of esmolol and lidocaine, both were found equally effective (2).

Based on the best evidence available at this time, the following recommendations can be made regarding the pharmacological mitigation of exacerbations of elevated ICP during emergency intubation:

- There is significant evidence that esmolol is consistently effective in doses of 1.4 to 3 mg/kg given 3 minutes before the induction and neuromuscular blocking agents. Esmolol, though, can cause or aggravate hypotension, especially in patients with hypovolemia, and should be used with great caution in trauma patients. In circumstances where blood pressure control and mitigation of RSRL are desired (e.g., spontaneous intracranial hemorrhage with hypertension), esmolol may be helpful.
- Evidence is mixed with respect to lidocaine's ability to mitigate RSRL, with some studies showing clear effect and others showing absence of effect. There is some evidence, although indirect, derived from tracheal suctioning of patients with elevated ICP under sedation or general anesthesia, that lidocaine can mitigate the ICP response to the stimulation of the trachea that is not mediated by catecholamine release. Overall, it would appear reasonable to administer lidocaine, 1.5 mg/kg intravenously, 3 minutes before induction and paralysis of patients with elevated ICP undergoing RSI.
- Fentanyl, in a dose of 3 mcg/kg, has some effect in mitigating the RSRL. Higher doses of fentanyl that are capable of inducing full sympathetic blockade are likely even more effective in blocking RSRL, but also carry a substantially higher risk of hypotension (especially in patients dependent on sympathetic drive) and hypoventilation or apnea. At present, it seems

appropriate to administer either fentanyl, 3 mcg/kg, or esmolol 2 mg/kg IV 3 minutes before the induction and neuromuscular blocking agents in patients with elevated ICP but without hypotension or shock.

- There is some controversy whether the increase in ICP caused by SCh is clinically significant, and whether a defasciculating dose of a competitive neuromuscular blocking agent is capable of mitigating this response. On balance, it seems reasonable to administer a defasciculating dose (one-tenth of the paralyzing dose) of a competitive neuromuscular blocking agent such as vecuronium (0.01 mg/kg) or rocuronium (0.06 mg/kg) 3 minutes before SCh is given. An alternative is to use either of these agents in a full RSI dose as the neuromuscular blocking agent for RSI, in which case, no defasciculating dose is required.

- There is a clear need for a well-controlled comparative study using a meaningful outcome measure to determine which, if any, of these interventions will decrease morbidity or mortality in patients with elevated ICP undergoing emergency RSI. Pending such a study, which will likely never be done because of logistical challenges, the approach outlined in Box 25-1 seems rational. Management of the patient at risk for elevated ICP should ensure cerebral perfusion and oxygenation. When intubation is indicated, pretreatment should be provided using lidocaine, 1.5 mg/kg, accompanied by a defasciculating dose of a competitive neuromuscular blocking agent if SCh is to be used, and either fentanyl 3 mcg/kg or esmolol 2 mg/kg if the patient is hemodynamically stable and not dependent on sympathetic drive to maintain his or her blood pressure.

REFERENCES

1. Abou-Madi MN, Keszler H, Yacoub JM. Cardiovascular reactions to laryngoscopy and tracheal intubation following small and large intravenous doses of lidocaine. *Can Anaesth Soc J* 1977;24(Jan):12–19.
2. Levitt M, Dresden G. The efficacy of esmolol versus lidocaine to attenuate the hemodynamic response to intubation in isolated head trauma patients. *Acad Emerg Med* 2001;8:19–24.
3. Tam S. Intravenous lidocaine: optimal time of injection before tracheal intubation. *Anesth Analg* 1987;66:1036–1038.
4. Miller CD, Warren SJ. IV lignocaine fails to attenuate the cardiovascular response to laryngoscopy and tracheal intubation. *Br J Anaesth* 1990;65:216–219.
5. Pathak D, Slater RM, Ping SS, et al. Effects of alfentanil and lidocaine on the hemodynamic responses to laryngoscopy and tracheal intubation. *J Clin Anesth* 1990;2:81–85.
6. Helfman SM, Gold MI, DeLisser EA, et al. Which drug prevents tachycardia and hypertension associated with tracheal intubation: lidocaine, fentanyl, or esmolol? *Anesth Analg* 1991;72:482–486.
7. Splinter WM, Cervenko F. Haemodynamic responses to laryngoscopy and tracheal intubation in geriatric patients: effects of fentanyl, lidocaine and thiopentone. *Can J Anaesth* 1989;36:370–376.
8. Chraemmer-Jorgensen B, Hoilund-Carlsen PF, Marving J, et al. Lack of effect of intravenous lidocaine on hemodynamic responses to rapid sequence induction of general anesthesia: a double-blind controlled clinical trial. *Anesth Analg* 1986;65:1037–1041.
9. Donegan MF, Bedford RF. Intravenously administered lidocaine prevents intracranial hypertension during endotracheal suctioning. *Anesthesiology* 1980;52:516–518.
10. Yano M, Nishiyama H, Yokota H, et al. Effect of lidocaine on ICP response to endotracheal suctioning. *Anesthesiology* 1986;64:651–653.
11. Adachi YU, Satomoto M, Higuchi H, et al. Fentanyl attenuates the hemodynamic response to endotracheal intubation more than the response to laryngoscopy. *Anesth Analg* 2002;95:233–237.
12. Payne KA, Murray WB, Oosthuizen JH. Obtunding the sympathetic response to intubation. Experience at 2 minutes after administration of the test agent in patients with cerebral aneurysms. *S Afr Med J* 1988;73:584–586.
13. Singh H, Vichitvejpaisal P. Comparative effects of lidocaine, esmolol, and nitroglycerin in modifying the hemodynamic response to laryngoscopy and intubation. *J Clin Anesth* 1995;7:5–8.
14. Feng CK, Chan KH, Liu KN, et al. A comparison of lidocaine, fentanyl, and esmolol for attenuation of cardiovascular response to laryngoscopy and tracheal intubation. *Acta Anaesthesiol Sin* 1996;34:61–67.

25

Reactive Airways Disease

Kerryann B. Broderick and Andy S. Jagoda

CLINICAL CHALLENGE

There are a number of confounders that make airway management of the patient with asthma or chronic obstructive pulmonary disease (COPD) a clinical challenge. These patients often have difficult anatomy, are hypoxic, desaturate quickly, and are hemodynamically unstable. Unlike many other clinical conditions, intubation itself, although challenging, does not resolve the primary problem, which is the obstruction of the small airways. In reality, the actual intubation may be the easiest part of the resuscitative sequence, because postintubation ventilation may be extremely difficult with persistent or worsening respiratory acidosis, barotrauma, or worsening hypotension caused by high intrathoracic pressures with diminished venous return. Thus the decision to intubate must be made carefully, and the appropriate technique must be chosen to facilitate the best possible outcome.

Severe asthma often presents one of the most difficult airway management cases encountered in the emergency department. Diaphoresis is a particularly ominous sign, and the diaphoretic asthmatic patient who cannot speak full sentences, appears anxious, or is sitting upright and leaning forward to augment the inspiratory effort must not be left unattended until stabilized.

Standard initial management of acute severe asthma exacerbation includes continuous beta$_2$-agonist nebulization therapy [albuterol (Ventolin) 15 to 20 mg/hr] for reversal of dynamic bronchospasm and an intravenous steroid [methylprednisolone (Solumedrol) 125 mg] for the treatment of the inflammatory component. If the patient is severely bronchospastic and cannot comply with a nebulized treatment, subcutaneous epinephrine or terbutaline (Brethine) 0.2 to 0.5 mg is indicated. The use of intravenous terbutaline is controversial but, if selected, should be initiated in the adult at 4 mcg/kg over 10 minutes followed by a continuous infusion of 0.04 to 0.2 mcg/kg/min; and in the child at 10 mcg/kg over 30 minutes followed by a continuous infusion of 0.1 mcg/kg/min. Intravenous albuterol (Salbutamol) can be administered at 3 mcg/kg over 10 minutes followed by an infusion of 0.04 to 0.2 mcg/kg/min in the adult. The addition of inhaled ipratropium bromide (Atrovent) or glycopyrrolate (Robinul), intravenous anticholinergic agents [atropine or glycopyrrolate (Robinul)], intravenous magnesium sulfate, intravenous ketamine (Ketalar), or inhalational helium/oxygen mixture is controversial and may be of benefit.

In COPD, much of the obstruction is fixed, comorbidity (especially cardiovascular disease) plays a greater role, and the prognosis, even with short-term mechanical ventilation, is worse. In the patient with COPD, anticholinergic therapy may be as important as beta$_2$-agonist therapy. Steroids again are important to attenuate underlying inflammation. Noninvasive ventilation

(BL-PAP) is of proven value in certain COPD patients and may help avoid intubation (see Chapter 35). By the time COPD patients have tired and require intubation, they have usually exhausted their catecholamine stores, are usually more hypoxic than one suspects clinically, and like the asthmatic patient, present significant clinical challenges after intubation. There have been recent reports in the literature of COPD patients *in extremis* who very shortly after intubation have become bradycardic and asystolic, and were unable to be resuscitated. The physiologic explanation is not apparent. It is proposed that these patients are profoundly hypoxic before intubation, are volume depleted because of their work of breathing and their asthenic body habitus, and after intubation experience a relative sympathectomy. This condition vasodilates them globally, contributing to a decrease in cardiac output, which eventually results in cardiac arrest. As in the asthmatic patient (see later), it is recommended that empiric incremental infusions of 500 mL of normal saline to a maximum of 1 to 2 L be started as soon as intubation is contemplated and that atropine and catecholamine infusions be available before intubation. These case reports, while of concern, do not reflect experience with the many COPD patients who are intubated annually and do not constitute scientific evidence regarding the incidence, cause, or treatment of this uncommon occurrence.

There is no role for intravenous aminophylline in the management of either acute severe asthma or acute severe COPD exacerbation.

APPROACH TO THE AIRWAY

Despite this vast array of treatment modalities, 1% to 3% of acute severe asthma exacerbations will require intubation. These patients are usually fatigued and have reduced functional residual capacity, so it is very difficult, if not impossible, to preoxygenate them optimally, and rapid desaturation must be anticipated. As most of these patients have been struggling to breathe against severe resistance, usually for hours, they have little if any residual physical reserve, and mechanical ventilation will be required. In fact, the need for mechanical ventilation is the indication for tracheal intubation; the airway itself is almost invariably patent and protected. This fact argues strongly against awake intubation techniques, such as blind nasotracheal intubation, which take longer, exacerbate hypoxemia, and carry higher complication rates and lower success rates than rapid sequence intubation (RSI).

TECHNIQUE

The single most important tenet in managing the status asthmaticus patient who requires intubation is to take total control of the airway as expeditiously as possible. Preoxygenation should be achieved to the greatest extent possible (see Chapters 3 and 5). The RSI drugs chosen should be administered to the patient in their position of comfort, often sitting upright. Once the patient loses consciousness, apply cricoid pressure, place the patient supine, and perform laryngoscopy and intubation, preferably with an 8.0- to 9.0-mm endotracheal tube to decrease resistance and facilitate aggressive pulmonary toilette.

DRUG DOSING AND ADMINISTRATION

If time permits, patients with reactive airways disease or obstructive lung disease should be pretreated with 1.5 mg/kg of intravenous lidocaine (Xylocaine) 3 minutes before induction to attenuate the reflexive bronchospasm in response to airway manipulation. Ketamine (Ketalar) is the induction agent of choice in the asthmatic patient because it stimulates the release of catecholamines and also has a direct bronchial smooth muscle relaxing effect that may be important in this clinical setting. Ketamine 1.5 mg/kg is given intravenously immediately before the administration of 1.5 mg/kg of succinylcholine (Anectine).

POSTINTUBATION MANAGEMENT

After the patient is successfully intubated and proper tube position has been confirmed, sedation, paralysis, and meticulous ventilator management are critical in improving patient outcome. Continuous sedation and paralysis for at least the next 4 to 6 hours with an appropriate benzodiazepine for amnesia and a competitive muscle relaxant will prevent asynchronous respirations, promote total relaxation of fatigued respiratory muscles, decrease the production of carbon dioxide, and allow optimum ventilator settings. Additional ketamine as well as continuous in-line albuterol and other pharmocologic adjuncts may also be given.

Mechanical Ventilation

All asthmatic patients have obstructed small airways and dynamic alveolar hyperinflation with varying amounts of end-expiratory residual intraalveolar gas and pressure (auto-PEEP or intrinsic PEEP). Elevations in auto-PEEP increase the risk for baro/volutrauma. Reversal of airflow obstruction and decompression of end-expiratory filled alveoli are the primary goals of early mechanical ventilation in the asthmatic. The former requires continuous in-line nebulization with increasingly higher doses of beta$_2$-agonists until reversal is objectively measured (decrease in peak and plateau airway pressures) or unacceptable side effects are produced. Safe, uncomplicated alveolar decompression requires prolonged expiratory time [inspiration/expiration (I/E) of 1:4 to 1:5], which is achieved by using smaller tidal volumes than usual, with a high inspiratory flow rate to shorten the inspiratory cycle time, permitting a longer expiratory phase. A general discussion of ventilation parameters can be found in Chapter 34.

The initial goal of ventilator therapy in the asthmatic patient is to improve arterial oxygen tension to adequate levels without inflicting barotrauma on the lungs or increasing auto-PEEP. Initial tidal volume should be reduced to 6 to 8 mL/kg to avoid barotrauma and air trapping. The speed at which a mechanical breath is delivered in liters per minute, typically 60 L/min, is called the *inspiratory flow* (IF) *rate*. In asthma the initial IF should be increased to 80 to 100 L/min with a decelerating flow pattern. Pressure control is preferred to volume control; in volume control, the operater selects the flow waveform to use square (constant) or ramp (decelerating), which is preferred. The ventilation rate should be determined in conjunction with the tidal volume, and initial rates of 8 to 10 breaths per minute (bpm) with a high inspiratory flow rate promote a prolonged expiratory phase that allows sufficient time for alveolar decompression. It is acceptable to permit the maintenance or gradual development of hypercapnia through reduced minute ventilation (the product of tidal volume and ventilatory rate) in the asthmatic patient, as this approach reduces peak inspiratory pressure and thus minimizes the potential for barotrauma. High intrathoracic pressure may compromise cardiac output and produce hypotension; therefore it is to be avoided.

The highest measured pressure at peak inspiration is the peak inspiratory pressure (PIP). The patient's lungs, chest wall, endotracheal tube, ventilatory circuit, ventilator, and mucus plugs all contribute to the PIP. This reading has an inconsistent predictive value for baro/volutrauma but ideally should be kept under 50 cm H_2O. A sudden rise in PIP should be interpreted as indicating tube blockage, mucus plugging, or pneumothorax until proven otherwise. A sudden, dramatic fall in PIP may indicate extubation.

The measured intraalveolar pressure during a 0.2- to 0.4-second end-inspiratory pause is referred to as the *plateau pressure* (P_{plat}). Values less than 30 cm H_2O are best and are not usually associated with baro/volutrauma. Measurement and trending of P_{plat} is an excellent objective tool to confirm optimal ventilator settings and the patient's response as well as the reversal of airflow obstruction. If initial ventilator settings disclose a P_{plat} of more than 30 cm H_2O, consider lowering minute ventilation and increasing inspiratory flow, both of which will prolong expiratory time and attenuate hyperinflation. If P_{plat} is unavailable, PIP may be used as a surrogate.

Most status asthmaticus patients who require intubation are hypercapnic. The concept of controlled hypoventilation (permissive hypercapnia) promotes *gradual* development (over three to four hours) and maintenance of hypercapnia (P_{CO_2} up to 90 mm Hg) and acidemia (pH as low as 7.2). This treatment is done primarily to decrease the risk of ventilator-related lung injury and prevent hemodynamic compromise as a result of increasing intrathoracic pressure from auto-PEEP or intrinsic PEEP ($PEEP_i$). Permissive hypercapnia is usually accomplished by reducing minute ventilation, increasing inspiratory flow rate to 80 to 120 L/min, and paralyzing and heavily sedating (and usually paralyzing) patients who otherwise would not tolerate these settings. Permissive hypercapnia may be instrumental in promoting prolonged expiratory times and reducing auto-PEEP.

Summary for Initial Ventilator Settings

1. Determine the patient's ideal body weight.
2. Set a tidal volume of 6 to 8 mL/kg with an F_iO_2 of 1.0 (100% oxygen).
3. Set a respiratory rate of 8 to 10 bpm.
4. Set an inspiratory to expiratory ratio of 1:4 to 1:5. Pressure control is preferred. If using the pressure control, the I/E ratio is adjusted directly by the I/E ratio parameter, or, by adjusting the inspiratory time parameter. If using volume control, the I/E ratio can be adjusted by increasing the peak flow rate, and the ramp inspiratory waveform should be selected. Peak inspiratory flow can be as high as 80 to 100 L/min.
5. Measure and maintain the plateau pressure at less than 30 cm H_2O; try to keep PIP at less than 50 cm H_2O.
6. Focus on the oxygenation and pulmonary pressures initially. If necessary, allow maintenance or gradual development of hypercapnia to avoid high plateau pressures and increasing auto-PEEP.
7. Ensure continuous sedation with a benzodiazepine and paralysis with a nondepolarizing muscle relaxant.
8. Continue in-line beta$_2$-agonist therapy and additional pharmacologic adjunctive treatment based on the severity of the patient's illness and objective response to treatment.

Complications of Mechanical Ventilation

Two of the more common complications seen in mechanically ventilated asthmatic patients are lung injury (baro/volutrauma) and hypotension. Lung injury is exemplified by tension pneumothorax. In those patients without tension pneumothorax, hypotension is usually related to either absolute volume depletion or relative hypovolemia caused by decreased venous return from increasing auto-PEEP and intrathoracic pressure. The inherent risks of developing either one of these complications are directly related to the degree of pulmonary hyperinflation. Of the two, hypotension occurs much more frequently than tension pneumothorax. Most asthmatic patients will have intravascular volume depletion because of the increased work of breathing, decreased oral intake following the onset of asthmatic exacerbation, and generalized increased metabolic state. It is appropriate for these reasons to infuse up to 2 L of normal saline (NS) either before the initiation of RSI or early during mechanical ventilation.

The differential diagnosis for hypotension in the mechanically ventilated patient is discussed in Chapter 3. A trial of hypoventilation (apnea test) may be used to distinguish tension pneumothorax from volume depletion. The patient is disconnected from the ventilator and allowed to be apneic up to 1 minute as long as adequate oxygenation is ensured by pulse oximetry. In volume depletion, the mean intrathoracic pressure will fall quickly, blood pressure should begin to rise, pulse pressure will widen, and pulse rate will fall within 30 to 60 seconds. If auto-PEEP is high, reductions in tidal volume and increases in inspiratory flow and I/E times will be required to reduce auto-PEEP. If auto-PEEP is not an issue, then an empiric volume infusion of 500 mL NS should be instituted and may be repeated based on the patient's response to the additional volume. With tension pneumothoraces, cardiopulmonary stability will not correct during the apnea time. This result should prompt the immediate insertion of bilateral chest tubes and reevaluation of the patient. Obviously, lower ventilatory pressure settings will be required thereafter. The initial ventilator settings and potential ventilator complications of the asthma patient are shared by the COPD patient.

EVIDENCE

1. Lidocaine in asthma. Intravenous lidocaine has been recommended in the literature to attenuate airway reflexes during intubation in patients with reactive airway disease (1,2). Stimulation of the airway in asthmatic patients is reported to result in bronchoconstriction, which is thought to be mediated via the vagus nerve (3). The recommendation to use intravenous lidocaine in RSI protocols for the severe asthmatic is extrapolated from the results of studies using healthy volunteers with a history of bronchospastic disease (4–6). In one placebo-controlled double-blind randomized study, volunteers who had a demonstrated decrease in forced expiratory volume (FEV_1) in response to histamine inhalation were shown to have a significant attenuation of response when pretreated with intravenous lidocaine (5). Unfortunately, there is also evidence that intravenous lidocaine does not protect against intubation-induced bronchoconstriction in asthma: In a prospective randomized double-blind placebo-controlled trial of 60 patients, lidocaine and placebo groups were not different in their transpulmonary pressure and airflow immediately after intubation and at 5-minute intervals (7). The same study evaluated inhaled albuterol (four puffs from a metered dose inhaler (MDI) 20 minutes before intubation), which showed significant mitigation of intubation-induced bronchospasm. There are no studies that have demonstrated that premedicating with intravenous lidocaine in RSI changes outcome; conversely, there is no evidence that premedication with intravenous lidocaine is harmful. Until better data are available, it seems reasonable to minimize the risk of intubation-induced bronchoconstriction by using lidocaine premedication in the asthmatic.

2. Ketamine in asthma. Theoretically, ketamine is a logical choice in managing the airway of the severe asthmatic because it increases circulating catecholamines, it is a direct smooth muscle dilator, it inhibits vagal outflow, and it does not cause histamine release (8). Case reports of dramatic improvement in pulmonary function with ketamine have driven its popularity (9,10), but no randomized studies have been performed to demonstrate ketamine's superiority over other agents. In a case series, 19 of 22 actively wheezing asthmatics had a decrease in bronchospasm during ketamine-induced anesthesia (11). In one prospective placebo-controlled double-blind trial of 14 mechanically ventilated patients with bronchospasm, the 7 patients treated with ketamine, 1 mg/kg, had a significant improvement in oxygenation but no improvement in PCO_2 or lung compliance; outcome (discharge from the intensive care unit) was the same in both groups. The study population was heterogeneous, making conclusions of the benefit of ketamine difficult at best (12). A randomized double-blind placebo-controlled trial of low-dose intravenous ketamine, 0.2 mg/kg bolus followed by an infusion of 0.5 mg/kg/hr, in nonintubated patients with acute asthma failed to demonstrate a benefit from intravenous ketamine (note that the incidence of dysphoric reactions led the investigators to decrease the bolus to 0.1 mg/kg) (13). At the present time, based on its mechanism of action and safety profile, ketamine appears to be the best agent available for RSI in the asthmatic.

3. Magnesium in asthma. Two metaanalyses have been performed analyzing the effect of intravenous magnesium on patients with asthma (14,15). Seven trials were identified and the authors conclude that magnesium has no identified role in the management of mild or moderate asthma. In severe asthma, there is evidence that magnesium improves pulmonary functions and admission rates. There is no good evidence that in severe asthma, magnesium decreases the need for intubation.

4. Anticholinergics in asthma. A metaanalysis of the role of ipratropium bromide in the emergency management of acute asthma exacerbation concluded that there is a modest benefit when it is used in conjunction with beta agonists (16). The metaanalysis recommended the use of inhaled ipratropium bromide because the benefit appears to outweigh any risks. Theoretically, in status asthmaticus where inhaled agents have limited delivery, intravenous anticholinergic agents may have benefit (17). However, other than case reports, there is no evidence at this time supporting their use. *COPD* studies are variable; one study of 356 patients in a randomized double-blind study using tiotropium, examining one-year health outcome measures, found that the peak expiratory flow rate (PEFR), St. Georges's Respiratory Questionnaire (SGRQ), and transition dyspnea index (TDI) focal scores were improved (18). A study of 623 patients, comparing salmeterol, titropium, and placebo at 6 months, found a statistically improved SGRQ over placebo and was found to be superior to salmeterol in the TDI category (19). In a second study of the same set of patients, the authors report that there was a tolerance that developed in the beta-agonist group that was not found in the anticholinergic group (20).

Most interesting is the study published March 2003, which was a longitudinal cohort study examining anticholinergics and mortality. Ipratropium was started in 827 patients with COPD and 273 with asthma. The study has reported a relative risk ratio for death for COPD of 1.6 (1.2 to 2.1) and for asthma of 2.4 (1.2 to 5.0) (21).

5. Heliox. A Cochrane Database review of the literature of heliox in the standard medical care during ventilated and nonventilated acute exacerbations of COPD failed to identify sufficient evidence to support its use (22). The reviewers identified four studies that met their inclusion criteria, only one of which involved intubated patients. Likewise, a systemic overview of heliox versus air/oxygen mixtures for the treatment of patients with acute asthma failed to find a clinically significant advantage to using heliox: The review did not identify well-done studies on intubated asthmatics (23). There is one case series of seven intubated patients with elevated airway pressures who had remarkable turnarounds in their clinical course with a 60 to 40 helium/oxygen mixture; however, this is a case series and thus suffers from inherent bias, making recommendations not possible (24).

REFERENCES

1. Walls R. Lidocaine and rapid sequence intubation. *Ann Emerg Med* 1996;27:528–529.
2. Gal T. Bronchial hyperresponsiveness and anesthesia: physiologic and therapeutic perspectives. *Anesth Analg* 1994;78:559–573.
3. Gold M. Anesthesia, bronchospasm, and death. *Semin Anesth* 1989;8:291–306.

4. Groeben H, Foster W, Brown R. Intravenous lidocaine and oral mexiletine block reflex bronchoconstriction in asthmatic subjects. *Am J Respir Crit Care Med* 1997;156:1703–1704.
5. Groeben H, Silvanus M, Beste M, et al. Both intravenous and inhaled lidocaine attenuate reflex bronchoconstriction but at different plasma concentrations. *Am J Respir Crit Care Med* 1999;159:530–535.
6. Downes H, Gerber N, Hirshman C. IV lignocaine in reflex and allergic bronchoconstriction. *Br J Anaesth* 1980;52:873–880.
7. Maslow A, Regan M, Israel E, et al. Inhaled albuterol, but not intravenous lidocaine, protects against intubation-induced bronchoconstriction in asthma. *Anesthesiology* 2000;93:1198–1204.
8. Huber F, Reeves J, Gutierrez J, et al. Ketamine: its effect on airway resistance in man. *South Med J* 1972;65:1176–1180.
9. Hommedieu C, Arens J. The use of ketamine for the emergency intubation of patients with status asthmaticus. *Ann Emerg Med* 1987;16:568–571.
10. Rock M, de la Roca S, Hommedieu C, et al. Use of ketamine in asthmatic children to treat respiratory failure refractory to conventional therapy. *Crit Care Med* 1986;14:514–516.
11. Corssen G, Gutierrez J, Reves J, et al. Ketamine in the anesthetic management of asthmatic patients. *Anesth Analg* 1972;51:588–596.
12. Hemmingsen C, Nielsen P, Odorica J. Ketamine in the treatment of bronchospasm during mechanical ventilation. *Am J Emerg Med* 1994;12:417–420.
13. Howton J, Rose J, Duffy S, et al. Randomized, double-blind, placebo controlled trial of intravenous ketamine in acute asthma. *Ann Emerg Med* 1996;27:170–175.
14. Alter H, Koopsell T, Hilty W. Intravenous magnesium as an adjuvant in acute bronchospasm: A meta-analysis. *Ann Emerg Med* 2000;36:191–197.
15. Rowe B, Bretzlaff J, Bourdon C, et al. Intravenous magnesium sulfate treatment for acute asthma in the emergency department: a systemic review of the literature. *Ann Emerg Med* 2000;36:181–190.
16. Stoodley R, Aaron S, Dales R. The role of ipatropium bromide in the emergency management of acute asthma exacerbation: a metaanalysis of randomized clinical trials. *Ann Emerg Med* 1999;34:8–18.
17. Slovis C, Daniels G, Wharton D. Intravenous use of glycopyrrolate in acute respiratory distress due to bronchospastic pulmonary disease. *Ann Emerg Med* 1987;16:898–900.
18. Vincken W, van Noord JA, Greefhorst AP. Improved health outcomes in patients with COPD during 1 yr's treatment with tiotropium. *Eur Respir J* 2002;19:205–206.
19. Donohue JF, van Noord JA, Batemane ED, et al. A 6-month, placebo-controlled study comparing lung function and health status changes in COPD patients treated with tiotropium and salmeterol. *Chest* 2002;122:47–55.
20. Donohue JF, Menojoge S, Kesten S. Tolerance to bronchodilating effects of salmeterol in COPD. *Respir Med* 2003;97:1014–1020.
21. Ringbaek T, Viskum K. Is there any association between inhaled ipatropium and mortality in patients with COPD and asthma? *Respir Med* 2003;97:264–272.
22. Rodrigo G, Pollack C, Rodrigo C, et al. Heliox for treatment of exacerbations of chronic obstructive pulmonary disease. *Cochrane Database Syst Rev* 2002; CD003571.
23. Ho A, Lee A, Karmakar M, et al. Heliox vs Air-oxygen mixtures for the treatment of patients with acute asthma. *Chest* 2003;123:882–890.
24. Gluck E, Onorato D, Castriotta R. Helium-oxygen mixtures in intubated patients with status asthmaticus and respiratory acidosis. *Chest* 1990;98:693–698.

26

Distorted Airways
and Upper Airway Obstruction

Michael F. Murphy and Erik D. Barton

CLINICAL CHALLENGE

Anatomically, the term *upper airway* refers to that portion of the anatomy that extends from the lips and nares to the first tracheal ring. Thus the first portion of the upper airway has two redundant pathways: a nasal pathway and an oral pathway. However, at the level of the oropharynx, the two pathways merge and that unique feature of redundancy is lost. The most common, life-threatening causes of upper-airway distortion and obstruction occur in the region of this common channel and are typically laryngeal. Additionally, disorders of the base of the tongue and the pharynx can cause obstruction. See Box 26-1.

APPROACH TO THE AIRWAY

The signs of upper-airway distortion and obstruction may be occult or subtle. Deadly deterioration may occur suddenly and unexpectedly. Seemingly innocuous interventions, such as small doses of sedative hypnotic agents to alleviate anxiety, may precipitate sudden and total airway obstruction. Rescue devices may not be successful and may even be contraindicated in some circumstances. The goal in these patients is to proceed rapidly in a sensible, controlled manner to manage the airway before complete airway obstruction occurs, focusing on the following:

1. When should an intervention be performed? Chapter 1 deals with the important question of when to intubate. If airway obstruction is severe, progressive, or potentially imminent, then immediate action (often cricothyrotomy) is required without further consideration of moving the patient to another venue (e.g., the operating room). Failing such an indication for an *immediate* cricothyrotomy, the question becomes more difficult: What is the expected clinical course?

   Penetrating wounds to the neck and airway are notoriously unpredictable. Some advocate securing the airway regardless of warning signs, whereas others advocate a watch and see posture. The problem with the second strategy is that obstruction is often sudden and unexpected, resulting in an airway (and patient) that cannot be rescued. Thus, if there is any evidence of significant vascular injury (hematoma, significant external bleeding), acting earlier rather than later is the most prudent course.

   Most nontraumatic causes of upper airway obstruction have less dramatic clinical courses. There are three cardinal signs of upper airway obstruction:

Box 26-1. Causes of Upper Airway Obstruction

A. Infectious
  a. Viral and bacterial laryngotracheobronchitis (e.g., croup)
  b. Parapharyngeal and retropharyngeal abscesses
  c. Lingual tonsillitis (a lingual tonsil is a rare but real congenital anomaly and a
    well-recognized cause of failed intubation)
  d. Infections, hematomas, or abscesses of the tongue or floor of the mouth (e.g., Ludwig's
    angina)
  e. Epiglottitis (also known as supraglottitis)
B. Neoplastic
  a. Laryngeal carcinomas
  b. Hypopharyngeal and lingual (tongue) carcinomas
C. Physical and chemical agents
  a. Foreign bodies
  b. Thermal injuries (heat and cold)
  c. Caustic injuries (acids and alkalis)
  d. Inhaled toxins
D. Allergic/idiopathic: including angiotensin-converting enzyme inhibitors (ACEI) angioedema
E. Traumatic: blunt and penetrating neck and upper-airway trauma

---

- "Hot potato" voice: the muffled voice one often hears in patients with mononucleosis and very large tonsils
- Difficulty in swallowing secretions, either because of pain or obstruction. The patient is typically sitting up, leaning forward, and spitting or drooling secretions.
- Stridor

The first two signs do not necessarily suggest that total upper-airway obstruction is imminent; however, stridor does. The patient presenting with stridor has already lost at least 90% of the airway caliber and requires immediate intervention. In the case of children below the age of 8 to 10 with croup, medical therapy may suffice. In older children and adults, the presence of stridor typically mandates a surgical airway, or at the very least a double setup. This technique uses an awake attempt (e.g., using ketamine sedation) from above with the capability, prepared in advance, to move to a surgical airway if needed. Positive pressure by bag and mask or other noninvasive ventilatory devices has been described as one method to help open an obstructed airway and may buy some time; however, this technique should not be relied on as more than a temporizing maneuver.

2. What options in addition to a cricothyrotomy exist if the airway deteriorates or obstructs either here in the emergency department (ED) or during transport? The answer to the second question needs to incorporate the following considerations:
  - *Is rescue bag and mask ventilation possible?* Will a mask seal be possible to achieve, or is the lower face disrupted? Has a penetrating neck wound rendered the upper airway incompetent to high airway pressures? As mentioned in Chapter 6, the bag and mask devices most commonly used in resuscitation settings are capable of generating 50 to 100 centimeters of water pressure (CWP) in the upper airway, provided that they do not have positive pressure relief valves and that an adequate mask seal can be obtained. Pediatric and neonatal devices often incorporate positive pressure relief valves that can be easily defeated if needed. This degree of positive pressure is often sufficient to overcome

the moderate degree of upper-airway obstruction offered by redundant tissue (e.g., the obese) or edematous tissue (e.g., angioedema, croup, or epiglottitis). Lesions that are hard and fixed, such as hematomas, abscesses, cancers, and foreign bodies, produce an obstruction that usually cannot be reliably overcome with bag and mask ventilation, even with high upper-airway pressures.

- *Where is the airway problem?* If the lesion is well above the level of the larynx and orotracheal intubation is judged to be impossible (for whatever reason), then supralaryngeal rescue devices such as LMAs and Combitubes may be considered and ought to be immediately at hand to attempt rescue of the airway.

3. What are the advantages and risks of an awake look? In most instances, unless the patient is in crisis or deteriorating rapidly, an awake direct laryngoscopy is possible. If the tip of the employing is visible without paralysis (grade 3 view) and is in the midline, orotracheal intubation employing rapid sequence intubation (RSI) is probably possible, unless the working diagnosis is a primary laryngeal disorder. If a primary laryngeal disorder is suspected, complete visualization of the larynx is mandatory (e.g., fiberoptic visualization). Attempting direct laryngoscopy in an awake, struggling patient with a laryngeal disorder is potentially dangerous and ill-advised.

4. Is rapid sequence intubation reasonable? If one is confident that orotracheal intubation is possible and highly confident that the patient can be successfully ventilated using bag/mask ventilation (BMV) intubation, then it is reasonable to proceed with RSI (e.g., early in the course of a penetrating neck injury). A double setup with readiness for a surgical airway is still advised. Often RSI is not considered advisable, and a controlled, urgent surgical or fiberoptic airway is appropriate, especially if patient cooperation and time are limited.

TIPS AND PEARLS

- Be very reluctant to transfer patients with upper-airway obstruction and unsecured airways, even short distances. Always secure the airways of patients with significant acute penetrating neck wounds before transport.
- The patient with upper-airway obstruction, a disrupted airway, or a distorted airway who *can* protect and maintain the airway and *can* maintain oxygenation and ventilation should be considered a *difficult airway,* and the difficult airway algorithm should be used.
- The patient with upper airway obstruction, a disrupted airway, or a distorted airway who *cannot* maintain oxygenation or ventilation should be considered a *failed airway,* and the failed airway algorithm should be used.
- Blind techniques (e.g., blind nasotracheal intubation) of airway management in these situations are contraindicated and should not be attempted.
- Bag/mask ventilation alone cannot be relied on to rescue the airway, particularly if the lesion is a fixed lesion.
- RSI is usually contraindicated unless the awake look proves otherwise.
- Contemplate a cricothyrotomy early and prepare for it before the awake look.
- Titrate ketamine rather than sedative/hypnotic drugs (e.g., midazolam, propofol, thiopental, etomidate) to get an adequate awake look. Topical anesthesia of the airway will not be particularly successful and will not be adequate unless accompanied by sedation.
- If the awake look indicates that orotracheal intubation is not possible or is equivocal, proceed directly to a cricothyrotomy or fiberoptic intubation.
- If the patient suddenly crashes and the lesion is above the level of the larynx, do two-handed bag and mask ventilation and try a Combitube or LMA while setting up for a cricothyrotomy.

If the lesion is at the larynx, do two-handed bag and mask ventilation and proceed immediately to a cricothyrotomy.

- Heliox may buy time. Helium is less dense than nitrogen, reducing turbulent flow and resistance through tight orifices, as is the case with some causes of upper-airway obstruction. The commercial preparations are usually 80% helium and 20% oxygen, and provided lung function is adequate, this mix will produce acceptable oxygen saturations. Other concentrations may be prepared.

- Crush injuries to the larynx and laryngeal fractures are best managed with tracheostomy rather than cricothyrotomy, or gently performed RSI if circumstances permit.

- In the event of a tracheal separation (e.g., clothesline-type injury to the neck) when one is performing a surgical airway, grasp the distal stump with an instrument before opening the pretracheal fascia.

- The patient with a bulky pharyngeal or laryngeal tumor may be intubated using a fiberoptic technique. While this technique typically requires more time to perform, it is preferable to surgically invading an airway that may hemorrhage or be subject to subsequent operative resection.

EVIDENCE

The evidence with respect to the emergency management of the patient with airways that are potentially or actually disrupted, distorted, or obstructed is essentially anecdotal. Most of the literature dealing with the topic comes either from the surgical or anesthesia literature: primarily small series or case reports. There are no controlled studies comparing intervention with expectant observation. In the surgical literature, cricothyrotomy, as might be expected, is typically overrecommended. In the anesthesia literature, intubation under deep-inhalation anesthesia and spontaneous ventilation has been the standard and, as might be expected, cricothyrotomy is underrecommended. Despite the lack of scientifically sound studies, the following additional reading is recommended.

REFERENCES

1. Crosby E, Reid D. Acute epiglottitis in the adult: is intubation mandatory? *Can J Anaesth* 1991;38:914–918.
2. Donald PJ. Emergency management of the patient with upper airway obstruction. *Clin Rev Allergy* 1985;3:25–36.
3. Halvorson DJ, Merritt RM, Mann C, et al. Management of subglottic foreign bodies. *Ann Otol Rhinol Laryngol* 1996;105:541–544.
4. Jacobson S. Upper airway obstruction. *Emerg Med Clin North Am* 1989;7:205–217.
5. Tong MC, Chu MC, Leighton SE, et al. Adult croup. *Chest* 1996;109:1659–1662.

27

The Critically Ill Patient

Michael F. Murphy

CLINICAL CHALLENGE

The three most important organ systems affected by endotracheal intubation are the brain, the heart, and the lungs. The LOAD mnemonic introduced in Chapter 3 identifies patients with disorders of these three organ systems as the primary targets of strategies to attenuate the adverse responses to intubation.

Patients with limited cardiopulmonary and central nervous system (CNS) reserve present a complex challenge when it comes to endotracheal intubation. The job of the intubator is to *assess the reserve* of each of these organ systems to evaluate how the act of intubation might adversely affect them and then select the best combination of medications and technique to mitigate these adverse effects.

Appropriate decision making and actions depend on a detailed understanding of the organ system responses to intubation, the effects of pharmacologic agents to be used to facilitate intubation, and the balance to be sought in each individual patient. This is a crucial decision in the patient who is critically ill, as small variations in technique or drug doses may have significant consequences.

TECHNIQUE

Organ System Responses to Endotracheal Intubation

As described in Chapter 4, the larynx is the most heavily innervated sensory structure in the body. Laryngoscopy and endotracheal intubation stimulate these sensory organs and produce adverse physiologic effects. The intensity of these physiologic responses is related to the intensity of stimulation, which depends on:

- The duration of laryngoscopy
- The aggressiveness of laryngoscopy
- The degree of attendant hypoxemia/hypercarbia
- Stimulation of the carina by the endotracheal tube
- The use of alternative placement techniques (e.g., lightwand) that produce less stimulation

These stimuli, if unchecked, have the potential to produce significant responses and, potentially, adverse end organ consequences. Depending on which organ systems are involved in a particular critically ill patient, the following organ system responses to endotracheal intubation may be the most important to consider:

- Increased intracranial pressure (ICP) and cerebral blood flow, particularly if autoregulation is disturbed
- increased airways resistance
- The autonomic nervous system
  - Adrenergic responses: Endotracheal intubation causes increased adrenergic activity with activation of the sympathetic nervous system and elevated circulating catecholamines. This in turn results in:
    - An increased systolic blood pressure (SBP) and mean arterial blood pressure (MAP) (up to two times normal)
    - Increased diastolic blood pressure (DBP) (up to 50% increase)
    - Increased heart rate (HR) (up to 50% increase)
    - Increased cardiac work and myocardial oxygen consumption (MVO_2)
    - Ventricular dysrhythmias (increased automaticity/irritability due to increased circulating catecholamines and increased blood pressure)
    - Decreased gastric emptying (increased gastric volume and risk of aspiration)
    - Decreased gut motility (ileus)
  - Cholinergic responses:
    - Bronchoconstriction and bronchorrhea
    - Bradycardia: rarely but occasionally in children and infants, especially if hypoxemic

Patients at Risk

Critically ill patients are especially at risk from the adverse cardiovascular and pulmonary responses to endotracheal intubation. The most important underlying conditions that place the patient at higher risk of adverse effects are listed in Box 27-1.

Box 27-1. High Risk Conditions

- The upper airway and respiratory system
  - Reactive airways disease
- The cardiovascular system
  - Major vessel aneurysm rupture (congenital, traumatic, or atherosclerotic)
  - Aortic or major vessel dissection and rupture
  - Ischemic heart disease (IHD)
  - Left ventricular systolic or diastolic dysfunction ("failure") due to any etiology (e.g., ischemic, hypertensive, congestive, etc.)
  - Valvular heart disease: Stenotic lesions limit the heart's ability to provide an adequate cardiac output to meet the needs of the body; regurgitant lesions may see increased regurgitant flow in the face of increased systemic vascular resistance (SVR).
  - L to R shunts [e.g., ventricular septal defect (VSD)] will increase as SVR and LV systolic pressure increases.
  - Cor pulmonale: The stress of intubation increases pulmonary vascular resistance (PVR) and in the face of cor pulmonale, may produce acute right heart failure.
  - Ventricular and atrial arrhythmias may be induced.
- The brain
  - Patients with intracranial hypertension or increased intracranial pressure (ICP)

Mitigating and Preventing the Adverse Physiologic Responses to Intubation

- Nonpharmacologic methods

  Increasing stimulation of the larynx proportionately increases the adrenergic and ICP responses to intubation. Thus, limiting the time and forcefulness of laryngoscopy reduces the magnitude of adverse physiologic responses. Preoxygenation (Chapter 3) limits the possibility of desaturation during intubation, avoiding the adrenergic response resulting from hypoxemia. There is also some evidence that the laryngeal stimulation during intubation with a lighted stylet is less compared to conventional laryngoscopy.

  In summary, the nonpharmacologic methods of limiting the adverse physiologic responses to intubation include the following:
  - Limit the time of laryngoscopy
  - Preoxygenate and use a pulse oximeter
  - Hyperventilate by bag and mask to prevent hypercapnia, especially if increased ICP or impaired autoregulation is suspected
  - Use an alternative technique that is associated with less stimulation, if reasonable (e.g., lighted stylet or ILM)
  - Place the endotracheal tube in an atraumatic way
  - Avoid ETT contact with the carina
- Pharmacologic methods

  Pharmacologic interventions are a double-edged sword in the critically ill patient. Although they may mitigate many of the adverse effects outlined earlier, the agents themselves may cause adverse effects, especially hypotension, respiratory depression (during the pretreatment interval), and hypercapnia. Consider the following:
  - The additive or potentiating effects of one technique or drug on another (e.g., the obtunded overdose patient may need less induction agent)
  - The patient's physiologic reserve: Patients with reduced cardiac reserve [decreased left ventricular (LV) function and valvular heart disease] are more sensitive to myocardial depressants such as induction agents; as are patients who are hypovolemic, such as those with uncontrolled hypertension, blood loss, or dehydration.
  - The potential of an adverse outcome related to the physiologic response to intubation: The physiologic response to intubation may be especially detrimental in patients with severe asthma, ischemic heart disease (IHD), elevated ICP, intracranial hemorrhage, and aneurysm rupture or major vessel dissection.
  - Underlying sympathetic tone: If the sympathetic nervous system is already maximally stimulated (e.g., hemorrhagic shock) and the patient is barely compensated, one must be cautious with any drug that can reduce sympathetic tone. This includes all sedative hypnotic agents (alcohol, benzodiazepines, barbiturates), neuroleptics (haloperidol and droperidol), opioids, lidocaine, and histamine releasers. Etomidate, ketamine, succinylcholine, vecuronium, and rocuronium are the safest choices. For sedation, small titrated doses of ketamine or haloperidol are probably safer than benzodiazepines or barbiturates.

When using medications to mitigate the adverse physiologic responses to intubation in patients with marginal pulmonary or cardiovascular reserve (e.g., those who are critically ill), administer conservative doses and err on the side of too little rather than too much. If postintubation hypertension and tachycardia occur, they can be managed by administering small doses of the induction agent or by titrating a benzodiazepine or opioid (e.g., fentanyl).

Specific Clinical Syndromes

Acute Pulmonary Edema

- **The clinical challenge**

  The patient with acute pulmonary edema due to LV failure who requires intubation presents several challenges to the physician performing the intubation:

  - Preoxygenation will provide little in the way of oxygen reserve, as these patients have little or no functional residual capacity (FRC). Oxyhemoglobin desaturation will occur rapidly.
  - The patient may be unable to lie flat and is often struggling and uncooperative, presenting airway access difficulties.
  - Foamy secretions may obscure visualization of the airway.
  - High airway resistance and low pulmonary compliance are likely to render bag and mask ventilation difficult or ineffective.
  - Cardiac reserve varies. The patient who is hypertensive is more likely to tolerate opioids and induction agents than one who is normotensive, who in turn is more likely to tolerate opioids and induction agents than a hypotensive patient.
  - Intubation is likely to exacerbate any element of bronchospasm.

  All these points emphasize the fact that there is little margin for error in these patients and that intubation should be atraumatic, swift, and successful on the first attempt whenever possible. This argues strongly for the superior pharmacologic and physical control, and success rates provided by rapid sequence intubation (RSI).

- **Approach to airway management**

  - Attempt to preoxygenate with 100% oxygen, even though it may not be as effective as in patients with normal lungs. Assist ventilation to maintain oxygen saturation if at all possible. The patient may require positive pressure ventilation throughout the intubation sequence to maintain adequate oxygen saturation.
  - Positioning: The cardiovascular system will tolerate the procedure, medications, and ventilation better in the supine position, but the patient usually prefers to be erect. It may be best to administer drugs with the patient erect and then to place the patient in a supine position for intubation.
  - Assess cardiovascular reserve. Patients who are hypertensive and hyperdynamic have the capacity to respond aggressively to intubation and may require medications to attenuate this response. Use caution in patients who are normotensive and extreme caution in those who are hypotensive.
  - Have intravenous nitroglycerine available. Pressors such as dobutamine or dopamine should be available. Alpha agent pressors such as phenylephrine and methoxamine are inappropriate, as they increase blood pressure at the expense of increased LV MVO_2. An exception is the patient with significant aortic or mitral stenosis and a fixed cardiac output, in which case alpha-adrenergic agonists may be preferable.
  - Use the largest endotracheal tube possible to minimize resistance to ventilation and facilitate pulmonary toilette [8 mm inner diameter (ID) in an adult female; 9 mm ID in an adult male]. Place a stylet in the tube.

- **Recommended intubation sequence**

  - Leave the patient upright with the head of the bed elevated.
    - Preparation
    - Preoxygenation
    - Pretreatment

- fentanyl 3 mcg/kg intravenously (IV) if the patient is hypertensive; reduced to 1 to 1.5 mcg/kg if normotensive; avoid altogether if hypotensive.
  - Paralysis with induction
    - Etomidate 0.3 mg/kg if hypertensive or normotensive; reduce to 0.2 mg/kg if hypotensive.
    - Succinylcholine 1.5 mg/kg
  - Protection and positioning
    - Sellick's maneuver
    - Place patient supine.
  - Placement with proof
    - Gentle intubation
    - Confirm tube placement with end-tidal carbon dioxide ($ETCO_2$).
  - Postintubation management
    - Titrate diazepam to ensure the patient is sedated (0.1 to 0.2 mg/kg IV to start).
    - Administer 0.1 mg/kg pancuronium or vecuronium to facilitate mechanical ventilation.
- **Initiating mechanical ventilation**
  - Immediately after intubation, bag ventilate the patient to assess compliance and resistance. Appreciate the time needed to complete expiration. Note the effect of positive pressure ventilation on blood pressure. Obtain a chest x-ray and look especially carefully for a right mainstem intubation, as one lung ventilation is even less well tolerated when the patient has pulmonary edema.
  - Set the inspired fraction of oxygen (F_iO_2) at 100%. A tidal volume of 10 mL/kg at a rate of 10 breaths per min, as usual, is a good place to start.
  - An elevated mean intrathoracic pressure due to positive pressure ventilation may impede venous return and improve LV function in the setting of acute LV failure, though peak airway pressures exceeding 35 to 40 cm of water pressure (CWP) are associated with an increased risk of pneumothorax. In the event that the lungs are very stiff and high airway pressures are compromising venous return and cardiac output, faster rates at lower tidal volumes may be required.
  - If there is significant bronchospasm, the rate may have to be decreased to extend the expiratory time and the tidal volume increased, if possible, to maintain minute volume.
  - Positive end-expiratory pressure (PEEP) beginning at 5 CWP or other forms of pressure support may be introduced to enhance FRC and oxygenation if the cardiac output will tolerate it. Increase the PEEP as needed and as tolerated.
  - Treat the pulmonary edema aggressively according to its cause.
- **Tips and pearls**
  - Dramatic falls in blood pressure caused by drugs (especially nitrates and histamine releasers) and ventilation may provide clues to underlying significant valvular heart disease.
  - The patient who has worrisome hypertension caused by the intubation will respond to small repeated doses of thiopental (25 to 50 mg) or propofol (10 to 20 mg), which may be used to both sedate and lower the blood pressure. However, postintubation hypertension that persists is the result of inadequate sedation and excessive sympathetic tone. Diazepam, supplemented with morphine or fentanyl, and nitrates constitute a good approach.
  - Circulation times are slowed in these patients and medication onset time may be considerably delayed.

Cardiogenic Shock

- **The clinical challenge**
  The patient in cardiogenic shock is gravely ill with a high mortality rate. This fact serves to emphasize the attention to detail that is required in managing the intubation.
  - Provided the patient is not in pulmonary edema, the FRC is probably intact and preoxygenation is useful.
  - By definition, there is no cardiac reserve, and medications that reduce cardiovascular performance are contraindicated. Induction agents, in particular, must be carefully selected. An amnestic agent, such as midazolam 1 to 2 mg may be well tolerated. Etomidate and ketamine in much-reduced doses (e.g., etomidate 0.1 mg/kg or ketamine 0.5 mg/kg) also are reasonable, though either may depress cardiac function.
  - Long-term sedation with diazepam in small titrated doses of 1 to 2 mg may be tolerated.
  - Circulation times are prolonged, so drug effects are substantially delayed.
- **Approach to airway management**
  - Evaluate the airway.
  - As with the patient in pulmonary edema, there is little margin for error in this patient and intubation should be atraumatic, swift, and successful on the first attempt.
  - Be prepared to handle surges in blood pressure and myocardial oxygen demand after intubation, rather than preemptively.
- **Recommended intubation sequence**
  - Preparation
  - Preoxygenation
  - Pretreatment: none
  - Paralysis with induction
    - Depending on the patient's circulatory status, either no induction agent or a greatly reduced dosage, such as:
      - 1 to 2 mg of midazolam *or* 40 mg of ketamine *or* 8 mg of etomidate
    - Succinylcholine 1.5 mg/kg
  - Protection and positioning: Sellick's maneuver
  - Position patient for intubation
  - Placement with proof: gentle, atraumatic intubation
  - Postintubation management: Diazepam 1 to 2 mg increments; pancuronium 0.1 mg/kg *or* vecuronium 0.1 mg/kg
- **Initiating mechanical ventilation**
  - Be cautious of impeding venous return and cardiac filling
- **Tips and pearls**
  - Paralytic agents such as succinylcholine do not have substantial cardiovascular activity. Pancuronium has sympathomimetic activity, though it is unlikely to be evident in the setting of cardiogenic shock, where sympathetic activity is already maximal. Histamine-releasing agents such as sodium thiopental or the benzylisoquinoline neuromuscular blocking agents (NMBAs) should be avoided.

Septic Shock

- **The clinical challenge**
  - Septic shock may be hyperdynamic or hypodynamic; myocardial contractility and systemic vascular resistance are compromised. The challenge is to maintain cardiac output and oxygen delivery to the tissues.

○ Any agent that may compromise myocardial contractility or systemic vascular resistance must be considered with great caution, and alternatives should be sought, if at all possible.
- **Approach to airway management**
  ○ Evaluate the airway.
  ○ The approach to airway management in the patient with septic shock is no different from that in the patient in cardiogenic shock (see recommended sequence earlier).
- **Initiating mechanical ventilation**
  ○ Ventilation should be initiated at 10 mL/kg at 10 breaths/minute. However, as most patients in septic shock are also acidemic, consideration should be given to increasing minute ventilation by 20% to 30%, if the cardiac output will tolerate it, until arterial blood gases (ABGs) can be obtained.
  ○ Pressure support may reduce shunt fraction and improve oxygenation, provided cardiac output is maintained.
- **Tips and pearls**
  ○ Be cautious with ventilation. Any reduction in venous return will not be tolerated.
  ○ Be meticulous in ensuring that an endobronchial intubation is avoided.

Anaphylaxis

- **The clinical challenge**
  ○ The patient suffering from a systemic anaphylactic reaction demonstrates hypotension due to release of vasoactive mediators, intense bronchoconstriction, and upper-airway edema.
  ○ The patient may be profoundly acidemic (respiratory and metabolic).
  ○ Orotracheal intubation may be difficult because of upper-airway edema, and a small-diameter endotracheal tube and surgical airway equipment should be readily at hand. Needle ventilation and other supralaryngeal rescue airway devices such as the Combitube or laryngeal mask airway will be ineffective because of the combination of upper-airway obstruction and bronchospasm.
  ○ Hypotension limits the spectrum of pharmacologic options for sedation.
  ○ Intense bronchospasm will challenge the ability to ventilate the patient effectively and attenuate the mixed acidosis that is present.
- **Approach to airway management**
  ○ Intense bronchospasm and hypotension will limit the effectiveness of preoxygenation and gas exchange in the preintubation period. Therefore expeditious intubation is desirable.
  ○ Be prepared to perform a surgical airway.
  ○ If you are confident in your ability to intubate the patient, maximize the success rate by using RSI, with cricothyroidotomy prepared as backup. If severe upper-airway edema or stridor is present, an awake technique or primary cricothyrotomy is recommended.
  ○ Treat the anaphylaxis aggressively with epinephrine during preparation for intubation. Steroids and antihistamines may be helpful, but epinephrine is the primary agent.
  ○ Ketamine provides the best blood pressure support and is a bronchodilator.
- **Recommended Sequence**
  ○ Preparation
  ○ Preoxygenation
  ○ Pretreatment: lidocaine 1.0 mg/kg
  ○ Paralysis with induction:
    - ketamine 1.5 mg/kg
    - succinylcholine 1.5 mg/kg
  ○ Protection and positioning

- ○ Placement with proof: Perform intubation.
- ○ Postintubation management: Confirm tube placement.
- ○ Continue to treat anaphylaxis.
- **Initiating mechanical ventilation**
  - ○ The substantial increase in airways resistance will mandate slow rates and moderate tidal volumes with permissive hypercapnia to achieve acceptable oxygenation, minimal barotrauma, and optimum cardiac output, as for asthma (see Chapter 25).
  - ○ Excessive mean intrathoracic pressure is likely to compromise venous return and cardiac output.
- **Tips and pearls**
  - ○ Avoid pure alpha-adrenergic agents to manage hypotension, as there is the theoretical potential of augmenting bronchospasm.
  - ○ Pancuronium or vecuronium are preferred for paralysis after intubation. Benzylisoquinoline derivatives (e.g., curare, cisatracurium) are to be avoided because of their ability to release histamine.

EVIDENCE

There is substantial evidence that orotracheal intubation produces adverse responses, and that those responses lead to adverse patient outcomes (1–7). Some of that literature is specific to emergency medicine and the patients we care for (1,6). It is also clear from the literature that obtunding those adverse responses results in an improved outcome (5–7). The critically ill patient has the most to lose and the most to gain from obtunding the responses.

The mainstays of controlling the responses are the technique chosen (8–10) and medications. Less stimulating techniques such as the lighted stylet and nontracheal devices (e.g., LMA) produce less response than traditional laryngoscopic intubation. Opioids such as fentanyl, alfentanil, sufentanil, and recently, remifentanil are the mainstays of the pharmacologic strategy. However, induction agents, nitrates, beta-blockers (e.g., esmolol), and others have also been used successfully (4,5,7,11–18).

REFERENCES

1. Schwab TM, Greaves TH. Cardiac arrest as a possible sequela of critical airway management and intubation. *Am J Emerg Med* 1998;16:609–612.
2. Bishop MJ, Bedford RF, Kil HK. Physiologic and pathophysiologic responses to intubation. In: Benumof JL, ed. *Airway management: principles and practice.* St Louis: Mosby, 1996.
3. Fox EJ, Sklar GS, Hill CH, et al: Complications related to the pressor response to endotracheal intubation. *Anaesthesiology* 1977;47:524–525.
4. Horak J, Weiss S. Emergent management of the airway. New pharmacology and the control of comorbidities in cardiac disease, ischemia, and valvular heart disease. *Crit Care Clin* 2000;16:411–427.
5. Bruder N, Ortega D, Granthil C. Consequences and prevention methods of hemodynamic changes during laryngoscopy and intratracheal intubation. *Ann Fr Anesth Reanim* 1992;11:57–71.
6. Rodricks MB, Deutschman CS. Emergent airway management. Indications and methods in the face of confounding conditions. *Crit Care Clin* 2000;16:389–409.
7. Kovac AL. Controlling the hemodynamic response to laryngoscopy and endotracheal intubation. *J Clin Anesth* 1996;8:63–79.
8. Habib MP. Physiologic implications of artificial airways. *Chest* 1989;96:180.
9. Nishikawa K, Kawamata M, Namiki A. Lightwand intubation is associated with less hemodynamic changes than fibreoptic intubation in normotensive, but not in hypertensive patients over the age of 60. *Can J Anaesth* 2001;48:1148–1154.
10. Kitamura T, Yamada Y, Chinzei M, et al. Attenuation of haemodynamic responses to tracheal intubation by the styletscope. *Br J Anaesth* 2001;86:275–277.
11. Adachi YU, Satomoto M, Higuchi H, et al. Fentanyl attenuates the hemodynamic response to endotracheal intubation more than the response to laryngoscopy. *Anesth Analg* 2002;95:233–237.

12. Habib AS, Parker JL, Maguire AM, et al. Effects of remifentanil and alfentanil on the cardiovascular responses to induction of anaesthesia and tracheal intubation in the elderly. *Br J Anaesth* 2000;88:430–433.

13. Maguire AM, Kumar N, Parker JL, et al. Comparison of effects of remifentanil and alfentanil on cardiovascular response to tracheal intubation in hypertensive patients. *Br J Anaesth* 2001;8690–8693.

14. Casati A, Fanelli G, Albertin A, et al. Small doses of remifentanil or sufentanil for blunting cardiovascular changes induced by tracheal intubation: a double-blind comparison. *Eur J Anaesthesiol* 2001;18:108–112.

15. Albertin A, Casati A, Deni F, et al. Clinical comparison of either small doses of fentanyl or remifentanil for blunting cardiovascular changes induced by tracheal intubation. *Minerva Anestesiol* 2000;66:691–696.

16. Salihoglu Z, Demiroluk S, Demirkiran et al. Comparison of effects of remifentanil, alfentanil and fentanyl on cardiovascular responses to tracheal intubation in morbidly obese patients. *Eur J Anaesthesiol* 2002;19:125–128.

17. Bensky KP, Donahue-Spencer L, Hertz GE, et al. The dose-related effects of bolus esmolol on heart rate and blood pressure following laryngoscopy and intubation. *AANA J* 2000;68:437–442.

18. Figueredo E, Garcia-Fuentes EM. Assessment of the efficacy of esmolol on the haemodynamic changes induced by laryngoscopy and tracheal intubation: a meta-analysis. *Acta Anaesthesiol Scand* 2001;45:1011–1022.

28

The Pregnant Patient

Michael F. Murphy and Richard D. Zane

THE CLINICAL CHALLENGE

Complications related to airway management represent the most significant cause of anesthetic-related maternal mortality. In fact, the incidence of airway management failure in the parturient at term is *ten times higher* than in an age-matched, nonpregnant population.

Airway management in the pregnant patient must take into account the stage of the pregnancy as well as anatomic and pathophysiologic conditions that antedate the pregnancy. Physiologic changes in the mother accommodate the increasing metabolic demands of a growing fetus. Importantly, the expiratory reserve volume, residual volume, and functional residual capacity (FRC) decrease by approximately 20% during pregnancy.

The unique features of the pregnant patient to be considered in airway management, especially in the last trimester and particularly near term, include the following:

- Difficult intubation is more common in the pregnant patient at or near term because of several contributing factors:
  - Weight gain during pregnancy
  - Larger breasts, which may obstruct access to the anterior neck for Sellick's maneuver or a surgical airway
  - Upper-airway edema and mucosal congestion (especially in preeclampsia)
  - A reduced FRC and increased rate of oxygen consumption results in more rapid desaturation.
- Increased risk of regurgitation and aspiration of gastric contents caused by:
  - Increased gastric volume and lower pH
  - Delayed gastric emptying
  - Increased incidence of gastroesophageal reflux (increased intraabdominal pressure, reduced lower esophageal sphincter tone)
- Vena caval compression in the supine position results in decreased venous return and cardiac output in the last trimester. The administration of induction agents may substantially reduce cardiac output and placental perfusion.
- Peripheral and pulmonary vascular resistance is decreased throughout pregnancy; blood pressure is decreased and pulse pressure is increased.
- Bag and mask ventilation may be more difficult because of the weight of the breasts on the chest wall and the increase in intraabdominal pressure caused by the gravid uterus, restricting diaphragmatic excursion.

- Capillary engorgement of the nasal and oropharyngeal mucosa and larynx predisposes to easy bleeding with manipulation.

With each maneuver or intervention, placental perfusion and oxygen delivery to the fetus must be considered. As a general rule, "What's good for the mother is good for the fetus, and what is bad for the mother is even worse for the fetus."

APPROACH TO AIRWAY MANAGEMENT

The sequence of events in managing the airway of the pregnant patient is no different from that of any other intubation in the emergency department, except for the unique features of pregnancy as described earlier:

1. Assemble rescue airway equipment and be prepared for the difficult airway. Remember that the mucosa may be engorged, edematous, and friable. Nasotracheal intubation is more likely to lead to mucosal damage and bleeding.
2. Preoxygenate, remembering that the FRC is reduced, oxygen consumption is increased, and apnea leads to desaturation more rapidly.
3. Attenuating the autonomic and cardiovascular responses to intubation with opioids and induction agents may lead to a reduction in maternal cardiac output and placental perfusion and must be weighed carefully in the context of the clinical situation. In addition, opioids and induction agents cross the placental barrier and may depress the neonate in the event that delivery is imminent. Muscle relaxants do not cross the placenta. In general, keep the intubation sequence as simple as possible.
4. An assistant trained in the application of cricoid pressure is essential in this situation.
5. Although rescue airway devices such as the intubating laryngeal mask (ILM) and the Combitube fill a similar role in the event that intubation fails, the enhanced risk of aspiration must be appreciated and definitive airway control expedited. However, the use of these devices as rescue devices is consistent with the standard of care, and provided adequate gas exchange is achieved, there is no need to move to more heroic measures such as cricothyrotomy.

RECOMMENDED INTUBATION SEQUENCE

- Preparation
- Preoxygenation
  - 100% oxygen
  - Tilt the abdomen slightly to the left with a wedge or pillow under the right hip to displace the gravid uterus from the inferior vena cava (IVC) and prevent the supine hypotensive syndrome of pregnancy.
- Pretreatment
  - Avoid pretreatment drugs unless there is a compelling reason to use them.
- Paralysis with induction
  - Etomidate 0.3 mg/kg
  - Succinylcholine 1.5 mg/kg
- Protection and positioning
  - Sellick's maneuver
- Placement with proof
  - Be gentle; the tissues may be friable

○ Ensure tracheal placement of the tube with a carbon dioxide detection device *before* releasing Sellick's maneuver.
• Postintubation management (see next section)

POSTINTUBATION MANAGEMENT

Pregnancy is associated with an increased metabolic rate, with the need to increase minute ventilation as the pregnancy progresses. At term, this translates into a 30% to 50% increase in minute ventilation. Arterial blood gases or pulse oximetry and end-tidal carbon dioxide monitoring will aid in adjusting the ventilation parameters. Modest adjustments of both rate (start at 12 per minute) and tidal volume (start at 12 cc/kg) will meet the ventilatory need. If ventilation pressures are high, placing the patient in reverse Trendelenburg position to move the abdominal contents down off the diaphragm may bring some improvement.

TIPS AND PEARLS

• Pregnant patients are hard to ventilate with a bag and mask. Be prepared to use a two-handed technique and achieve a definitive airway (endotracheal intubation) as rapidly as possible.
• Because of the glottic edema, a smaller-than-usual endotracheal tube size may be required.

EVIDENCE

There is no evidence specific to emergency medicine with respect to emergency airway but the following additional reading is suggested.

ADDITIONAL READINGS

1. Crosby ET. The difficult airway in obstetric anaesthesia. In: Benumof JL, ed. Airway management: principles and practice. St Louis: Mosby, 1996.
2. Dennehy KC, Pian-Smith MC. Airway management of the parturient. *Int Anesthesiol Clin* 2000;38:147–159.
3. Lewin SB, Cheek TG, Deutschman CS. Airway Management in the Obstetric Patient. *Crit Care Clin* 2000;16:505–513.

29

Prolonged Seizure Activity

Robert J. Vissers

I. The clinical challenge

A general discussion of the diagnosis and treatment of seizure disorder is beyond the scope of this book. This chapter focuses primarily on the considerations of airway management in the seizure patient. In the simple, self-limited, grand mal seizure, airway management is directed at termination of the seizure and prevention of hypoxia from airway obstruction. Paralysis and intubation should be considered when SpO_2 falls below 90% or when typical first-line measures fail to terminate the seizure in a reasonable time. For the simple seizure, basic airway maneuvers, expectant observation (most seizures end spontaneously), supplemental high-flow oxygen, and vigilance are usually all that is necessary. Airway protection from aspiration is rarely required in the simple, self-limited seizure because the uncoordinated motor activity precludes coordinated expulsion of gastric contents.

Determining when to proceed from supportive measures to intubation is one of the clinical challenges in the airway management of the seizing patient. *Status epilepticus* is defined as continuous seizure activity for 30 minutes or multiple seizures without recovery of consciousness in between. Although useful in discussions of seizure management, status epilepticus is less precise with regard to indications for airway management. Therefore the discussion focuses on when intubation may be indicated in the patient with prolonged seizure activity. The absolute and relative indications for intubation in the seizing patient are listed in Box 29-1.

II. Approach to the airway

A. Self-limited seizure

Most seizures terminate rapidly, either spontaneously or in response to medication, and require only supportive measures. Positioning the patient on his or her side, providing oxygen by face mask, suctioning secretions and blood carefully, and occasionally using the jaw thrust to relieve obstruction from the tongue are usually all that is necessary to prevent hypoxia and aspiration. Bite-blocks should not be placed in the mouths of seizing patients. They are not indicated and will only serve to increase the likelihood of injury. Attempts to ventilate during a seizure are usually ineffective and rarely necessary.

B. Prolonged seizure activity

Although most self-limited seizures do not require intubation, there are several indications for intubation in the prolonged seizure. Extensive generalized motor activity will eventually cause hypoxia, significant acidosis, rhabdomyolysis, and hyperthermia.

Box 29-1. Indications for Endotracheal Intubation

Absolute indications

1. Hypoxemia ($SpO_2 < 90\%$) secondary to hypoventilation or airway obstruction
2. Treatment of underlying etiology (e.g., intracranial bleed with elevated intracranial pressure)
3. Cessation of a prolonged seizure refractory to anticonvulsants to prevent accumulating metabolic debt (acidosis, rhabdomyolysis)
4. Generalized status epilepticus

Relative indications

1. Prophylaxis for the respiratory depressant effect of anticonvulsants (e.g., benzodiazepines, barbiturates)
2. Termination of seizure activity to facilitate diagnostic workup (e.g., computed tomography scanning)
3. Airway protection in prolonged seizures

Respiratory depression may result from high doses or combinations of anticonvulsants. Oxygen saturation of less than 90%, despite supplemental high-flow oxygen, is an indication for immediate intubation.

There is no clear guideline that specifically defines the duration of seizure activity requiring intubation. A good rule of thumb is that seizures lasting more than 10 minutes despite appropriate anticonvulsant therapy should be considered for intubation. Generally, when first-line (benzodiazepine) anticonvulsants fail to terminate grand mal seizure activity, rapid sequence intubation (RSI) is indicated. Phosphenytoin, which has a relatively short loading time, may be initiated as a second-line agent before intubation, if time allows. Other second-line anticonvulsants (phenytoin, phenobarbital) require at least 20 more minutes for a loading dose; therefore, at the time of initiation of such a load, intubation is advisable.

III. Technique

RSI is the method of choice in the seizing patient. In addition to its technical superiority, RSI ends all motor activity, allowing the body to begin to correct the metabolic debt. However, cessation of motor activity while the patient is paralyzed does not represent termination of the seizure, and fully effective loading doses of appropriate anticonvulsants (e.g., phenytoin) are required immediately after intubation. The recommended technique for the seizure patient is described in Box 29-2.

Standard RSI technique is appropriate in the seizing patient with the following modifications:

1. Preoxygenation may be suboptimal because of uncoordinated respiratory effort; therefore pulse oximetry is critical. After giving succinylcholine, it is more likely that the patient may desaturate below 90% before complete relaxation and therefore may require oxygenation using a bag and mask before attempts at intubation.
2. Sodium pentothal shares anticonvulsant activity with other barbiturates and may be the best choice for induction in the absence of hypotension. Midazolam is an equally efficacious alternative and preferred in the hemodynamically compromised patient. The induction dose of midazolam for an actively seizing patient is 0.3 mg/kg, but can be reduced to 0.1 to 0.2 mg/kg if the patient is hemodynamically compromised. Etomidate has an unclear effect on seizure activity and therefore should be considered

---

Box 29-2. RSI for Patients with Prolonged Seizure Activity

Time	Action	
Zero minus 10 minutes	Preparation	
Zero minus 5 minutes	Preoxygenation	Continue anticonvulsant Rx
Zero minus 3 minutes	Pretreatment	Continue anticonvulsant Rx
Zero	Paralysis with induction:	Sodium thiopental 3 mg/kg or Midazolam 0.3 mg/kg
Zero plus 20 to 30 seconds	Protection and positioning	Succinylcholine 1.5 mg/kg
Zero plus 45 seconds	Placement with proof:	Perform intubation
Zero plus 60 seconds	Postintubation management	Continue anticonvulsant Rx Vecuronium 0.1 mg/kg IV Lorazepam 0.02 mg/kg IV Consider midazolam drip

---

only if associated hypotension precludes the use of pentothal or midazolam. Although etomidate may raise the seizure threshold (and therefore inhibit seizure activity) in generalized seizures, it lowers the threshold in focal seizures. Little data exist on propofol as an induction agent in patients with seizures; however, EEG activity may actually be increased in lower doses.

3. Prolonged paralysis with vecuronium, and sedation with an agent that also suppresses seizures, is desirable for the first hour after intubation to facilitate investigations [e.g., computed tomography (CT) scan] and to allow acidosis to correct with controlled ventilation.

4. Continuous bedside electroencephalogram (EEG) monitoring is necessary in the paralyzed patient to assess for ongoing seizure activity. If this is not immediately available, motor paralysis should frequently be allowed to wear off to evaluate the effectiveness of anticonvulsant therapy.

5. If elevated intracranial pressure (ICP), head injury, known central nervous system pathology, or suspected meningitis is present, ICP intubation technique should be used.

IV. Drugs and dosages

1. Preintubation seizure management
   - Lorazepam 0.02 mg/kg IV *or*
   - Diazepam 0.1 mg/kg IV or 0.5 mg/kg per rectum
   with
   - Phosphenytoin 20 mg/kg (as mg of phenytoin equivalent)

2. Induction agents
   - Sodium thiopental 3 mg/kg *or*
   - Midazolam 0.3 mg/kg

3. Postintubation sedation and therapy
   - Midazolam 0.05 to 0.1 mg/kg/hr IV infusion
   - Propofol 4 to 12 mg/kg/hr IV infusion
   - Pentobarbital 1 to 4 mg/kg/hr IV infusion

V. Tips and pearls

1. Always ensure that hypoglycemia is not the cause of the seizure. Check glucose or administer intravenous dextrose solution in all cases.

2. Even in the difficult airway, RSI is generally preferred for airway management in the actively seizing patient. If the airway is assessed to be difficult, a double setup may be desirable.

3. The paralyzed patient may still be seizing, possibly causing neurological injury despite the lack of motor activity. Administer effective doses of long-acting anticonvulsants and use benzodiazepines for long-term sedation. Arrange continuous EEG monitoring, if possible, or allow motor recovery frequently (at least every hour) to assess response to therapy.

4. Prolonged seizure activity almost always represents a significant change in seizure pattern for the patient. A careful search for an underlying cause, including head CT scan, is indicated.

EVIDENCE

1. Which benzodiazepine is best? The answer depends on the setting in which it is being used. In one multicenter study, 570 patients with status epilepticus were randomized to lorazepam (0.1 mg/kg), phenytoin (18 mg/kg), diazepam (0.15 mg/kg) and phenytoin, or phenobarbital (15 mg/kg) (1). Lorazepam alone was most effective in terminating seizures within 20 minutes and maintaining a seizure-free state in the first 60 minutes after treatment. There was no difference in 30-day outcome and adverse events (1). Lorazepam also performed better than diazepam or placebo in a double-blind prehospital study of 205 patients with status epilepticus where termination of seizures occurred in 59% of patients versus 43% and 21%, respectively (2). Diazepam still remains a popular agent in the emergency setting because of its rapid onset (less than 20 seconds, compared to 1 minute for midazolam and 2 minutes for lorazepam) (3). Diazepam is stable at room temperature, in a premixed form, and is readily absorbed rectally; therefore it is often the benzodiazepine of choice stocked on a resuscitation cart.

There are no data on the ideal benzodiazepine as an induction agent in status epilepticus; however, the relatively rapid onset, combined with the familiarity of midazolam, suggests this may be the best choice.

2. Midazolam, propofol, or pentobarbital for postintubation therapy? For postintubation care, the patient should be sedated using a drug that not only provides amnesia and anxiolysis, but also optimizes antiepileptic therapy. Benzodiazepines have all these properties and are readily available in the acute care setting. Midazolam is preferred over diazepam and lorazepam as a continuous intravenous infusion because of its shorter half-life, water solubility, hemodynamic stability, and greater clinical experience in refractory status epilepticus (3,4).

Recent reports suggest midazolam or propofol being preferred as a first agent, then thiopental as a second line drug; however, no prospective randomized trial exists comparing these therapies directly (5,6). A systematic review to evaluate the efficacy and outcomes of these three agents in refractory status epilepticus found 28 studies that described a total of 193 patients (5). Pentobarbital was more effective at preventing breakthrough seizures; however, it was also associated with more episodes of hypotension and there was no difference in outcomes between any of the agents.

Despite the popularity of propofol for refractory seizure management in the intensive care unit setting, there is little experience in the emergency setting, and the ICU studies are too small to draw any conclusions (7–11).

REFERENCES

1. Treiman DM, et al. A comparison of four treatments for generalized convulsive status epilepticus. *N Engl J Med* 1998;339:792–798.
2. Alldredge BK, et al. A comparison of lorazepam, diazepam and placebo for the treatment of out-of-hospital status epilepticus. *N Engl J Med* 2001;345:631–637.
3. Treiman DM. Pharmacokinetics and clinical use of benzodiazepines in the management of status epilepticus. *Epilepsia* 1989;30:4–15.
4. Kumar A, Bleck TP. Intravenous midazolam for the treatment of refractory status epilepticus. *Crit Care Med* 1992;20:483.
5. Claassen J, et al. Treatment of refractory status epilepticus with pentobarbital, propofol, or midazolam: a systematic review. *Epilepsia* 2002;43:146–153.
6. Claassen J, et al. Continuous EEG monitoring and midazolam infusion for refractory nonconvulsive status epilepticus. *Neurology* 2001;57:1036–1042.
7. Prassad A, et al. Propofol and midazolam in the treatment of refractory status epilepticus. *Epilepsia* 2001;42:380–386.
8. Stecker MM, et al. Treatment of refractory status epilepticus with propofol: clinical and pharmacokinetic findings. *Epilepsia* 1998;39:18–26.
9. Bradford JC, Kyriakedes CG. Evaluation of the patient with seizures: an evidence-based approach. *Emerg Med Clinic North Am* 1999;17:203–220.
10. Pollack CV, Pollack ES. Seizures. In: Rosen P, Barkin R, Danzl DF, et al., eds. *Emergency medicine: concepts and clinical practice,* 4th ed. St Louis: Mosby, 1998.
11. Willmore LJ. Epilepsy emergencies: the first seizure and status epileptics. *Neurology* 1998;51:534–538.

30

The Geriatric Patient

Diane M. Birnbaumer

Advanced age is characterized by a loss of physiologic reserve. Aspects of aging affect virtually every consideration in airway management from the decision to intubate to the choice and doses of pharmacologic agents.

I. The clinical challenge

Aging affects the decision to intubate in three primary areas. First, the elderly patient may not have the respiratory reserve and energy to continue breathing effectively against the resistance caused by the respiratory threat. The work of breathing in this setting can be substantially increased and can rapidly deplete the patient's muscular energy stores. The patient may already have underlying medical conditions, such a chronic lung disease, that compromise oxygenation even at baseline. Comorbidity, such as ischemic heart disease, may reduce the patient's tolerance of hypoxemia. In addition, medications, especially psychotropic medications, may further compromise the patient's ability to generate an adequate respiratory effort. All these elements combine to make the elderly patient less able to sustain or overcome prolonged or severe respiratory compromise. Thus the decision to intubate may occur at an earlier point in the course of the respiratory or airway emergency as compared to the course in younger patients.

Second, elderly patients have a disproportionately increased incidence of difficult airways, primarily because of reduced mobility in the cervical spine and temporomandibular joints, caused by degenerative processes. Thus, one might start planning the approach to the airway earlier than in a younger patient to permit time to assess the airway adequately and to plan for contingencies.

The third, and potentially most challenging, effect of aging is on the ethical considerations regarding intubation. Many elderly patients, especially those with debilitating, chronic disease (including chronic obstructive pulmonary disease), have expressed their wish not to be intubated. When such expression is manifested on a properly executed, recently (less than 6 months) dated, legal advance directive, and when the patient can verbalize his or her agreement with this directive, the physician may confidently abstain from intubation. When one or more of these criteria are not met or when the patient cannot verbalize but family members state that the patient has recanted and would desire intubation, the decision is much more complex. A full discussion of these issues is beyond the scope of this manual. In general, when information is contradictory or incomplete, the physician or provider must take such action as he or she believes the patient would want. It is widely advocated that a provider forced to choose between aggressive intervention and potentially fatal inaction in the context of incomplete information should choose the course most likely to keep the patient alive until more information is available.

II. Approach to the airway

The standard approach to airway management involves several steps. First, the patient should be assessed to determine if a potentially difficult airway exists. In the absence of a difficult airway, rapid sequence intubation (RSI) should be performed. In cases of difficult or failed airways, rescue devices may be needed. Each of these areas may be affected by the changes seen in aging.

Elderly patients may be more likely to require use of the difficult airway algorithm. Elderly patients often have dentures, which may interfere with laryngoscopy and should be removed before laryngoscopy. However, if bagging is necessary in these edentulous patients, this lack of teeth may impair mask seal and interfere with effective ventilation, so unless dentures are obstructing the airway, they should remain in place until immediately before laryngoscopy. Temporomandibular joint arthritis that limits mouth opening will be detected when evaluating the 3-3-2 rule. This disorder will also worsen the Mallampati score and make laryngoscopy more difficult. When evaluating for airway obstruction, elderly patients are more likely than younger patients to have a history or airway surgery or irradiation. Neck mobility may be affected by cervical spine arthritis. This condition can limit the ability to line up the airway axes, making intubation and visualization more problematic and at times frankly impossible.

Despite the preceding problems, most elderly patients are candidates for RSI. RSI may require modification because of the changes seen with aging, and these modifications are outlined in the following section.

III. Technique

A. Preparation

Preparation should always include easy access to suctioning and readiness to turn the patient into the lateral decubitus position, as aspiration risk and morbidity are higher in the elderly. Aging leads to decreased lower esophageal sphincter tone, which increases the risk of aspiration. If aspiration occurs, outcome is worse in the elderly patient than in a younger patient, with more severe morbidity and increased mortality.

Orotracheal intubation using RSI is the usual method used for intubating the elderly patient. Blind nasotracheal intubation in the elderly has a higher morbidity rate, particularly from bleeding and posterior pharyngeal perforation; therefore, this technique should be used with caution, if at all, in the elderly. When elderly patients have a failed airway, alternatives are similar to those for younger patients. Intubation over a gum elastic bougie may facilitate orotracheal intubation. Devices such as the Combitube or laryngeal mask airway (classic, unique, or intubating) are reasonable alternatives in failed-airway situations, as are lighted stylets and fiberoptic devices. Finally, if necessary, surgical cricothyrotomy is always an alternative in the failed-airway situation in any adult, regardless of age.

B. Preoxygenation

Preoxygenation, a critical step for maximizing oxygen reserve during intubation, may be less effective in the elderly. Underlying heart and lung disease and decreased reserve often limit the amount of preoxygenation achievable in these patients. Oxygen desaturation will occur more quickly in the elderly, whose desaturation characteristics will mimic those of the moderately ill adult (see Chapter 3, Fig. 3-1.) Oxygen saturation should be meticulously monitored, and bag-mask ventilation should be initiated if oxygen saturation falls below 90%.

IV. Drug dosage and administration
   A. Pretreatment
   The pretreatment agents most frequently considered when intubating the elderly are lidocaine, opioids (fentanyl), and defasciculating doses of paralytic agents. As with other patients, lidocaine is indicated in elderly patients being intubated for elevated intracranial pressure or those with significant reactive airways disease. Defasciculation is rarely necessary and should be used with caution, as in the elderly the use of these smaller doses of paralytic agents runs the risk of inadvertent paralysis with hypercapnia, an undesirable situation in a patient with potentially compromised cerebral perfusion. Pretreatment with fentanyl can be very important in the elderly, as it will blunt the catecholamine response to intubation, which may be detrimental in this population with a high rate of cardiovascular and cerebrovascular disease. On the other hand, fentanyl should be used cautiously, as elderly patients may be particularly sensitive to the respiratory depressant effect of opioids. Use of fentanyl in lower doses (1 to 2 mcg/kg) is prudent, and the fentanyl should be given slowly, over 2 to 3 minutes.
   B. Paralysis and induction
   Paralytic use should not be affected by age, and the use of paralytic agents to achieve muscle relaxation is as important in the elderly as it is in younger patients. Although in most cases succinylcholine is the agent of choice, elderly patients are more likely to have suffered a recent stroke, a contraindication to administration of this agent if the stroke was between 3 days and 6 months before the intubation, because of the risk of inducing hyperkalemia. A careful review of medical records and examination of the patient for a preexisting stroke should be done in all elderly patients in whom RSI is considered. If there is concern about the possibility of a prior stroke with muscular weakness, a nondepolarizing agent (preferably rocuronium) should be used instead of succinylcholine.
   When etomidate is used as the induction agent, no changes are necessary in the elderly. However, when midazolam is used, the dose should be reduced to one-third to one-half, as the elderly may become hypotensive with typical induction doses of 0.3 mg/kg. In general, a dose of midazolam 0.1 mg/kg is appropriate in the elderly patient, 0.05 mg/kg if the patient is compromised by severe comorbid disease.
V. Postintubation management
   Typically, ventilator settings are not significantly affected by age. If the patient has obstructive lung disease and develops air stacking, permissive hypercapnia may be used, but this treatment should be used cautiously in the elderly, as the resultant acidosis may be detrimental if the patient also has heart disease. Postintubation sedation is as important in the elderly as in younger patients, but care should be exercised in dosing these agents, as elderly patients are more prone to hypotension from sedatives and opioids, compounded by the diminished venous return caused by positive pressure ventilation. The best method in administering these agents is to "start low, go slow," keeping in mind that adequate sedation is the ultimate goal.
VI. Tips and pearls
   Although preparation is critical in all patients requiring airway management, certain aspects are even more crucial in the elderly. Preoxygenation should be maximized, and bag and mask ventilation with the Sellick maneuver may be necessary to maintain adequate oxygenation when intubating the elderly. Drug choices and doses should be considered carefully, keeping in mind the higher likelihood of preexisting conditions such as prior stroke and cardiovascular and cerebrovascular diseases.

EVIDENCE

1. Reducing the doses of induction and sedation agents in the elderly. Most studies of the pharmacokinetics and pharmacodynamics of induction agents in the elderly show an increased tendency for hypotension and hypoventilation to usual doses when these agents are used in the elderly. Although this effect is less pronounced with etomidate, it can still occur, despite etomidate's excellent cardiovascular stability (1–5).

2. Desaturation and oxygenation in the elderly. Baseline oxygenation saturation falls with aging, and preoxygenation is particularly important in these patients. With adequate preoxygenation, elderly patients do not desaturate more rapidly than younger patients, but when inadequate preoxygenation is provided, desaturation is common (6,7).

REFERENCES

1. Cressey DM, Claydon P, Bhaskaran NC, et al. Effect of midazolam pretreatment on induction dose requirements of propofol in combination with fentanyl in younger and older adults. *Anaesthesia* 2002;56:108–113.
2. Jones NA, Elliott S, Knight J. A comparison between midazolam co-induction and propofol predosing for the induction of anaesthesia in the elderly. *Anaesthesia* 2002;57:649–653.
3. Martin G, Glass PSA, Breslin DS, et al. A study of anesthetic drug utilization in different age groups. *J Clin Anesth* 2003;15:194–200.
4. McCarthy G, Elliott P, Mirakhur RK, et al. A comparison of different pre-oxygenation techniques in the elderly. *Anaesthesia* 1991;46:824–827.
5. Valentine SJ, Marjot R, Monk CR. Preoxygentation in the elderly: a comparison of the four-maximal-breath and three-minute techniques. *Anesth Analg* 1990;71:516–519.
6. Vinson DR, Bradbury DR. Etomidate for procedural sedation in emergency medicine. *Ann Emerg Med* 2002;39:592–598.
7. Yano H, Iishi H, Tatsuta M, et al. Oxygen desaturation during sedation for colonoscopy in elderly patients. *Hepatogastroenterology* 1998;45:2138–2141.

31

The Morbidly Obese Patient

Richard D. Zane

THE CLINICAL CHALLENGE

Although simple visual inspection is often sufficient to diagnose obesity as it may relate to airway management, the World Health Organization (WHO) and the National Institutes of Health (NIH) define obesity using body mass index (BMI). Even though morbidity and mortality rises as BMI increases above 25, both the WHO and NIH define obesity as a BMI of 30 or higher, morbid or severe obesity as a BMI of 40 or higher, and superobesity as a BMI in excess of 50.

APPROACH TO THE AIRWAY

As for all patients, the approach to managing the airway of a morbidly obese patient requires a structured, careful method, making sure to identify the specific predictors of difficult bag/mask ventilation (BMV), cricothyroidotomy, laryngoscopy, and tracheal intubation. Morbidly obese patients develop both physiologic and anatomic changes that can complicate all aspects of airway management. Obviously, not all obese patients are alike as some may have multiple risk factors for a difficult airway and others may not.

The degree of obesity is correlative to the level of physiologic and anatomic changes that may make airway management more challenging. Physiologic and anatomic changes associated with morbid obesity are listed in Box 31-1. The principle effects of obesity on airway management are more rapid oxyhemoglobin desaturation, difficult BMV, and, often, difficult laryngoscopy and intubation.

The severity of obesity, age, and anatomic distribution of body fat affects almost every aspect of normal physiology with dramatic effect on the respiratory and cardiovascular systems. In general, patients with severe obesity tend to be hypoxemic at baseline and have a widened alveolar–arterial oxygen gradient caused primarily by ventilation-perfusion mismatching. Also, in obese patients the expiratory reserve volume (ERV) is often decreased and the forced expiratory volume to forced vital capacity (FEV_1 to FVC) ratio is increased, and these indices change in direct proportion to the degree of obesity. This fall in ERV has been ascribed to closure of the small airways predominately at the lung bases. The functional residual capacity (FRC) falls even further when the individual assumes a supine position, which increases ventilation-perfusion mismatching. Even though the vital capacity (VC), total lung capacity (TLC), and functional residual volume (FRV) are generally maintained in otherwise normal individuals with mild to moderate obesity, they may be reduced by up to 30% in morbidly obese patients and 50% in severe or superobese patients. Additionally, the work of

---

Box 31-1. Physiologic and Anatomic Changes Associated with Obesity

Physiologic changes associated with obesity are:

- Degenerative joint disease
- Hyperkinetic circulation
- Increased blood volume
- Increased renal blood flow
- Increased intraabdominal pressure
- Increased intrathoracic pressure with a restrictive pattern
- Decubital changes

Anatomic changes associated with obesity are:

- Increased facial girth
- Increased tongue size
- Smaller pharyngeal area
- Redundant pharyngeal tissue
- Increased neck circumference
- Increased chest girth
- Increased breast size
- Increased abdominal girth
- Increased intraabdominal and intrathoracic pressure

---

breathing is increased in morbidly obese patients because of increased chest wall resistance, increased airway resistance, and abnormal diaphragmatic position as well as other changes including a higher minute ventilation (Vm) because of a need to expel a higher daily production of carbon dioxide.

These significant alterations in normal physiology combined with the fact that obese patients have a higher metabolic rate of oxygen consumption make the preoxygenation phase of rapid sequence intubation (RSI) significantly more difficult, leading to a shorter period of safe apnea time after administration of neuromuscular blockade (see Chapter 3). The degree to which the apnea time is decreased is directly proportional to the degree of obesity and severity of associated comorbidity.

When evaluating the obese patient for a difficult airway, it is essential to consider all aspects of airway management: BMV, laryngoscopy with tracheal intubation, and cricothyrotomy. Increased chest wall weight, increased facial girth, redundant pharyngeal tissue, and the tendency of obese men to wear facial hair can make BMV difficult, virtually always requiring use of a two-person technique with both oral and nasopharyngeal airways in place. In severe or super-obese patients, BMV may simply be impossible as the mask seal pressure required to overcome the increased weight and resistance may be far in excess of that possible with a bag and mask. Cricothyrotomy is more difficult because of the increase in neck circumference, the thickness of the subcutaneous tissues, anatomical distortions, and adipose tissue obscuring landmarks, often requiring deeper and longer incisions. Obesity alone has been shown to predict difficult tracheal intubation and is associated with higher Mallampati scores (greater than or equal to three). There is also an inverse relationship between the degree of obesity and pharyngeal area, further complicating tracheal intubation. Obese patients tend to have smaller pharyngeal area caused by deposition of adipose tissue into pharyngeal structures. Virtually every pharyngeal structure increases in size with deposition of adipose tissue, including the tongue, tonsillar pillars, and aryepiglottic folds.

The smaller pharynx due to fat deposition results not only in decreased patency of the pharynx, but also increases the likelihood that relaxation of the upper airway muscles during RSI will cause collapse of the soft-walled pharynx between the uvula and epiglottis, making BMV and tracheal intubation more difficult and greatly reinforcing the need to use oral and nasal airways.

TECHNIQUE

In addition to assuming that the patient's airway will be intrinsically difficult because of the obesity, a careful LEMON assessment should also be done to anticipate and plan for possible difficulty. As described in Chapter 6, it would be prudent to gather rescue airway devices and airway adjuncts, call for assistance if indicated, and, using the difficult airway algorithm as a guide, strongly consider awake laryngoscopy or a fiberoptic approach with topical anesthesia and systemic sedation if the airway appears particularly difficult. Positioning is very important when attempting direct laryngoscopy on the morbidly obese. Two approaches are advocated. The first is to elevate the shoulders by placing folded blankets under the shoulders and upper back, and then raise the head even higher by placing towels under the occiput. The second method is to hyperextend the neck by pulling the patient's head off the top of the stretcher, aided by Trendelenberg position. A short-handled ("stubby") laryngoscope may also help by avoiding interference by the patient's chest tissues. If tracheal intubation is difficult or impossible, a laryngeal mask airway (LMA) has been shown to be an effective, temporary ventilatory device in morbidly obese patients and provides an excellent conduit for flexible fiberoptic bronchoscopy. In the superobese patient, the pressure required to overcome the weight of the chest will likely overcome the seal pressure of the LMA, making ventilation difficult or impossible. An intubating LMA is useful under these circumstances as well as a lighted stylet. The insertion technique for the lighted stylet is the same as in the nonobese patient, although one may encounter a greater diffusion of light depending on the degree of obesity, and room lighting may need to be dimmed. As obesity tends to obscure normal laryngeal anatomy, having a gum elastic bougie readily available may make tracheal intubation possible when only the epiglottis is visible on direct laryngoscopy.

In the obese patient, BMV can be difficult and must be performed optimally, which may require two providers using two- or three-handed bilateral jaw thrust and mask seal, with oropharyngeal and nasopharyngeal airways in place and the airway pressure relief valve and mask seal set so that continuous positive airway pressure (CPAP; 5 to 15 cm H_2O) is delivered to the pharynx. Cricothyroidotomy may be virtually impossible in the severely obese patient as the chin may be directly contiguous with the chest wall, making identification of and access to anatomic landmarks difficult. In the moderately obese patient, care must be taken to ensure that landmarks are found, and this step may require one or two assistants whose sole role is to hold or retract neck, facial, and chest fat folds.

DRUG DOSAGE AND ADMINISTRATION

The physiologic changes associated with obesity change many of the pharmacokinetic properties of drugs including absorption, distribution, metabolism, protein binding, and clearance. These changes may differ with the degree of obesity as well as the patient's underlying disease, making the final pharmacologic modification in the obese patient difficult to determine. The volume of distribution (Vd) of a particular drug is an important factor in determining dosing, and in the obese patient, the lipophilicity of the drug is the largest contributor to Vd. In obese patients, the Vd of drugs that are weakly lipophilic is somewhat increased when compared with normal patients, whereas Vd is significantly increased for many, but not all, lipophilic drugs. Hepatic metabolism of drugs is largely unchanged in the obese patient, and renal excretion, as in the normal patient, depends on the creatinine clearance although obese patients tend to have a higher glomerular filtration rate (GFR). For many drugs, it is unclear if weight-related dosage adjustments should be made and whether these adjustments should be based on the actual body weight, ideal body weight (IBW), or a percentage of the actual body weight. See Table 31-1.

TABLE 31-1. *Dosing recommendations for drugs commonly used in airway management*

Drug	Loading dose	Maintenance dose
Benzodiazepines[a]	IBW	IBW
Fentanyl	TBW	0.8 × IBW
Ketamine	IBW	IBW
Lidocaine	IBW	IBW
Morphine	IBW	IBW
Pancuronium	IBW	IBW
Propofol[b]	IBW	DW[c]
Rapacuronium	IBW	—
Succinylcholine	TBW	—
Thiopental	IBW	IBW
Vecuronium	IBW	IBW

[a]Midazolam may have a prolonged sedative effect as it accumulates in adipose tissue and inhibition of cytochrome P450 3A4 by other drugs or obesity itself.
[b]Propofol may have a prolonged recovery time in the obese patient.
[c]Dosing weight (DW) = IBW + 0.4 (TBW − IBW).
TBW, total body weight; IBW, ideal body weight.

POSTINTUBATION MANAGEMENT

The changes in the anatomy and physiology of obese patients have important implications in ventilator management. Depending on the degree of obesity, patients tend to have reduced lung volumes and increased airway resistance; calculating tidal volume according to the patient's actual body weight will result in high airway pressures and may lead to barotrauma. The initial tidal volume should be calculated based on IBW and then adjusted according to airway pressures and the success of oxygenation and ventilation. Generally, the use of positive end-expiratory pressure (PEEP) is recommended as it may prevent end-expiratory airway closure and atelectasis, particularly in the posterior lung regions. In severe or superobesity, it may be necessary to ventilate the patient in the semierect position to move the weight of the breasts, abdominal fat, or panus off the chest wall.

Portable bedside radiographs are usually of very poor quality in the obese patient, limiting their value although one can usually determine if the endotracheal tube (ETT) is in the correct position.

TIPS AND PEARLS

- The predicted difficulty in intubation combined with the decreased physiologic reserve in obese patients makes timely airway management important, and the decision to intubate cannot be delayed.
- Most tracheostomy tubes will not be appropriate for the morbidly obese patient; a 6-mm inner diameter (ID) ETT that is advanced through the cricothyroidotomy incision may serve as a temporary measure.
- Applying surgical lubricant to the mask to improve the seal may augment BMV in obese patients with facial hair.

ADDITIONAL READING

1. Behringer EC. Anatomic changes associated with obesity. Approaches to managing the upper airway. *Anesthesiol Clin North America* 2002;20:vi,813–832.

2. Ogunnaike BO. Rapid desaturation of the morbidly obese after pre-oxygenation. Anesthetic management of morbidly obese patients. *Semin Anesth* 2002;21(Mar):46–58.
3. Varon J. Drug dosing in the critically ill obese patient. Management of the obese critically ill patient. *Crit Care Clin* 2001 Jan17(1):187–200.
4. Butler KH, Clyne B. Management of the difficult airway: alternative airway techniques and adjuncts. *Emer Med Clin North Am* 2003 May;21(2):259–289.
5. Ray RM. Airway management in the obese child. *Pediatr Clin North Am* 2001 Aug;48(4):1055–1063.

32

Foreign Body in the Adult Airway

Ron M. Walls

Management of the suspected or known foreign body in the adult airway follows similar rationale to that used in the pediatric patient. The path chosen will depend on the patient's presentation, especially whether the foreign body is causing complete or only partial obstruction.

THE CLINICAL CHALLENGE

Airway obstruction caused by a foreign body presents a unique series of challenges to the provider. First, when incomplete obstruction is present, there exists the distinct possibility that a particular action or the failure to take specific action could drastically worsen the situation by converting a partial obstruction to a complete obstruction. Second, when complete obstruction is present, instinctive and habitual interventions, such as bag/mask ventilation, have the potential to make the situation significantly worse, for example, by helping to move a supraglottic obstruction below the cords, making retrieval more difficult (or impossible). Third, a common maneuver, like endotracheal intubation with bag ventilation, may meet with an unexpected result, such as the complete inability to move any air, defying the provider to find a solution to a problem perhaps never before encountered. Finally, the completely or partially obstructed airway is a unique clinical situation, requiring a specific set of evaluations and interventions, often in a very compressed period of time.

The patient with a foreign body in the airway may present with signs of upper-airway obstruction or may present comatose and apneic, with only the history of onset to provide clues as to the cause of the crisis. The obstruction may be complete, as in the patient who typically has been eating, aspirates a food bolus, and is unable to move any air or to phonate. Although these patients usually receive treatment in the prehospital setting, they may occasionally present at the emergency department (ED). In addition, a partially obstructing foreign body may be transformed to a completely obstructing foreign body just before ED arrival or during ED assessment. A partially obstructing foreign body will cause symptoms of partial upper-airway obstruction, specifically stridor, subjective difficulty breathing, and often a sense of fear, panic, or impending doom on the part of the patient. In many cases there will be a preceding condition that has increased the risk of aspiration. Many patients who aspirate food are physically or mentally impaired, or intoxicated with drugs or alcohol.

TECHNIQUE

Management of the foreign body in the adult airway depends on the location of the foreign body and whether the obstruction is incomplete or complete. Location may be supraglottic, infraglottic, or distal to the carina. Obstruction may be complete or incomplete. Because the precise location of the foreign body is usually not known, the following discussion focuses on the approach to the foreign body whose location is uncertain.

1. Incomplete obstruction by a foreign body

   When the patient presents with an incompletely obstructing foreign body, the most important step is to prevent the conversion of a partial obstruction into a complete obstruction. If the patient is breathing spontaneously and oxygen saturation is adequate (possibly with supplemental oxygen), then the best approach is usually to observe the patient closely for signs of complete obstruction while mobilizing the necessary providers for prompt removal in the operating room (OR). If there is an incompletely obstructing foreign body just proximal to the glottis, attempts at removal in the ED might result in displacement of the foreign body into the trachea, where it is no longer amenable to removal with common ED instruments. If transfer to the OR is not an option, for example, because it would require transfer to another hospital, a decision must be made as to whether the foreign body should be removed in the ED. If so, the best approach is to handle the airway much as one would handle awake laryngoscopy for a difficult intubation (see Chapter 7). Appropriate equipment should be assembled, the patient should be fully preoxygenated, and then following explanation of the procedure to the patient, titrated sedation and topical anesthesia are administered. With the patient sedated, the operator carefully begins to insert the laryngoscope with the left hand, inspecting at each level of insertion before advancing to ensure that the foreign body is not pushed farther down by the tip of the laryngoscope. The technique is one of "lift and look" followed by a small advance (perhaps one centimeter), then another lift and look, and so on. It may be necessary to take a break to allow the patient to reoxygenate or to administer more sedation or anesthesia. When the foreign body is identified, the best instrument for removal (Magill forceps, tenaculum, towel clip) is selected. Some foreign bodies, especially balls, cannot be grasped well with the Magill forceps. After the object is grasped and successfully removed, laryngoscopy should again be performed to ensure that no foreign body remains in the airway if there is any doubt that the foreign body was not removed intact. The patient should then be observed for several hours (depending on patient condition) to ensure that there are no further complications and that no foreign body moved distally in the airway.

   Upper-airway foreign body without complete obstruction should be considered a genuine emergency and all attempts must be made to expedite the patient's transfer to the OR for definitive management of the foreign body. If, while waiting for definitive therapy, the airway becomes completely obstructed, then the patient will be managed in a manner identical with that described in the following section.

2. Complete obstruction of the airway

   When airway obstruction is complete, the patient will be unable to breathe or to phonate and may hold his or her entire neck with one or both hands in the universal choking sign. The patient will appear terrified and will be making attempts at inspiration. In general, after complete obstruction of the airway with ensuing apnea, oxygen saturation will rapidly fall to levels incompatible with consciousness within seconds to minutes.

   Initial management is dictated by whether the patient is conscious or unconscious. If the patient is conscious, the Heimlich maneuver should be immediately and repeatedly applied until either the foreign body is expelled or the patient loses consciousness. (See algorithm, Fig. 32-1.) There is no point in attempting instrumented removal of an upper-airway foreign body while the patient is still conscious. If the Heimlich maneuver is successful in removing the foreign body, and the patient can phonate and breath normally, then observation for

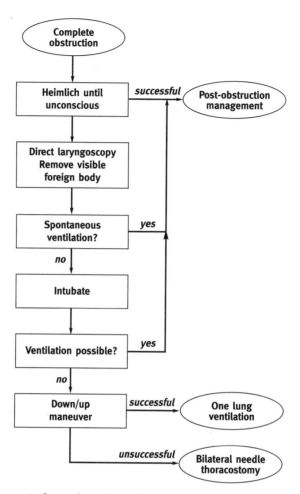

FIG. 32-1. Management of complete obstruction by a foreign body. See text for explanation.

12 to 24 hours is sufficient and it is not mandatory to visualize the airway if the patient remains asymptomatic. If the Heimlich maneuver is unsuccessful in removing the foreign body and the patient loses consciousness, or if the patient presents unconscious with an upper-airway foreign body, then the first step is immediate direct laryngoscopy *before any attempts at bag and mask ventilation, which may cause the foreign body to move from a supraglottic to an infraglottic position.* Generally, the patient will be flaccid and it will not be necessary to administer a neuromuscular blocking agent. However, this presentation is analogous to the crash airway and rarely, it may be necessary to administer a single dose of succinylcholine to achieve sufficient relaxation to identify and remove the foreign body. In any case, under direct laryngoscopy, a foreign body above the glottis should be easily identifiable. Again, Magill forceps, a tenaculum, a towel clip, or any other suitable device can be used to attempt to remove the foreign body. After removal of the foreign body, direct laryngoscopy is again performed to ensure that there is no residual foreign body in the upper airway. As the foreign body is removed, the patient may begin spontaneous ventilation immediately. If so, a repeat laryngoscopy may be advisable to ensure that no residual foreign body is present. If the patient does not begin to breath spontaneously,

immediate intubation and initiation of positive pressure ventilation is indicated and can be performed during the same laryngoscopy (Fig. 32-1).

The laryngoscopy to remove the foreign body should be performed quickly and efficiently. If no foreign body is identified and if the glottis is clearly visualized, then either there is no foreign body or the foreign body is below the vocal cords. In this case, the patient should immediately be intubated and ventilated. If ventilation is successful, it should be continued and resuscitation proceeds as for any other patient. If bag ventilation via the endotracheal tube meets with total resistance (no air movement, negative end-tidal CO_2 detection), then the trachea must be assumed to be completely obstructed. The stylet should immediately be replaced into the endotracheal tube, the cuff deflated, and the tube advanced all the way to its hilt in an attempt to push a tracheal foreign body into the right (or left) mainstem bronchus. The tube is then withdrawn to its normal level and ventilation is attempted. The strategy here is to try to convert an obstructing tracheal foreign body (which will be lethal) to an obstructing mainstem bronchial foreign body (which can be removed in the OR). Thus, the patient can be kept alive by ventilating one good lung while the other lung is obstructed.

If the down-then-up maneuver just described is not successful in establishing one lung ventilation, there are two clinical possibilities. The first is that the patient has one obstructed mainstem bronchus and a tension pneumothorax on the other side. Pneumothorax can occur in foreign body cases because of the abnormally high pressures generated both by the patient while conscious and by the rescue maneuvers. Because the operator has no way of knowing into which mainstem bronchus the foreign body was advanced (most commonly the right, but may be the left), bilateral needle thoracostomy should be performed, in hopes of relieving a tension pneumothorax. If a pneumothorax is not identified, the second clinical possibility is unfortunately present: complete bilateral mainstem obstruction, a condition from which survival is not possible, regardless of treatment.

POSTINTUBATION MANAGEMENT

Postintubation management depends on the clinical circumstances. If the foreign body has been successfully removed and the patient remains obtunded, perhaps from posthypoxemic encephalopathy, then ventilation and general management is as for any other postarrest patient. If the foreign body has been pushed down into one mainstem bronchus, the other lung must be ventilated carefully while waiting for the OR. Frequently, the patient receives excessive tidal volume at an excessive rate, an approach distinctly likely to lead to pneumothorax with immediate and severe compromise, because the lung that sustains the pneumothorax is the only functional lung the patient has.

TIPS AND PEARLS

1. If the obstruction is incomplete, the best approach is to wait for definitive removal in the OR under a double setup. If you are forced to act, move slowly and deliberately to ensure that you do not convert an incomplete obstruction into a complete obstruction.
2. Call for help early.
3. If the obstructing foreign body is above the vocal cords and cannot be removed, immediate cricothyrotomy is indicated.
4. If the obstructed foreign body is distal to the vocal cords and cannot be seen from above by direct laryngoscopy, cricothyrotomy will be of little or no benefit and should not be performed.

5. The Heimlich maneuver is a reasonable first step in any case of complete obstruction and is the only maneuver that can be performed on a patient with a complete obstruction who is awake and responsive.

EVIDENCE

There have been no randomized prospective trials evaluating various approaches to the obstructed airway. Advanced life support courses have endorsed the Heimlich maneuver as a first step, but this endorsement similarly is not supported by level one evidence.

33

Airway Management in the Prehospital Setting

Richard D. Zane and Ron M. Walls

THE CLINICAL CHALLENGE

Many of the principles of prehospital airway management are similar to those in the emergency department (ED), with the very obvious exception that the prehospital environment is necessarily austere. Patient management in the prehospital setting is done without many of the resources and backup assistance that are readily available in the ED. In addition, patient care must often be provided in awkward circumstances such as in private homes, in stairwells, in the seat of a damaged automobile, or on the street, where lighting and position are often not ideal. Local protocols, regional and topographic differences in transport time, the availability or unavailability of neuromuscular blocking agents, limited and varied equipment, limited backup, and mandatory transport of the patient all introduce considerations and issues that are not only different from those in the ED but also different from one prehospital system to another.

APPROACH TO THE AIRWAY

The decision to intubate the patient in the prehospital setting is based on the same principles as those applied in the ED (Chapter 1). A prehospital algorithm for the decision to intubate is shown in Fig. 33-1. The initial step is a quick evaluation of the patient, with a particular focus on assessment of the airway and ventilation. If the patient is maintaining the airway, protecting the airway, and ventilating and oxygenating adequately, then intubation is rarely indicated in the prehospital setting. However, failure to maintain or protect the airway or to exchange gases adequately mandates intubation unless the problem can be corrected by other means or transport is very short.

TECHNIQUE

If the patient is not maintaining his or her own airway, as evidenced by obstructed or noisy breathing, deep coma with unresponsiveness, or apnea, then the jaw-thrust maneuver should be immediately applied to attempt to establish a patent upper airway. Unless the patient has a contraindication to manipulation of the head and neck (e.g., blunt trauma with possible cervical spine injury), the head should be extended on the neck and the mandible should be thrust forward by pressure applied bilaterally at the angles of the mandible. This is best done using the ring or small fingers of the rescuer's hands, so that the remaining fingers can be free to apply and

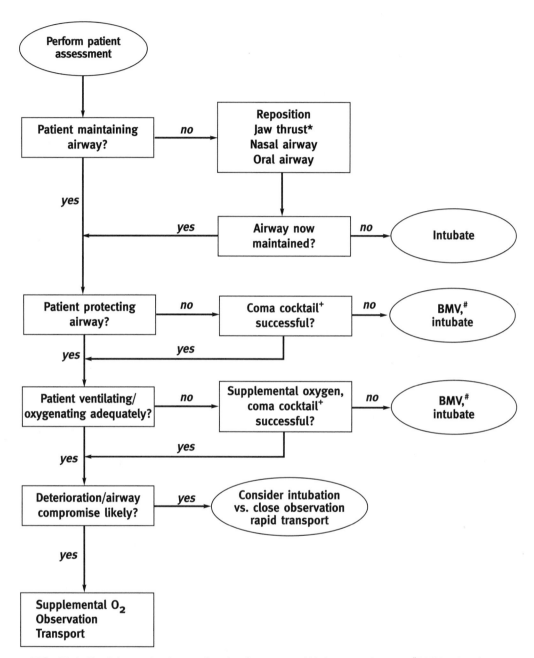

FIG. 33-1. Decision to intubate. *Caution in trauma; +Naloxone, glucose; #BMV = bag/mask ventilation.

properly seal a mask for ventilation. If the patient does not begin breathing spontaneously when the jaw-thrust maneuver is applied, then bag and mask ventilation (BMV) should be initiated, with placement of nasal and oral airways (see Chapter 5). In most circumstances, BMV in this setting should be followed by endotracheal intubation as soon as adequate preparations have been made, and providing the EMT is trained and licensed to intubate. If BMV is unsuccessful, despite careful attention to proper technique, then immediate intubation or placement of an alternate airway device, such as a Combitube or LMA, is indicated (see Chapters 9,10).

After a patient airway has been established, the next evaluation should determine whether the patient is protecting the airway from aspiration. Aspiration of gastric contents is a serious adverse event and must be prevented. Failure to maintain a patent airway usually indicates loss of protective airway reflexes. It is appropriate to administer a coma cocktail, which typically includes naloxone in doses of 0.4 to 2 mg as a specific reversal agent for opioid-induced respiratory depression, and glucose, 25 g IV, for possible hypoglycemia. In some systems, point-of-care glucose testing is performed rather than empiric glucose administration. If the coma cocktail is unsuccessful in reversing the patient's coma sufficient to permit self-protection of the airway, then BMV and intubation are indicated.

If the patient is maintaining and protecting the airway, the next assessment is of the adequacy of ventilation and oxygenation. If the patient is hypoventilating and a coma cocktail has not already been administered, this should now be done. Oxygenation failure, such as in pulmonary edema, may respond simply to supplemental oxygen via a nonrebreather mask or via bag and mask with assisted respirations. If neither supplemental oxygen nor administration of reversal agents can establish adequate oxygenation, then BMV is indicated, followed by intubation.

Finally, there is a population of patients for whom intubation may be indicated despite adequate airway maintenance and protection and acceptable levels of oxygenation and ventilation. An example is a pulmonary edema patient who is rapidly tiring but is maintaining oxygen saturations at 90%. If long transport time to the hospital is anticipated and the patient is not responding to other interventions, such that it is anticipated that the patient likely will deteriorate and require intubation before arrival at hospital, then early, anticipatory intubation may be appropriate before development of frank hypoxemia with worsening metabolic and respiratory acidosis. Other examples include a patient with drug overdose and rapidly decreasing level of consciousness, the cyclic antidepressant overdose patient who has had a generalized seizure, or certain cases of upper-airway trauma in which ongoing airway bleeding or expansion of a hematoma might threaten the patient. In such cases, careful evaluation and consultation with medical control is essential. In most circumstances, expeditious transport of the patient with supplemental oxygen via a nonrebreather mask is the appropriate course of action. Nevertheless, in certain circumstances, intubation may be both prudent and indicated (Fig. 33-1).

Once a decision to intubate is made, the next step is to choose the best method for intubation, based on individual patient circumstances and the attributes of the emergency medical services (EMS) system and the intubator. The choice will depend on whether neuromuscular blockade is available in the system, the availability of airway adjuncts and rescue devices, and whether prehospital cricothyrotomy is possible and permitted, along with a number of individual operator attributes.

If the patient is unresponsive and exhibits agonal cardiac or respiratory activity, the situation is analogous to the crash airway scenario depicted in Chapter 2. The choice here is between BMV, insertion of an alternate airway device (Combitube or LMA), oral tracheal intubation, and blind nasotracheal intubation. Regardless, the patient should have an airway established and oxygenation maintained using a bag and mask until intubation is attempted. If the patient has a relatively clear upper airway (no trauma, no foreign body, and no obstruction) and is breathing spontaneously, then blind nasotracheal intubation may be reasonable (see Chapter 8). However, apnea is a strong contraindication to blind nasotracheal intubation because the patient's breath sounds are used to guide the tube into place. Similarly, either abnormal anatomy or a foreign body in the upper airway is a strong relative contraindication to this technique. In addition, blind nasotracheal intubation has a lower success rate and higher complication rate than oral intubation. Nevertheless, in some systems and in certain patients, blind nasotracheal intubation may be the preferable method. This may be especially true if the patient's jaw is clenched and the use of neuromuscular blockade is not an option. Also, blind nasotracheal intubation may be a better choice if the patient is relatively inaccessible (e.g., trapped in an automobile) and neither LMA or Combitube is available (see later).

Oral intubation via direct laryngoscopy is also an acceptable method for the unresponsive patient and is the method of choice if the patient's jaw is not clenched. In the case of the unresponsive patient, intubation proceeds exactly as described earlier in discussions of the crash airway scenario. Direct laryngoscopy is performed, and the tracheal tube is placed under direct vision. If direct laryngoscopy is unsuccessful in visualizing the vocal cords, then a drug-assisted intubation is required. In some settings, drug-assisted intubation will include both induction (sedative) agent and neuromuscular blockade. In other settings, where neuromuscular blockade is not permitted, drug-assisted intubation will be done with sedation alone. In either case, drug-assisted intubation may be preferable to blind nasotracheal intubation, even in the clenched-jaw patient.

If the patient is conscious and combative and requires intubation, then drug-assisted intubation is required. At the outset, though, the benefits and risks of intubation should be weighed against the benefits and risks of rapid transport without intubation. Combative or uncooperative behavior is a strong relative contraindication to blind nasotracheal intubation because of the increased risk of complications in attempting to insert the tube in a patient who is resisting. If the patient is not frankly comatose and is not uncooperative or combative, then assessment must be made as to whether the patient would tolerate laryngoscopy. If the patient is sufficiently cooperative or obtunded to permit oral laryngoscopy without medications, then this treatment may be attempted. Again, preference is expressed for oral intubation over nasal intubation except in circumstances in which the jaw is clenched, thus preventing oral access. Even in such cases, oral intubation with medication may be preferable to blind nasotracheal intubation.

Blind nasotracheal intubation is discussed in detail in Chapter 8. In general, although blind nasotracheal intubation has been very widely used in prehospital care, it is rapidly falling out of favor as medications are being introduced to facilitate intubation in the prehospital setting. Blind nasotracheal intubation has two main uses. First, in circumstances in which direct laryngoscopy and visualization of the glottis are impossible, blind nasotracheal intubation may be the method of choice. An example is the patient who is trapped in the automobile after a motor vehicle crash and requires intubation before extrication can be accomplished. In such cases, blind nasotracheal intubation may be the only method that can be used by an operator either from inside or outside the vehicle. The second circumstance is the patient with a clenched jaw. A small number of patients will have increased masseter tone and hence a clenched mandible, even when they are deeply unconscious and breathing inadequately. In such cases, the choice is between administering medications for oral intubation or performing blind nasotracheal intubation. Even though RSI is clearly the method of choice under these circumstances, many prehospital care providers do not have this option, and blind nasotracheal intubation may be preferable or may be the procedure of choice for the individual operator.

In general, blind nasotracheal intubation should not be performed in patients with asthma, chronic obstructive pulmonary disease, or pulmonary edema unless drug-assisted intubation is impossible. In such patients, prolonged attempts at nasotracheal intubation impair oxygenation and can worsen existing hypoxemia and lead to full-scale respiratory arrest. Again, this is a judgment call and an individual provider might choose to attempt nasotracheal intubation on the patient with status asthmaticus; however, great caution must be exercised, as prolonged or traumatic attempts may significantly worsen the patient's condition.

The prehospital environment is unique in that a provider may be very far from assistance and rescue airway techniques and devices have a very important role. Although several new devices have been developed that may be useful for airway management in the prehospital setting, providers should become very facile with one or perhaps two rescue techniques and devices:

1. *Laryngeal mask airway (LMA)*. The LMA is described in detail in Chapter 9. The LMA is rapidly becoming the rescue device of choice for many prehospital systems and has gained some traction as a primary airway device in lieu of endotracheal intubation. The LMA is inserted blindly through the oropharynx, and the skill is fairly easy to acquire. Although the LMA does not protect the airway against aspiration, it does provide effective ventilation in virtually every patient into whom it is placed properly. In certain circumstances, the patient can be intubated through the LMA, but this approach is better left for the ED and probably should not be attempted in the field. The standard LMA is available in both reusable and disposable models for prehospital systems. The disposable model is preferable because the LMA will likely stay with the patient once the patient arrives in the receiving hospital. However, the disposable LMA (LMA-Unique) is available only in adult sizes; the reusable LMA (LMA-Classic) has sizes ranging from neonate to large adult.
2. *The Combitube*. The Combitube is widely used both as a rescue device and for elective anesthesia. The insertion technique is described in Chapter 10. The Combitube is also relatively easily learned, has a high ventilation success rate, and can be inserted into a patient in difficult circumstances, such as from the outside of a vehicle. The Combitube should not be confused with the esophageal obturator airway (EOA), which is a dangerous device that has no place in modern airway management.
3. *Lighted stylet*. The lighted stylet is a method of light-assisted intubation that is discussed in detail in Chapter 11. There has been limited experience with the lighted stylet in the prehospital setting, but the technique is relatively easy to learn and may be a helpful adjunct to direct laryngoscopy for oral tracheal intubation in the field.
4. *Continuous positive airway pressure (CPAP)*. Noninvasive ventilatory support (NVS) is addressed in detail in Chapter 35. NVS, specifically CPAP, is slowly becoming more common in the out-of-hospital setting especially in ground or air critical care transport. CPAP is most useful in treating patients who require minimal to moderate additional ventilatory support like those with congestive heart failure or an exacerbation of chronic obstructive pulmonary disease (COPD).

FAILED INTUBATION

Occasionally, the prehospital provider will be faced with a failed intubation. Failed intubation in the field should be anticipated by evaluation of the patient for difficult airway attributes as discussed in Chapter 6. If a difficult airway is anticipated, it may be most prudent to transport the patient rapidly to the ED for definitive care rather than to spend a long time attempting to intubate in the field, perhaps ending in a failed intubation and further damaging the airway, making intubation ultimately more difficult. Transport time should also be considered when determining whether it is appropriate to perform drug-assisted intubation. Again, in many settings, especially urban systems with short transport times, transport to the ED may be preferable to struggling with a difficult airway in the prehospital setting.

The primary rescue device for failed intubation is BMV. Prehospital providers must be expert at BMV using both one-handed and two-handed techniques, supplemented by oral and nasal pharyngeal airways. If BMV is inadequate at providing effective oxygenation, the patient should be repositioned, the jaw thrust should be applied vigorously, oral and nasal airways should be placed (if not already), a two-handed technique should be used to seal the mask to the patient, and any other steps should be taken that the operator determines might be helpful (Chapter 5). Again, meticulous BMV and rapid transport might be the appropriate action if oxygenation is adequate and intubation appears difficult or impossible.

If intubation is unsuccessful, it is important to try to determine why. Chapter 5 describes the sequence of steps involved in successful direct laryngoscopy. Repositioning of the patient, a change in equipment, or even a change in operator may help. In addition, prehospital providers should be familiar with techniques such as the BURP (backward, upward, rightward pressure on the larynx) maneuver that may facilitate direct laryngoscopy and intubation.

When laryngoscopy fails, digital or tactile intubation may be an option. This is a blind technique that uses anatomical landmarks where the endotracheal tube is passed by sliding the end of the tube along the tongue to the undersurface of the epiglottis and through the glottic opening. By palpating the epiglottis with the index and long fingers, the epiglottis can be picked up by the long finger and directed anteriorly. The tube is guided by the index finger under the epiglottis and into the trachea. A stylet bent at a 90-degree angle 4 to 6 cm from the tip of the tube should be used to assist in placement. Although exceedingly rare, some advantages of digital intubation include relatively fast placement with experienced providers, no need for special equipment, and no movement of the head and neck. The major significant limitation is that the patient must be unconscious.

Some systems allow cricothyrotomy to be performed in the prehospital setting. If this is the case, adequate training and skill maintenance are important. Cricothyrotomy in the field should be an exceedingly rare event. Cricothyrotomy accounts for only approximately 1% of all ED intubations, and although use has varied in reports among various systems, one might anticipate a similar or lower percentage in the field.

DRUG DOSAGE AND ADMINISTRATION

The use of rapid sequence intubation (RSI), paralytics, and sedatives is highly variable from one EMS system to another. As in the ED setting, RSI is clearly associated with a higher first-pass success rate of intubation when compared to non-RSI intubations, except in totally unresponsive patients. An ever-growing number of prehospital systems are using neuromuscular blockade to facilitate intubation in the field, but many EMS systems have not instituted RSI for myriad reasons including training and supervision issues, skill degradation, short transport times, and sometimes, antiquated attitudes toward EMS providers and a lack of understanding and familiarity with the prehospital environment.

Medication administration for prehospital airway management can occur in two forms:

1. Sedation alone
2. Sedation with neuromuscular blockade

Helicopter flight systems and critical care and specialized transport teams are usually trained and experienced in the use of neuromuscular blockade for intubation and encounter sufficient numbers of cases to maintain skills and knowledge. Field protocols for sedation or sedation with neuromuscular blockade vary from system to system. In general, sedation is used when the patient is not sufficiently cooperative for intubation, when mandibular relaxation is felt to be inadequate, or when the jaw is clenched. In such cases, sedative agents such as midazolam, diazepam, lorazepam, or others are administered and titrated until the patient can be intubated. In systems using neuromuscular blockade, typically a protocol dictates both the indications for and the manner of administration of neuromuscular blockade. In such cases,

---

Box 33-1. Simplified Rapid Sequence Intubation for Prehospital Care

1. Prepare equipment and ensure that the patient is in an appropriate area for intubation.
2. Preoxygenate the patient with nonrebreather mask for at least 3 minutes if possible.
3. Pretreatment drugs—infrequently used. Suggestion: lidocaine 1.5 mg/kg intravenously for head injury, reactive airways disease.
4. Paralysis with sedation—administer sedative drug in adequate dose (example: midazolam 0.2 mg/kg) and neuromuscular blocking agent (example: succinylcholine 1.5 mg/kg).
5. Protection—wait 20 seconds. Apply Sellick's maneuver.
6. Placement—45 seconds after drugs are given, intubate. Confirm endotracheal tube placement, secure tube, transport patient.

---

it is almost always mandatory to administer a sedative agent along with the neuromuscular blocking agent to ensure that the patient is optimized for intubation and that there is no undue physiological or psychological stress from the intubation attempts. Prehospital sequences are typically much simpler than those used in the ED and, with the exception of atropine in children receiving succinylcholine, pretreatment agents are rarely used (Chapters 3 and 16). A typical prehospital, drug-assisted intubation protocol using neuromuscular blockade is shown in Box 33-1.

The sequence is simplified in the prehospital setting because the options are fewer. Prehospital providers rarely carry a wide array of induction agents, and the circumstances are less controlled. Thus the complexity of training prehospital providers regarding the nuances of use of multiple pretreatment agents and the actual administration of these agents in the prehospital setting may present more problems rather than provide potential benefit for the patient.

POSTINTUBATION MANAGEMENT

The most common postintubation management in the prehospital environment, after securing an airway, is bag ventilation. As airway management is often a high-intensity situation, it is important to attempt to control respiratory rate and tidal volume, which are often inappropriately elevated because of the provider's excitement. As interfacility critical care and specialized care transport becomes more common, transport ventilators are getting more advanced and in-hospital techniques of postintubation management are now possible in the pre- or interhospital environment.

TIPS AND PEARLS

- Always weigh the risks and benefits of intubation in the prehospital setting against transport to the ED. In many circumstances, rapid transport might be the best way of managing the airway.
- Master BMV. There are very few airway emergencies in the prehospital setting that will not be temporized or managed adequately with proper BMV until the patient can be transported to hospital, particularly when transport times are short.
- If transport times are long, especially in systems with high rates of trauma, consider introducing neuromuscular blockade into the prehospital setting. This approach requires a comprehensive program, including quality oversight.

- Newer devices such as the LMA and Combitube may have a role in prehospital care. These should be evaluated on a system-by-system basis.
- All prehospital intubations should have their airway reassessed on arrival at the ED. Even though prehospital providers are extensively trained in acute airway management and are comfortable caring for patients in respiratory distress, up to 25% of prehospital intubations are found to be esophageal on arrival at the ED. Confirmation of endotracheal tube placement with end-tidal carbon dioxide ($ETCO_2$) detector should be a first priority both in the field and on arrival.
- Air-medical, critical care, and specialized transport programs are frequently asked to transport patients from a community hospital ED or intensive care unit to a tertiary care facility. These teams are occasionally confronted with the situation where a patient has not had his or her airway definitively managed, but this is needed for safety in transport. It is always preferable to manage these airways while still in the sending health-care facility as opposed to en route in an ambulance or helicopter.

EVIDENCE

There is a paucity of evidence related to prehospital airway management. The Combitube is relatively easily learned, is reasonably reliable, and can be inserted into a patient in difficult circumstances (1). Both the Combitube and LMA appear reasonably easy to learn, even if the operator has little prior training (2). A large analysis of prehospital use of the Combitube in cardiac arrest patients found good results with minimal adverse events (3). Intubation, on the other hand, has been subjected to several studies. Although results vary widely by system, up to 25% of prehospital intubations are found to be esophageal (4). A pediatric study in a large urban center found that transport to hospital with bag/mask ventilation provided outcomes at least as good as intubation (and perhaps better) in children with head trauma (5). The LMA is rapidly becoming the rescue device of choice for many prehospital systems and is capable of providing both ventilation and intubation (6). The disposable LMA performs as well as the original reusable model, at least under conditions of general anesthesia (7). The intubating LMA appears to have a very high insertion and ventilation success rate when used as a rescue procedure after failed intubation by adequately trained personnel (8). Cricothyroidotomy can be learned by those previously inexperienced in its use, probably within five repetitions of the procedure, but little is known about skills retention (9).

REFERENCES

1. Davis DP. The Combitube as a salvage airway device for paramedic rapid sequence intubation. *Ann Emerg Med* 2003;42:697–704.
2. Yardy N. A comparison of two airway aids for emergency use by unskilled personnel. The Combitube and laryngeal mask. *Anaesthesia* 1999;54:179–183.
3. Vezina D, et al. Complications associated with the use of the esophageal-tracheal Combitube. *Can J Anaesth* 1998;45:76–80.
4. Wang HE. Failed prehospital intubations: an analysis of emergency department courses and outcomes. *Prehosp Emerg Care* 2001;5:134–141.
5. Gausche M, et al. Effect of out-of-hospital pediatric endotracheal intubation on survival and neurological outcome: a controlled clinical trial. JAMA 2000;283:783–790.
6. Young B. The intubating laryngeal-mask airway may be an ideal device for airway control in the rural trauma patient. *Am J Emerg Med* 2003;21:80–85.
7. Brimacombe J, et al. A comparison of the disposable versus the reusable laryngeal mask airway in paralyzed adult patients. *Anesth Analg* 1998;87:921–924.
8. Dimitriou V, et al. Flexible lightwand guided tracheal intubation with the intubating laryngeal mask Fastrach® in adults after unpredicted failed laryngoscope guided tracheal intubation. *Anesthesiology* 2002;96:296–299.
9. Wong DT, et al. What is the minimum training required for successful cricothyrotomy? *Anesthesiology* 2003;98:349–353.

34

Mechanical Ventilation

Michael F. Murphy and Gregory W. Murphy

Setting up a ventilator is a task that few emergency physicians do on a daily basis. However, emergency physicians must know how to order and modify ventilation parameters. This chapter introduces the lexicon of ventilator management. It also provides simple explanations of how mechanical ventilators interact with patients (the modes of mechanical ventilation) and the two primary ways ventilators deliver a breath: volume-control and pressure-control ventilation.

Spontaneous ventilation draws air into the lungs (negative pressure); mechanical ventilation pushes it in (positive pressure). In either case, the amount of negative or positive pressure required to deliver the breath (tidal volume) must overcome resistance (R) to airflow. The viscosity and density of the gas helps to determine resistance. Gases that are less viscous and less dense create less resistance and generally flow more easily. For instance, helium is less dense than nitrogen and produces better flow characteristics through tight orifices, as one might encounter in epiglottitis or laryngeal cancer. Other factors contributing to this resistance to airflow relate to the caliber, length, and degree of branching of the tube the gas is flowing through. In fact, caliber is the most powerful determinant of this resistance to gas flow, resistance being inversely proportional to the fourth power of the radius (r^4).

Gas flow through a branching network of straight tubes, such as the tracheobronchial tree, may be orderly (*laminar*) or disorderly (*turbulent*). Laminar flow produces less resistance than turbulent flow; therefore, it takes less pressure to move a similar volume of gas per unit of time when flow is laminar. It also takes less effort [work of breathing (WOB)] on the part of the person or the ventilator. Factors that enhance the likelihood of laminar flow include using gases with lower density and viscosity; shorter, wider tubes [e.g., endotracheal tubes (ETTs)]; and no branching. The tracheobronchial tree has many generations of branches, and so intrinsically promotes turbulent flow. Turbulent flow is also created when the speed or velocity of gas flow is increased. Turbulence is a significant factor in mechanical ventilation: The greater the turbulence, the higher the pressure needed to get the gas in, and in the case of mechanical ventilators, the greater the risk of pneumothorax and other untoward events.

When it comes to mechanical ventilation, the aim is to have the machine deliver each breath as fast as possible with the least amount of pressure, but not so fast as to create turbulent flow and high pressures. When one is initiating mechanical ventilation, the initial inspiratory flow rate (peak flow) is generally set at 50 to 60 L/min. As one turns the flow rate up gradually in sequential breaths, the peak pressure also increases gradually. However, at a certain point, called the critical flow, a small increase in flow rate produces a large jump in peak pressure, indicating that flow has just become turbulent. As the asthmatic on a ventilator improves (i.e., less bronchospasm; increased airways caliber), the amount of pressure the ventilator must generate to deliver the same tidal volume falls. This effect is due to two factors that reduce airway resistance: the increased caliber (radius) of the airways and the transition from turbulent to laminar flow.

VENTILATOR TERMINOLOGY

The following terms are used in mechanical ventilation:

A. *Tidal volume* (V_t). The tidal volume is the volume of a single breath. It is usually in the range of 10 to 15 mL/kg. Smaller tidal volumes and more rapid rates are often used in restrictive lung diseases because higher tidal volumes in stiff lungs lead to excessive airway pressure. In obstructive lung diseases, one sometimes attempts to increase the tidal volume and decrease the rate (i.e., constant minute volume) to allow more time for expiration. The problem is that this approach often leads to unacceptably high airway pressures, impeding venous return to the heart, lowering cardiac output, and risking pneumothorax. The trade-off is pressure versus volume.

B. *Respiratory rate* (RR) or *frequency* (f). The usual starting respiratory rate is 10 breaths per minute in the adult. It is much higher in neonates, infants, and small children, and in those conditions where carbon dioxide production is accelerated (e.g., fever, acidosis, and other hypermetabolic conditions). The non–gas-exchanging parts of the respiratory system (dead space) constitute a fixed volume of each tidal breath. The remainder of the volume in each breath participates in gas exchange and constitutes alveolar ventilation. Rapid respiratory rates and small tidal volumes risk ventilating little more than dead space, a particular risk in infants and small children. The trade-off here is rate versus volume (alveolar ventilation).

C. *Fractional concentration of inspired oxygen* (F_iO_2). This ranges from the concentration of oxygen in room air (0.21 or 21%) to that of pure oxygen (1.0 or 100%). Though it is possible to administer hypoxic mixtures of gases (less than 21%), it is never done intentionally.

D. *Airways resistance* (R_{AW}). Multiple factors contribute to airways resistance and were described earlier. Subtle changes in peak inspiratory flow rates (peak flow) and endotracheal tube (ETT) diameter and length can contribute materially to airways resistance. The intubated, spontaneously breathing patient experiences a substantial increase in WOB as the ETT size is reduced. This effect is analogous to a healthy individual trying to breath through a drinking straw. After a short time, air hunger and fatigue become appreciable. The same thing happens to a patient breathing spontaneously through an ETT, especially a small one.

E. *Ventilation mode.* This term refers to the way the patient interacts with the ventilator and is of three types (pattern of breathing):
   • Continuous mechanical ventilation (CMV)
   • Synchronized intermittent mandatory ventilation (SIMV)
   • Continuous positive airway pressure (CPAP)

F. *Volume-control ventilation* (VCV) and *pressure-control ventilation* (PCV) describe how the ventilator controls and delivers a volume of gas, breath by breath.

VENTILATION MODES

Mechanical ventilators usually have three modes of ventilation to chose from: continuous mechanical ventilation (CMV), synchronized intermittent mandatory ventilation (SIMV), and continuous positive airway pressure (CPAP). The best mode in a given circumstance depends on the needs of the patient.

A. *CMV, or assist/control ventilation mode.* This mode is usually selected for patients who have no spontaneous respiratory activity of their own, such as overdoses and those given long-acting neuromuscular blocking drugs. The patient receives a minimum number of breaths each minute, at a predetermined tidal volume. This is called a *controlled* or *mandatory* breath. If the patient initiates his or her own inspiration, the negative pressure will trigger the ventilator to deliver a breath at the preset tidal volume, an *assisted* breath. The patient can choose whatever rate he or she prefers, but every breath is that of the preset tidal volume and the rate will not fall below the preset level.

B. *SIMV ventilation mode.* This mode is selected for patients who have some respiratory activity of their own, when it is desirable to ensure that they get a minimum minute ventilation. Patients receive a minimum number of breaths each minute at a predetermined tidal volume (mandatory or assisted breaths). They are also permitted to breathe spontaneously, at a rate greater than that set by the operator, at a volume of their own choosing (spontaneous breaths). This mode is often used when attempting to wean patients from mechanical ventilation. It allows the clinician to get some idea of how adequately the patient is ventilating on his or her own while allowing the patient to build strength in the respiratory muscles to enhance the success of weaning.

C. *CPAP ventilation mode.* This mode is selected for patients who are breathing spontaneously through an endotracheal or tracheostomy tube. It may be selected to predict whether the patient can be safely extubated. It is also used to decrease the WOB through a tube (drinking-straw concept) and in some forms of lung disease. Various forms of pressure support are used to augment ventilation and oxygenation (by optimizing functional residual capacity). Pressure-supported ventilation (PSV), also called *positive-pressure support* (PPS), can be used to decrease the WOB. When used in this manner, the operator selects an amount of pressure (PSV pressure) that the ventilator will supply at the instant the patient begins inspiration. This helps the patient overcome airways resistance and makes it easier to get a breath. The PSV pressure is usually titrated to a value that results in a normal spontaneous tidal volume (5 to 7 mL/kg) or until the patient appears to relax and arterial blood gases (ABGs) are within an acceptable range. Continuous positive airway pressure (CPAP) may also be called positive end-expiratory pressure (PEEP) when used this way.

HOW THE VENTILATOR DELIVERS A BREATH

A. **Volume-control ventilation**

In this method of delivering a breath, the operator sets the tidal volume of each breath. The pressure required to deliver this volume varies, depending on the compliance and resistance of the lungs, the flow rate selected, the size and length of the ETT, and other minor factors as discussed earlier. In adults, the initial peak flow is usually set to 50 to 60 liters per minute and then adjusted to the *critical flow point,* which is the maximum flow rate at which flow remains mostly laminar. As the flow rate is slowly and steadily increased, a sudden jump in pressure indicates that flow has become turbulent (i.e., the critical flow point). The flow rate is then reduced to just below this point. Pressure alarms are set [usually at 10 to 15 cm per H_2O greater than peak inspiratory pressure (PIP)] to warn of the risk of barotrauma and identify changes in compliance and resistance.

With VCV, one is also able to determine the flow characteristics of the delivered breaths. The waveform may be square or decelerating (Fig. 34-1). Choosing a square wave results in the tidal volume being delivered at the constant peak flow selected throughout inspiration. This waveform usually generates a higher peak pressure than the decelerating waveform but has the advantage of a shorter inspiratory time and more time for expiration. A decelerating flow wave causes inspiration to be initiated at the selected peak flow and then

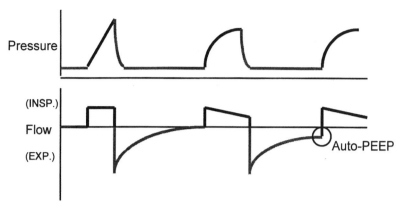

FIG. 34-1. Volume-control ventilation. The lower trace demonstrates a square flow waveform first. The next waveform is a decelerating waveform. Note that the peak pressure generated by the square waveform exceeds that of the decelerating waveform. The third waveform demonstrates inspiration being initiated before expiratory flow has reached zero. This is how breath stacking and auto-PEEP occur.

decelerates linearly as the breath is delivered. Because resistance to flow normally increases as the breath is delivered, the decelerating waveform generally results in lower peak inspiratory pressures. However, this approach increases the inspiratory time, at the expense of expiratory time, potentially trapping gas in the lung (stacking breaths), and leading to a continuous buildup of pressure called *auto-PEEP.* For this reason, the peak flow setting for decelerating flow wave is usually higher than that used in a square wave flow pattern. Auto-PEEP may lead to overdistension and rupture of alveoli (volutrauma) and decreased venous return and cardiac output. Most mechanical ventilators measure auto-PEEP. When setting up the ventilator, one can switch back and forth from one waveform to another in attempting to determine which is better for the patient.

B. **Pressure-control ventilation**

In this method of delivering a breath, the operator specifies an inspiratory pressure and an inspiratory time (I/E ratio) predicted to give a reasonable rate and tidal volume, based on the patient's expected resistance and compliance. The peak flow of the administered tidal breath and the flow waveform vary according to the patient's resistance and compliance. Early in inspiration the ventilator generates a flow rate that is sufficiently rapid to reach the preset pressure, automatically alters the flow rate to stay at that pressure, and cycles off at the end of the predetermined inspiratory time. The flow waveform created by this method is a decelerating pattern (Fig. 34-2). A normal I/E ratio is 1:2. If the respiratory rate is 10 breaths per minute evenly distributed over the minute, each cycle of inspiration and expiration is 6 seconds. With an I/E ratio of 1:2, inspiration is 2 seconds and expiration is 4 seconds.

The I/E ratio is usually determined by simply observing the pressure and flow waveforms on the ventilator monitor, especially the termination of flow at the end of expiration to avoid generating auto-PEEP (Fig. 34-3). The inspiratory pressure is selected and then the inspiratory time is adjusted by watching the monitor so that when the end inspiratory flow approaches zero, inspiration is terminated and expiration begins. Short inspiratory times lead to low tidal volumes and hypoventilation; long ones may increase mean intrathoracic pressure and compromise hemodynamic function.

In general, pressure-control ventilation imposes less WOB on the patient than volume-control ventilation. Newer ventilators allow the operator to select either option and

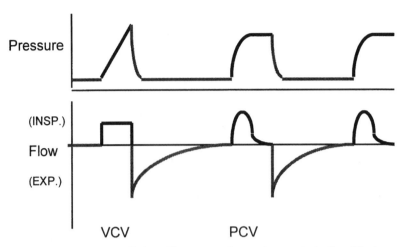

FIG. 34-2. Pressure-control ventilation. These waveforms demonstrate the differing waveform characteristics between VCV and PCV. Note that PCV generates lower peak pressures than VCV.

determine what is best in a given situation. Older ventilators may not. No matter which option is selected, alarms are set to warn of pressures and volumes that are too low or too high.

INITIATING MECHANICAL VENTILATION

Mechanical ventilators simply do for patients what they cannot do for themselves: breathe. The indication for mechanical ventilation is the failure of the patient to maintain adequate gas exchange.

The patient who is spontaneously breathing possesses a complex series of physiologic feedback loops that control the volume of gas moved into and out of the lungs each minute

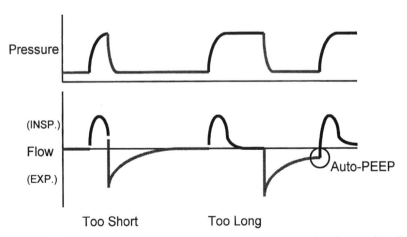

FIG. 34-3. PCV and I/E ratio. The first waveform set demonstrates an inspiratory time that is so short that the tidal volume is likely insufficient. The second and third waveform sets demonstrate how an inspiratory time that is too long may lead to breath stacking and auto-PEEP, as illustrated in Fig. 34-1.

(minute ventilation). They automatically determine the respiratory rate and the volume of each breath necessary to effect gas exchange and maintain homeostasis. The patient who is entirely dependent on a ventilator has no such "servocontrol" mechanism and must rely on the individuals setting the ventilatory parameters to meet their needs adequately. In the past, this meant frequent blood gas determinations. Now we rely on noninvasive techniques such as pulse oximetry and end-tidal carbon dioxide monitoring.

A certain amount of ventilation is required each minute (minute ventilation or minute volume) to remove the carbon dioxide produced by metabolism and delivered to the lungs by the circulatory system each minute. This minute volume approximates 100 mL/kg, provided the metabolic rate is normal. Febrile patients, for instance, produce 25% more carbon dioxide each minute than the same patients when they are afebrile. Minute ventilation would need to increase by 25% to accommodate for this increase, guided by arterial blood gases or end-tidal carbon dioxide monitoring.

In general, we use the rule of 10s in initiating ventilation in an adult:

- V_t—10 mL/kg
- f—10 breaths per minute
- F_iO_2—1.0

The vast majority of patients are easily ventilated, and this formula produces reasonable arterial blood gas tensions. Larger tidal volumes and lower rates delivering the same minute ventilation are acceptable, provided the volume/pressure trade-off is acceptable. Similarly, faster rates and smaller tidal volumes are acceptable, provided the rate/dead space ventilation trade-off is accounted for.

High airway pressure is a material enemy in mechanical ventilation. The many faces of barotrauma (pneumothorax, pneumomediastinum, etc.) are visible outcomes of high airway pressure. However, this airway pressure is also transmitted directly to the intrathoracic compartment compressing the great veins and the right atrium, and when averaged over the respiratory cycle is known as the *mean intrathoracic pressure*. This pressure compromises cardiac output and may in severe situations, such as that with the ventilated asthmatic, produce a pulseless electrical activity (PEA) rhythm. Airway pressure exceeding 35 to 40 centimeters of water pressure (CWP); by convention, airway pressures are measured in CWP, not millimeters of mercury is generally considered a barotrauma risk, though barotrauma is possible at lower pressures with some disorders. The same applies to mean intrathoracic pressure and venous return.

For some patients, the most perplexing task in establishing adequate mechanical ventilation is trading off rate, volume, and pressure. Ventilating the asthmatic is a good example. On the one hand, the tidal volume has to be sufficient, at a given rate, to provide reasonable minute ventilation. One wants the inspiratory part of the cycle to be short (i.e., high inspiratory flow rate) to allow maximum time for expiration and avoid starting the next inspiration before expiration is complete (stacking breaths). Meanwhile, the rate has to be slow enough to allow reasonable time for expiration. The dilemma is how to give a big enough tidal volume, quickly, and without developing excessive pressure. Deliberate hypoventilation (permissive hypercapnia) is one strategy used to attenuate the risks of high airway pressures. In some cases, one simply accepts the risks and acts accordingly. However, this is one case where attention to detail can make a material difference:

- Use as large an ETT as possible.
- Cut the ETT to minimize the length.
- Adjust the peak flow in an attempt to minimize turbulent flow.

Chapters in Section 5 deal with specific disorders and discuss initiating mechanical ventilation for those conditions.

TIPS AND PEARLS

- Have a respiratory therapist (RT) review the features of ventilators available for use in your particular ED.
- Know how to take a patient off the ventilator and resume bag ventilation until an RT can return. To do this, you must be able to turn the ventilator on and off and know how to silence the alarms. These minimal steps will preserve calm until the RT can respond. Bag ventilation can be used to deal with temporary problems and provides the additional feedback of "feel."
- Use the rule of 10s to initiate ventilation.
- Understand the typical resistance and compliance characteristics of the various respiratory disorders. This information may help predict if and how the rule of tens may need to be altered.
- Use CMV in totally apneic patients and SIMV for patients with some spontaneous respiratory effort.
- Always disconnect the patient from the breathing circuit when moving him or her. The circuit is heavy and may drag the ETT out, especially in infants and children.

35

Noninvasive Ventilation

Kerryann B. Broderick

DEFINITIONS

Intensive ventilatory support, both invasive (patient is intubated) and noninvasive (patient is not intubated; ventilatory support is delivered by mask), has become an accepted part of emergency department (ED) patient management. *Noninvasive ventilatory support* (NIVS) is defined as the provision of an oxygen mixture (often 100%) under controlled pressure using a mask as the physical interface between the ventilator and the patient's airway. Several variations of NIVS are potentially useful in the care of emergency patients: continuous positive airway pressure (CPAP), bi-level positive airway pressure (BL-PAP), and mask mechanical ventilation (MMV).

Most emergency physicians are comfortable initiating mechanical ventilation after intubating the patient with acute respiratory distress. Managing such patients *noninvasively,* however, is often more unfamiliar and challenging, and as a result, it is often not attempted, or abandoned too soon. The keys to successfully using NIVS in the ED are patient selection and appropriate aggressiveness of therapy—that is, before resorting to endotracheal intubation and mechanical ventilation.

Of the four modes of NIVS that are pertinent to emergency medicine, one is of historic interest only. The four modes are intermittent positive pressure breathing (IPPB), CPAP, MMV, and BL-PAP.

Intermittent Positive Pressure Breathing (IPPB)

Intermittent positive pressure breathing (IPPB) was emergency medicine's first foray into NIVS. IPPB ventilators are used with either a face mask or a mouthpiece and sense inspiratory effort to provide a quick burst of pressure to a preset level, augmenting tidal volume (V_t). This pressure is not sustained and inspiration assist is terminated when the preset pressure is reached. There is no CPAP, and the duration of each IPPB treatment is generally limited to 15 to 20 minutes.

Beta-adrenergic-agonist aerosols were given to patients with acute bronchospasm under the presumption that IPPB would (i) reduce the work of breathing (WOB), (ii) deliver aerosolized particles more deeply into the respiratory tree than by passive inhalation alone, and (iii) help clear mucoid secretions. In fact, in controlled studies, IPPB accomplished none of these objectives. It is also expensive in terms of initial equipment purchase, supplies, and personnel required, and its use was associated with a high incidence of induced barotrauma. Today, IPPB has no role in the ED.

Continuous Positive Airway Pressure (CPAP)

Continuous positive airway pressure (CPAP), as the name implies, delivers a constant, preset level of pressure support throughout the respiratory cycle. Unlike IPPB, CPAP has extensive and well-documented utility as a means of NIVS in the ED. Mask CPAP is efficacious as the sole ventilatory support in the treatment of pulmonary edema. Some authors have suggested that CPAP provides benefits during acute asthma exacerbation by reducing inspiratory WOB, mean airway pressures, and air trapping. When it is used in obstructive diseases, however, extrinsic CPAP [or positive end-expiratory pressure (PEEP)] must be provided at a level no higher than intrinsic or auto-PEEP (PEEP$_i$) to be potentially beneficial. Intrinsic PEEP exists at baseline in patients with chronic obstructive pulmonary disease (COPD) or acute asthma exacerbation and results acutely from improper assisted ventilation (when adequate time is not allowed between breaths for complete exhalation, sometimes referred to as breath stacking). The end-expiratory pressure in the alveoli becomes more positive than the positive pressure in the more proximal airways; this phenomenon further compromises hemodynamics, makes inspiratory efforts increasingly less effective, and may precipitate volu/barotrauma. Extrinsic PEEP is postulated to allow respiratory muscles previously used to maintain PEEP$_i$ to relax and be recruited to participate in inspiratory effort, thereby decreasing WOB.

Mask Mechanical Ventilation (MMV)

Mask mechanical ventilation (MMV) is the provision of mechanical ventilation using a mask instead of an endotracheal tube, and can be used with virtually any mechanical ventilator mode. Most patients tolerate MMV better than they do intubation with mechanical ventilation. The patient is, by definition, dependent on the ventilator, and so requires very close supervision and monitoring, something that is not always possible in the ED. If the patient cannot be monitored intensively to ensure that the MMV is adequately supporting ventilation, or if MMV fails, intubation is indicated.

Bi-Level Positive Airway Pressure (BL-PAP)

Bi-level PAP is correctly abbreviated BL-PAP, although it is sometimes imprecisely referred to as Bi-PAP, which is the name of one manufacturer's BL-PAP ventilator. Virtually all modern ventilators are capable of delivering BL-PAP, and it is no longer necessary to obtain a specialized device for this purpose. Conceptually, BL-PAP combines inspiratory pressure-supported ventilation (PSV) at one pressure level and CPAP at a second (lower) level. BL-PAP–capable ventilators provide differential preset support during spontaneous inspiration (inspiratory positive airway pressure, or IPAP) and expiration (expiratory positive airway pressure, or EPAP) to assist ventilation, but permit full exhalation while still providing continuous airway pressure. The IPAP is necessarily set higher than EPAP, and the difference between the two settings is equivalent to the amount of pressure support (PS) provided. BL-PAP is pressure limited and flow triggered; the machine senses the initiation of inspiration and immediately cycles to the preset IPAP, thereby increasing V_t with less WOB. IPAP levels are sustained for at least 200 milliseconds and for as long as 3 seconds (unlike IPPB), or until the patient ceases inspiratory effort or begins to exhale. The machine then cycles to the EPAP setting, below which it never drops, thereby maintaining supraatmospheric end-expiratory pressure. The EPAP reduces WOB analogously to PEEP/CPAP.

INDICATIONS AND CONTRAINDICATIONS

The indications for NIVS in the ED are straightforward: The eligible patient must have a patent, nonthreatened airway; be conscious and cooperative; and have an existing, although insufficient ventilatory drive. Patients who may benefit from NIVS may be hypercarbic, hypoxemic, or both. Typical ED patients who should be considered eligible include patients with chronic obstructive pulmonary disease (COPD), congestive heart failure (CHF) exacerbation, pneumonia, status asthmaticus, or mild postextubation stridor. NIVS is ***contraindicated*** if the patient has a threat to his or her airway, is unable to cooperate, or is apneic. If the patient is *in extremis*, with very poor oxygen tensions and severe and worsening ventilatory inadequacy, immediate intubation is usually indicated, and it is not appropriate to delay intubation for a trial of NIVS. This is a relative contraindication, though, and clinical judgment is required.

The objectives of NIVS are the same as those for invasive mechanical ventilation: to improve pulmonary gas exchange, alleviate respiratory distress, alter adverse pressure/volume relationships in the lungs, permit lung healing, and avoid complications. Patients on NIVS must be monitored at least as closely as those on ventilators, using familiar parameters (vital signs, arterial blood gases (ABGs), oximetry, chest radiograph, bedside spirometry, etc.).

TECHNIQUE

Recommended initial settings for BL-PAP machines in the noninvasive support of patients in respiratory distress or failure are IPAP of 8 cm H_2O and EPAP of 3 cm H_2O, for a pressure support (IPAP minus EPAP) of 5 cm H_2O. Either a face mask or a nose mask can be used, but a nose mask is generally better tolerated. There are different masks, and a respiratory therapist must measure the patient to ensure a good fit and seal. The level of supplemental oxygen flowing into the circuit should be governed by pulse oximetry and corroborated by ABG results as necessary; it is appropriate to initiate therapy with 2 to 5 liters per min, but this amount should be adjusted with each titration of IPAP or EPAP. The ventilator must be set in BL-PAP or spontaneous mode to support the patient's respiratory effort.

As the patient's response to ventilatory and other therapy is monitored (using cardiac and blood pressure monitors, oximetry, ABGs as indicated, and the patient's voiced assessment of tolerance and progress), support pressures are titrated. One approach that has been used successfully in hypoxemic patients in impending respiratory failure is to titrate by raising EPAP and IPAP in tandem in 2 cm H_2O steps, allowing a reasonable trial period (e.g., 5 minutes) at each level before increasing further. If the patient is hypercapneic, it may be better to raise the IPAP in 2 cm H_2O steps with the EPAP being increased in a ratio to IPAP of approximately 1:2.5. The $PEEP_i$ cannot be measured by a noninvasive ventilator; therefore, EPAP should generally be maintained below 8 to 10 cm H_2O to be certain that it does not exceed $PEEP_i$ in patients with obstructive lung disease. The IPAP must always be set higher than EPAP.

TIPS AND PEARLS

- Patients who need airway protection must be differentiated from those who need intensive ventilatory support. None of the modes of NIVS provide airway protection; When airway patency is not ensured, endotracheal intubation is indicated. Once intubated, the patient can be supported, if necessary, with a mechanical ventilator.
- Patients with both a patent airway and some preserved respiratory drive—even if that drive is clearly insufficient—may be candidates for NIVS. Patients most likely to respond to NIVS

in the ED (and therefore avoid intubation) are those with more readily reversible etiologies of their distress, such as COPD exacerbation with fatigue, pneumonia with hypoxemia-induced fatigue, or cardiogenic pulmonary edema.

- The ventilatory management of patients in frank or impending respiratory failure with NIVS is a *minute-to-minute*, ongoing strategic decision. Noninvasive ventilators (BL-PAP, CPAP) should be readily accessible to the ED, and physicians, nurses, and respiratory care personnel must be comfortable with their use and knowledgeable of their limitations.
- Patient selection must take into account the overall condition of the patient, the patient's tolerance of mask support versus intubation, and the anticipated degree of reversal of the underlying insult with ventilatory and pharmacologic support.
- One must be prepared for prompt intubation (i.e., difficult airway assessment done, drugs and equipment readily at hand) if therapeutic failure occurs.
- Nonventilatory therapy (e.g., ACE inhibitors, diuretics and nitrates for pulmonary edema, beta-adrenergic agonist aerosols and corticosteroids for COPD) must be pursued aggressively.
- Finally, the patient should be carefully monitored for progress of therapy, tolerance of the mode of support, and any signs of clinical deterioration that indicate a need for intubation with mechanical ventilation. In many patients, noninvasive MMV, mask CPAP, or BL-PAP provide sufficient support of the patient's own ventilatory drive so that more invasive management is unnecessary.
- Patients treated in the ED with NIVS generally should not be given sedatives or major analgesics, because preservation of respiratory drive is essential to the use of these modes. Anecdotally, some physicians who have used BL-PAP extensively report safe use of small, incremental doses of benzodiazepines for patients who have difficulty tolerating the face or nose mask.
- A trial of NIVS in the ED can be challenging, especially for physicians inexperienced in its use. Optimal results are usually obtained when autonomy is given to respiratory care personnel who are comfortable with this approach (e.g., "BL-PAP at 8/3, 4 L oxygen bleed-in, titrate to effect, and keep oxygen saturation = 95%"). It is preferred that a noninvasive ventilator be physically housed in the ED or be readily available from a nearby location; if delay ensues when NIVS is required, the patient probably will have improved significantly or be intubated by the time the machine is available.

SUMMARY

The keys to success with NIVS are to (i) be prepared with adequate equipment and trained personnel in the ED, (ii) select and then monitor patients carefully (blood pressure should preferably be normal to high to compensate for the decreased venous return to the heart that results from increased intrathoracic pressure when positive pressure ventilation is applied), (iii) treat the underlying condition aggressively and rapidly, and (iv) maintain immediate readiness to intubate the patient if NIVS fails.

When NIVS is successful (i.e., when intubation is avoided) several potential therapeutic, patient comfort, and fiscal benefits are derived. The advantages of NIVS over mechanical ventilation include preservation of speech, swallowing, and physiologic airway defense mechanisms; reduced risk of airway injury; reduced risk of nosocomial infection; and probably a decreased length of stay in the intensive care unit (ICU).

When compared with intubated and ventilated patients, patients treated with NIVS bear an increased risk of pulmonary barotrauma, aerophagia, and pressure stress to the face (regarding the latter, BL-PAP is a leak-tolerant system, so pressure sores are a much less frequent complication of extended BL-PAP support than of CPAP or MMV). In some published series, patients successfully supported in the ED with NIVS were frequently able to be admitted to telemetry units instead of ICUs, thereby incurring a significant cost savings. Uncontrolled studies without definitive inclusion criteria have found NIVS successful in avoiding intubation and mechanical ventilation in 60% to 90% of the variety of patients on whom it has been clinically tested. This broad range reflects in part the inconsistent inclusion criteria applied by the various studies.

Use of NIVS in the ED is likely to expand. These techniques are used commonly in ICUs, and are gaining increasing acceptance among emergency physicians. The most promise for benefit to ED patients from NIVS use is simply expanding its application (i.e., wider use of BL-PAP and CPAP to avoid intubation and its attendant complications). Fiscal pressure to avoid unnecessary intubation and ventilation, with attendant long ICU stays, may also drive expansion of this therapy.

EVIDENCE

Most of the studies done with NIVS compare NIVS to standard medical care (SMC) with outcome measures of intubation, ICU length of stay, and mortality. Unfortunately, most of the studies are quite small and have either enrollment criteria or endpoints that are somewhat subjective. Nonetheless, there is a considerable body of literature analyzing the use of NIVS.

1. NIVS and COPD. Two metaanalysis studies have been performed analyzing the use of NIVS in COPD. The most recent metaanalysis was by Peters in 2002 of 15 randomized control trials of NIVS versus standard medical treatment (SMC) (1). Eight trials enrolled patients with COPD and seven enrolled patients characterized as a mixed-disease group. NIVS was associated with an overall 8% reduction in mortality ($p = 0.03$), 19% reduced need for intubation ($p = 0.001$), and 2.74 days shorter hospital stay ($p = 0.004$). The COPD group had more significant reductions with 13% decrease in mortality ($p = 0.001$), 18% decreased need for MV ($p = 0.02$), and decrease in hospital stay by 5.66 days ($p = 0.01$). Keenan et al. in 1997, published a metaanalysis of such trials and identified only seven out of 212 that met rigorous inclusion criteria for analysis. The analysis showed NIVS to have a decreased mortality [odds ratio $= 0.29$; 95% confidence interval (CI), 0.15 to 0.59], and a decreased need for intubation (odds ratio, 0.20; 95% CI, 0.11 to 0.36) (2).

2. NIVS and asthma. Shivaram et al. demonstrated both a decreased WOB and an increased patient comfort level during CPAP support of acute asthma exacerbations (3,4). Meduri studied NIVS in 17 patients with asthma and acute respiratory failure over a 3-year period and demonstrated marked improvements in pH, P_aCO_2, and respiratory rates even at lower pressures of support (2.5 cm H_2O) (5). These small studies should not be considered to constitute evidence that NIVS is of benefit in acute asthma, and NIVS should be used in asthma only with extreme caution.

3. NIVS and pulmonary edema (PE). In small studies there appears to be a benefit to NIVS in the PE patients; however, larger prospective trials are needed before firm conclusions can be drawn. A randomized prospective study of 39 patients with PE compared CPAP to SMC and found a significant decrease in need for intubation ($p = 0.005$) in the CPAP group. Bersten reported no significant difference in mortality and hospital length of stay (6). An open nonrandomized study on 29 patients with NIVS found oxygen saturation increased from 73.8 ± 11 to $93 \pm 5\%$, mean pH increased from 7.22 ± 0.1 to $7.31 \pm .07$ ($p < 0.01$), and P_aCO_2 decreased from 62 ± 18.5 mm Hg to 48.4 ± 11.5 (7). A randomized, controlled, prospective clinical trial on 27 patients comparing nasal CPAP to nasal BL-PAP against historical controls for intubation rates and myocardial infarction (MI) found that BL-PAP improved ventilation and vital signs more rapidly than CPAP. However, intubation rates, hospital stay, and overall mortality between the two modes of NIVS showed no significant differences in this study. Mehta also reported a higher rate of MI in patients with BL-PAP (71%) as compared to CPAP (31%) and usual medical care from historical controls (38%) (8). A randomized prospective study of 40 patients comparing BL-PAP to high-dose isosorbide (HDI) reported that 80% of patients in the BL-PAP group required intubation as compared with 20% in the HDI group, MI rates of 55% and 10%, and death in two and zero patients, respectively (9). A metaanalysis of NIVS studies in pulmonary edema from 1983 through 1997 found that only 3 of 497 studies were sufficiently rigorous to fulfill their study criteria. These three randomized control trials showed NIVS patients to have a decreased need for intubation (−26%; 95% CI, −13% to −38%), but the decrease in hospital mortality was not significant (−6.6%; 95% CI, +3% to −16%) as compared to standard therapy alone (10). A more recent study compared BL-PAP to standard medical therapy in a mixed population of COPD and acute respiratory failure patients. The study ended prematurely after interim analysis of the first 20 patients, because the data showed clear benefit in the BL-PAP group (11).

REFERENCES

1. Peters JV. Noninvasive ventilation in acute respiratory failure—a meta-analysis update. *Crit Care Med* 2002;30:555–562.
2. Keenan SP, Kernerman PD, Cook DJ, et al. Effect of noninvasive positive pressure ventilation on mortality in patients admitted with acute respiratory failure: a meta-analysis. *Crit Care Med* 1997;25:1685.
3. Shivaram U, Donath J, Khan FA, et al. Effects of CPAP in acute asthma. *Respiration* 1987;52:157.
4. Shivaram U, Miro AM, Cash ME, et al. Cardiopulmonary responses to CPAP in acute asthma. *J Crit Care* 1993;8:87.
5. Meduri GM. Noninvasive positive-pressure ventilation in patients with acute respiratory failure. *Clin Chest Med* 1996;17:513.
6. Bersten AD. Treatment of severe cardiogenic pulmonary edema with continuous positive airway pressure delivered by face mask. *N Engl J Med* 1991;325:1825–1830.
7. Hoffman B. The use of noninvasive pressure support ventilation for severe respiratory insufficiency due to pulmonary oedema. *Intensive Care Med* 1999;25:15–20.
8. Mehta S. Randomized, prospective trial of bilevel versus continuous positive airway pressure in acute pulmonary edema. *Crit Care Med* 1997;25:620–628.
9. Sharon A. High-dose intravenous isorsorbide-dinitrate is safer and better than bi-pap ventilation combined with conventional treatment for severe pulmonary edema. *J Am Coll Cardiol* 2000;36:832–837.
10. Pang D. The effect of positive pressure airway support on mortality and the need for intubation in cardiogenic pulmonary edema: a systematic review. *Chest* 1998;114:1185–1192.
11. Thys F. Noninvasive ventilation for acute respiratory failure: a prospective randomised placebo-controlled trial. *Eur Respir J* 2002;20:545–555.

36

Pulse Oximetry

Michael F. Murphy

Pulse oximetry provides a noninvasive and continuous means of rapidly determining arterial oxygen saturation and its changes. The devices are easy to use and interpret, pose no risk to the patient, and are relatively inexpensive. However, reliable interpretation of the information provided by these devices requires an appreciation of their limitations in certain situations.

PRINCIPLES OF MEASUREMENT

Transmission oximetry is based on differences in the optical transmission spectrum of oxygenated and deoxygenated hemoglobin. Light absorption is related to the concentration of the solute, in this case oxy- and deoxyhemoglobin. At the wavelength of red light (660 nanometers), reduced hemoglobin absorbs about ten times as much light as oxyhemoglobin. In addition to arterial hemoglobin, other absorbers in the light path include skin, soft tissue, and venous and capillary blood. Pulse oximeters assess the pulsatile variation of red and infrared light transmitted through a tissue bed such as a finger, toe, earlobe, and so on. The light sources are light emitting diodes (LEDs) and the detectors are photodiodes. The light absorption is divided into a pulsatile (AC) component due to the pulsatile flow of arterial blood and a nonpulsatile (DC) component of the tissue bed that includes venous blood, capillary blood, and nonpulsatile arterial blood. Data averaged over several arterial pulse cycles are then presented as saturation (SpO_2). Studies have shown an excellent correlation between arterial hemoglobin (Hb) oxygen saturation and pulse oximeter saturation.

Reflection pulse oximetry uses reflected rather than transmitted light on a single-sided monitor. It can therefore be used more proximally anatomically (e.g., forehead, bowel), although it may be difficult to secure. Other than using specific reflection spectra, the principles are the same as for transmission oximetry.

INDICATIONS

Pulse oximetry is particularly useful in the emergency department (ED) evaluation of patients with acute cardiopulmonary disorders such as chest trauma, bronchiolitis, asthma, heart failure, and chronic obstructive pulmonary disease (COPD). It is a standard monitoring parameter for patients undergoing sedation and in patients with a decreased level of consciousness, such as intoxication, overdose, and head injury. Its ability to decrease the frequency with which arterial blood gases (ABGs) are done has also been demonstrated, particularly when used in conjunction with end-tidal carbon dioxide determination. Continuous monitoring may indicate the insidious development of shock as vasoconstriction develops.

Continuous oximetry is mandatory in patients requiring definitive airway management.

LIMITATIONS AND PRECAUTIONS

Limitations to the accuracy of pulse oximetry exist with severe vasoconstriction (e.g., shock, hypothermia), excessive movement, synthetic fingernails and nail polish, severe anaemia, or the presence of abnormal hemoglobins. Reflection oximetry has been demonstrated to reflect oxygen saturations more accurately in the setting of hypothermia and vasoconstriction. Carboxyhemoglobin (COHb) and methaemoglobin (MetHb) contribute to light absorption and cause errors in the pulse oximetry readings. The pulse oximeter sees COHb as though it were mostly OxyHb and gives a falsely high reading. MetHb produces a large pulsatile absorbance signal at both the red and infrared wavelengths. This effect forces the absorbance ratio toward unity, which corresponds to a SpO_2 of 85%. Thus, in the presence of high levels of MetHb, the SpO_2 is erroneously low when the arterial saturation is above 85% and erroneously high when the arterial saturation is below 85%. In dark-skinned patients, erroneously high readings (about 3% to 5%) and a higher incidence of failure to detect signal have been reported.

Pulse oximetry has been shown to be of limited accuracy and reliability during cardiopulmonary resuscitation and may be misleading. Nevertheless, its use is indicated during resuscitation as information useful to patient management may be gleaned.

In general, signals are weaker from ears than from fingers except in the face of hypotension or peripheral vasoconstriction, but ear responses are faster. Nasal bridge probes have been reported to read falsely high in some circumstances.

The pulse oximeter measures oxygen saturation, not the partial pressure of oxygen. This means that it is possible for the partial pressure of oxygen to fall substantially before the oxygen saturation starts to fall. The explanation lies in the sigmoid shape of the oxyhemoglobin dissociation curve. If a healthy adult patient is given 100% oxygen to breathe for a few minutes and then ventilation ceases for any reason, several minutes may elapse before the oxygen saturation starts to fall (see Chapter 3). The pulse oximeter in these circumstances therefore warns of a potentially fatal complication several minutes after it has begun. This is sometimes referred to as *monitor lag*.

Because the signal is averaged over 5 to 20 seconds, there is a delay in the correction of the reading after the actual oxygen saturation starts to drop. This is called *response delay* due to signal averaging.

Adequate oxygen saturation does not indicate that the patient is **ventilating** sufficiently. This is particularly important in patients with decreased levels of consciousness, such as during the performance of procedural sedation.

EVIDENCE

Monitor lag (the time taken for oxyhemoglobin saturation to reflect falling oxygen partial pressure) and response delay (the time taken to equilibrate because of intermittent sampling) are well described by Hill and Stoneham (1). Kellerman et al. demonstrated that ready availability of pulse oximetry in the ED reduces arterial blood gas sampling (2). Reflection oximetry has been demonstrated to more accurately reflect oxygen saturations in the setting of hypothermia and vasoconstriction (3). The limitations of pulse oximetry in reflecting the adequacy of oxygenation during cardiopulmonary resuscitation are well documented (4–6).

REFERENCES

1. Hill E, Stoneham MD. Practical applications of pulse oximetry. *Update in anaesthesia* 2000;11:1–2. http://www.nda.ox.ac.uk/wfsa/html/u11/u1104_01.htm
2. Kellerman AL, Cofer CA, Joseph S, et al. Impact of portable oximetry on arterial blood gas test ordering in an urban emergency department. *Ann Emerg Med* 1991;20:130–134.
3. Bebout DE, Mannheimer PD, Wun CCW. Site-dependent differences in the time to detect changes in saturation during low perfusion. *Crit Care Med* 2001;29:115a (abst).
4. Griffin M, Cooney C. Pulse oximetry during cardiopulmonary resuscitation. *Anaesthesia* 1995;50:1008.
5. Spittal MJ. Evaluation of pulse oximetry during cardiopulmonary resuscitation. *Anaesthesia* 1993;48:701–703.
6. Moorthy SS, Didorff SF, Schmidt SI. Erroneous pulse oximeter data during CPR. *Anesth Analg* 1990;70:339.

Subject Index

Pages followed by *f* indicate figures; pages followed by *t* indicate tables

AIRWAY MANAGEMENT AIDS

FROM THE EDITORS OF THE...

MANUAL OF EMERGENCY AIRWAY MANAGEMENT

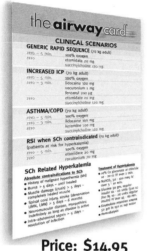

THE AIRWAY CARD

The definitive airway management pocket reference

The Airway Card, designed to fit into a lab coat pocket, is made of a durable synthetic material. The three-page, foldout card contains essential information for Emergency Airway Management, including Rapid Sequence Intubation. Drug doses are presented for standard RSI, with recommended modifications for special circumstances. Pediatric considerations include pre-calculated drug doses and equipment recommendations for children of different sizes.

Bulk Discounts available
1 to 9: $14.95 each
10-19: 10% discount – $13.46 each
20-24: 20% discount – $11.96 each
25 or more: 25% discount – $11.21 each
Price includes International shipping.

Price: $14.95

EMERGENCY ALGORITHMS POSTER SET

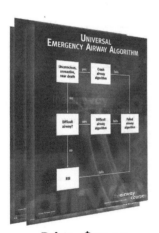

Improve individual and team performance!

A set of five posters comprises the Universal Algorithm, depicting an overview of the approach to the management of the airway in an emergency, and the four subtending algorithms: the Main (RSI), the Crash, the Difficult, and the Failed Airway Management Algorithms.

Each algorithm presents a step-by-step approach that is easy to follow and provides a ready reference in trauma resuscitation rooms, acute care ED rooms, the ICU, and other locations where emergency intubation might be necessary.

The 19" x 25" posters are designed to accommodate the limited wall space available in the typical resuscitation room and are offset printed on sturdy, coated material in an easy-to-read style.

The Emergency Airway Management Algorithms featured on the posters are those designed and taught by **The Airway Course**™, recognized internationally as a leader in Emergency Airway Management. The algorithms are identical to those featured in the *Manual of Emergency Airway Management*, 2nd edition, © 2004.

**Price: $79.95
per set of 5**

Bulk Discounts available
1 to 4: $79.95 per set of 5
5-9: 10% discount – $71.96 per set of 5
10-14: 20% discount – $63.96 per set of 5
15 or more: 25% discount – $59.96 per set of 5
Price includes International shipping.

Please see back for more information and order form.

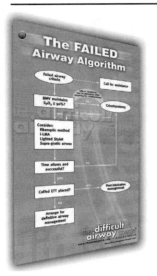

Price: $19.95

ANESTHESIA MACHINE CARD

The reliable reference for airway emergencies in the OR

The Anesthesia Card is a sturdy, $5\frac{1}{2}$" x $9\frac{1}{2}$" emergency resource with laminate coating and a grommet to enable it to hang on the anesthesia machine.

Dealing with The Difficult Airway in an emergency does not lend itself to the deliberate approach that we use in anesthesia when we predict a difficult airway in an elective surgical patient. Thinking and action must be preplanned and virtually reflexive. The same applies when we suddenly find ourselves in the situation where intubation has failed and is not likely to be successful (The Failed Airway). This quick reference resource provides the direction that is crucial to a positive outcome in emergency situations.

Bulk Discounts available
1 to 9: $19.95 each
10-19: 10% discount – $17.96 each
20-24: 20% discount – $15.96 each
25 or more: 25% discount – $14.96 each
Price includes International shipping.

AMEC ORDER FORM

	Quantity	Price	Total
The Airway Card			
Algorithm Poster Set			
Anesthesia Machine Card			
All Prices in US Dollars		**Amount Due:**	

Three ways to order:

Online: www.theairwaysite.com
Phone: Toll free in US and Canada
    1-866-9AIRWAY (1-866-924-7929)

Mail: Airway Management Education Center (AMEC)
    333 South State Street, Suite V-324
    Lake Oswego, OR 97034

First Name _____ Last Name _____

Home Address _____

City _____ State (Province) _____ Zip code (Postal) _____

Email _____ Home Phone _____ Work Phone _____

Hospital Affiliation _____

☐ Enclosed please find my check for $_____ USD. Made payable to "AMEC"

☐ Please charge $_____ USD to my ☐ VISA ☐ MasterCard
  Card # _____ Expiration date _____
  Signature _____